REVIEWS IN CANCER EPIDEMIOLOGY

REVIEWS IN CANCER EPIDEMIOLOGY

Volume 1

Edited by

Abraham M. Lilienfeld, M.D., M.P.H., D.Sc. (Hon.)
University Distinguished Service Professor
The Johns Hopkins University, School of Hygiene and Public Health,
Baltimore, Maryland, U.S.A.

ELSEVIER/NORTH-HOLLAND
New York • Amsterdam

Elsevier North Holland, Inc.
52 Vanderbilt Avenue, New York, New York 10017

Distributors outside the United States and Canada:
Elsevier/North-Holland Biomedical Press
335 Jan van Galenstraat, P.O. Box 211
Amsterdam, The Netherlands

ISSN: 0166-8544
ISBN: 0-444-00382-7

Editorial Services Barbara Conover
Design Edmée Froment
Art Editor Virginia Kudlak
Production Manager Joanne Jay
Compositor Typographic Services, Inc.
Printer Haddon Craftsmen

Manufactured in the United States of America

CONTENTS

PREFACE

Epidemiologic studies of various forms of cancer increased markedly in number after exogeneous or nongenetic factors were demonstrated to play an important etiologic role. Advances in those laboratory methods used in several epidemiologic studies to determine the role of such factors as hormones, and in statistical methods used in analyzing findings of such studies, have accelerated epidemiologic research. Because epidemiology is eclectic in nature, utilizing data obtained from biology, chemistry, physics, statistics, sociology, genetics, and other disciplines, methods and findings are reported in a wide variety of scientific periodicals and publications. It therefore becomes important periodically to collate and assess knowledge about various aspects and components of cancer epidemiology. From such evaluative reviews, it is hoped that suggestions for further research will emerge or be stimulated. It is for these reasons that this series of reviews, of which this is the first volume, was initiated.

Cancer epidemiology can be viewed from a variety of perspectives: the site of the malignancy, which is the most frequent approach; specific etiological agents that may result in different forms of malignancy; analytic methods used by the epidemiologist; and others. The series will contain reviews of cancer epidemiology from every possible perspective in order to provide the reader with both depth and breadth.

The present volume contains reviews regarding a variety of sites of cancer: prostate, pancreas, breast, and brain. Some of these sites have been the subject of extensive epidemiologic studies whereas others have only begun to be investigated. The role of two etiologic agents or classes of agents are reviewed: exogenous sex hormones and chromium chemicals.

A review of what is currently known about aplastic anemia, although it is not a malignant disorder, has been included since oncologists have to deal frequently with this problem; research on this problem is beginning.

This series of *Reviews of Cancer Epidemiology* is written to provide current information for epidemiologists, oncologists, and practicing physicians, by epidemiologists and other scientists who are conducting research in their area of expertise. It should prove useful to students, practicing physicians, epidemiologists and all those conducting research on this important disease.

Abraham M. Lilienfeld, M.D., M.P.H., D.Sc. (Hon.)

LIST OF CONTRIBUTORS

Valerie Beral, M.B., M.R.C.P.
Senior Lecturer, Department of Medical Statistics and Epidemiology, London School of Hygiene and Tropical Medicine, Kappel Street (Gower Street), London, WC1E 7HT, England

Ellen B. Gold, Ph.D.
Assistant Professor, Department of Epidemiology, School of Hygiene and Public Health, The Johns Hopkins University, 615 North Wolfe Street, Baltimore, Maryland 21205

Leon Gordis, M.D., Dr. P.H.
Professor and Chairman, Department of Epidemiology, School of Hygiene and Public Health, The Johns Hopkins University, 615 North Wolfe Street, Baltimore, Maryland 21205

Richard B. Hayes, D.D.S., M.P.H., Ph.D.
Epidemiologist at the Study Center of Social Oncology, Rotterdam, The Netherlands

Jack S. Mandel, M.P.H.
Assistant Director, Division of Epidemiology, School of Public Health, University of Minnesota, 1360 Mayo Memorial Building, 420 Delaware Street S.E., Minneapolis, Minnesota 55455

Leonard Schuman, M.D., M.S.
Professor and Director, Division of Epidemiology, School of Public Health, University of Minnesota, 1360 Mayo Memorial Building, 420 Delaware Street S.E., Minneapolis, Minnesota 55455

Moyses Szklo, M.D., Dr. P.H.
Associate Professor, Director of the Clinical and Chronic Diseases Epidemiology Program, Department of Epidemiology, School of Hygiene and Public Health, The Johns Hopkins University, 615 North Wolfe Street, Baltimore, Maryland 21205

David B. Thomas, M.D., Dr. P.H.
Associate Professor, University of Washington, and the Fred Hutchinson Cancer Research Center, Seattle, Washington 98104

EPIDEMIOLOGY OF CANCER OF THE PROSTATE

JACK S. MANDEL, M.P.H., and LEONARD M. SCHUMAN, M.D., M.S.

CONTENTS

INTRODUCTION

Early references to what might have been prostatic disorders can be traced back to 3400 B.C. and the tablet recordings of the Mesopotamian Society (1). "Choking" of the bladder and accompanying urinary difficulties have also been alluded to in early biblical and ancient Chinese and Egyptian writings. However, it is unclear whether these disorders involved cancer or merely hypertrophy of the prostate.

Descriptions of cancer of the prostate (scirrhus) appeared in the eighteenth and early nineteenth century writings of Morgagni, Sullivan, Varillie, Langstaff, and Brodie. Recent reviews of the history of prostatic cancer can be found in Murphy (2) and Bush and Bush (1). It was generally considered a rare disorder until 1900 when Albarran and Hallé reporting on a pathological study of 100 prostate glands, found that 14 percent showed malignant changes (2). It has since risen to its current position as the second leading site of cancer in United States males accounting for 16.3% of all incident cancer cases (3). It is estimated that for the United States, in 1980, 66,000 new cases of prostatic cancer will have been diagnosed and 21,500 deaths will have occurred (4).

Despite the magnitude of this problem, relatively few epidemiologic studies have been conducted, reasons for which are unclear. Perhaps, the neglect results from the fact that the disease occurs primarily among older men (average age at diagnosis is 73), or more likely, from the fact that relatively few promising etiologic clues have been suggested. In fact, most of the available data on prostatic cancer come from three sources: basic descriptive data on mortality and morbidity; studies whose prime objective was a disease other than prostatic cancer but which included it in an effort to describe all patterns of mortality or morbidity; or a few case-control studies each of which has some methodological fault.

Nevertheless, the available data warrant critical review in the hopes of gleaning factors of possible etiologic significance for further investigation. The purpose of this chapter is to examine data on prostatic cancer and extract from this labyrinth cogent hypotheses that may explain why as many as 75% of all men over the age of 70 develop this disease.

From the Division of Epidemiology, School of Public Health, University of Minnesota, Minneapolis, Minnesota.

GEOGRAPHIC DISTRIBUTION

Introduction

Variations in cancer morbidity and mortality rates both among and within countries may provide valuable etiologic insights. However, comparisons of such data on a world-wide basis must consider various artifacts that may account for the apparent differences in rates. Factors such as methods of data collection, availability, access and utilization of medical care, diagnostic acumen, certification of cause of death, completeness of death registration, and accuracy of the population census, make such comparisons difficult. Nevertheless, because many countries do have fairly complete and accurate enumerations of cases and deaths, an evaluation of their data may reveal real differences in disease rates. Variations in the rates for different countries may reflect differences in climate, geology, air quality, occupations, diet, socio—economic conditions, ethnicity or genetic background, which may in turn be helpful in the formulation of specific etiologic hypotheses.

International Variation

Mortality. A number of reports present age-adjusted mortality rates for cancer of the prostate (5–8). Figure 1 presents the prostatic cancer mortality rates in 1973 for 52 countries (8). Overall, the rates varied by about 150-fold from a high of 19.84 per 100,000 population in Switzerland to a low of 0.13 in Thailand. The highest rates occurred in northern European countries, New Zealand, Australia, United States, and Canada and the lowest rates were found among South and Southeast Asians, Latin Americans, and Southeastern Europeans. Within Europe, rates were generally lower among eastern than among western countries. The low rates among Orientals is a consistent finding in all reports on mortality and morbidity.

Morbidity. An excellent compilation of cancer incidence rates in five continents is available from a report by the International Agency for Research on Cancer, data for which were contributed by 28 countries from population-based registries utilizing a "reliable" system for reporting cancer cases (9). The adequacy and completeness of reporting was assessed by use of a number of factors. Included were the proportion of cases verified histologically, the proportion of cases registered for which no information was available other than a death certificate statement that death was due to cancer and a comparison of the number of site-specific cancers registered during a period of time with the number of deaths attributed to those cancers in the same period. Table 1 presents a ranking within three categories, of the age–adjusted incidence rates from 78 registries reporting to the International Agency for Research on Cancer.

Prostatic cancer accounted for between 1.0% of all male cancers in Osaka, Japan to 22.2% of all male cancers among Spanish New Mexicans. The ranking of the countries on proportional incidence, although not presented here, was similar to the rankings on age-adjusted incidence rates in Table 1.

The low rates (< 5 per 100,000 population) among the Orientals noted in the mortality data (Figure 1) are also apparent here (Table 1). However, mem-

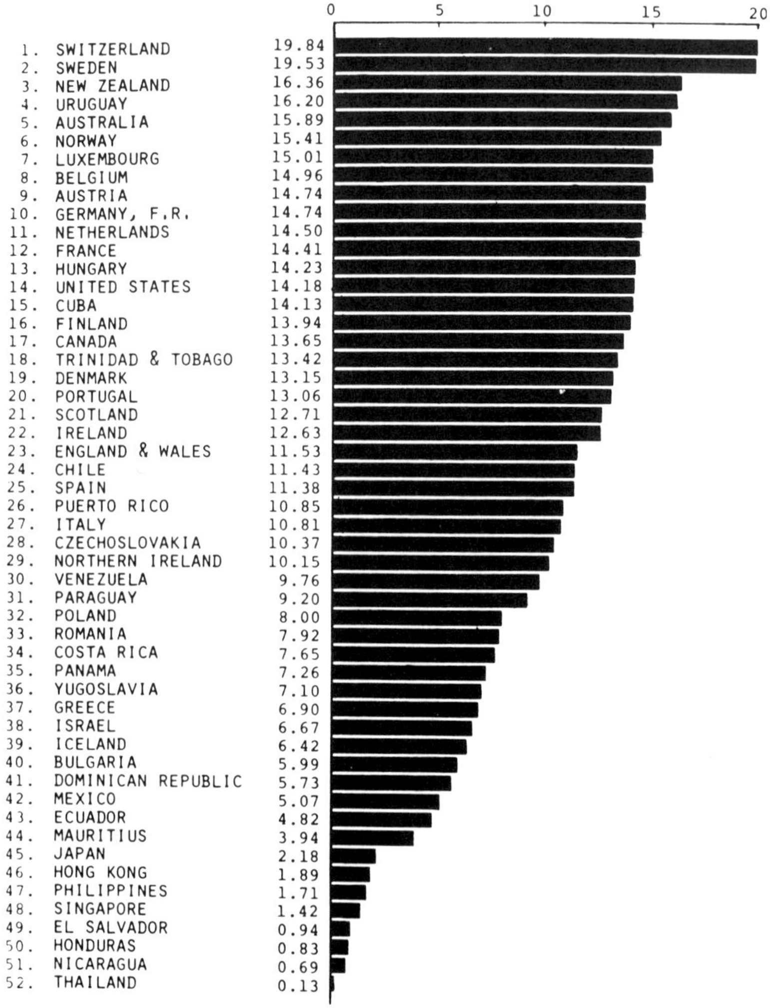

FIGURE 1. Age-Adjusted Death Rates For Cancer of the Prostate in 52 Countries in 1973. Rates per 100,000 population.

Source: Segi, M., Age-Adjusted Death Rates For Cancer For Selected Sites (A-Classification) in 52 Countries in 1973, Segi Institute of Cancer Epidemiology, Japan, 1978.

bers of these races living in Hawaii and the San Francisco area have substantially higher rates. The highest incidence rates (> 65 per 100,000 population) were noted among U.S. blacks, although African blacks did not show similar high rates.

There appears to be a slight east–west gradient with higher rates noted for western areas. For example, in Canada, rates were higher for the western provinces of British Columbia, Alberta, Saskatchewan and Manitoba, and lower in the eastern provinces of Newfoundland, the Maritime Provinces and

TABLE 1. Age-Adjusted Incidence Rates[a] for Cancer of the Prostate for 78 Registries from 28 Countries

High (>30.0)	
San Francisco Bay Area: blacks	77.0
Alameda County: blacks	75.0
Detroit: blacks	67.1
New Mexico: Anglo/other white	50.1
San Francisco Bay Area: whites	44.6
El Paso: Spanish/Latin	43.5
Hawaii: Caucasian	42.3
Utah	41.0
British Columbia	40.8
Alameda County: white	40.4
Saskatchewan	39.0
Sweden	38.8
Iowa	38.6
Connecticut	37.7
Manitoba	37.6
Norway: Urban	36.3
Detroit: white	36.1
New Zealand: Maori	34.6
New Mexico: Spanish/Latin	34.3
Norway	33.1
Alberta	32.4
Rhodesia: Bulawayo	32.3
Norway: Rural	31.0
Medium (15.0–29.9)	
Switzerland: Geneva	29.9
Maritime Provinces, Canada	29.7
New York State	29.4
Quebec	28.2
New Mexico: American Indian	27.5
El Paso: Anglo/other white	26.8
Iceland	26.7
New Zealand: Non-Maori	25.9
Hawaii: Japanese	24.6
Federal Republic of Germany: Hamburg	22.9
Finland	22.7
Brazil; Pernambuco; Recife	22.6
United Kingdom; South Western Region	22.2
Denmark	21.8
Newfoundland	21.6
Puerto Rico	21.4
Federal Republic of Germany; Saarland	21.1
Kingston; Jamaica	20.7
Colombia; Cali	19.8
Hawaii: Hawaiian	19.8
United Kingdom; Oxford	19.2
United Kingdom; Ayrshire	19.2
San Francisco Bay Area: Chinese	18.2
Cuba	18.0
Hawaii: Chinese	17.8
Spain; Zaragoza	17.7
United Kingdom; Birmingham	17.7
United Kingdom; Liverpool	17.5
Yugoslavia; Slovenia	16.8
United Kingdom; South Metro Region	16.4
Brazil; Sao Paulo	16.3
Hungary; County Vas	16.1
Poland; Warsaw City	15.6
Low <15.0)	
German Democratic Republic	14.6
Israel: All Jews	14.3
United Kingdom; Sheffield Region	14.1
Hawaii: Filipino	14.0
Romania; County Timis	13.5
Israel: Jews Born Africa or Asia	13.2
Israel: Jews Born Europe or America	12.6
Poland; Cieszyn Area and Nowy Sacz	12.0
Nigeria; Ibadan	10.0
Israel: Jews Born in Israel	9.7
Poland; Warsaw Rural Areas	9.4
Hungary; County Szabolcs	9.1
India; Bombay	8.0
Poland; Cracow City and District	8.0
Poland; Katowice District	7.1
Malta	7.0
Singapore: Malay	4.8
Israel: Non-Jews	4.3
Singapore: Indians	4.0
Singapore: Chinese	3.6
Japan; Okayama Prefecture	2.8
Japan; Miyagi Prefecture	2.7
Japan; Osaka Prefecture	2.7

Source: Waterhouse, J., Muir C., Correa, P., Powell, J. Cancer Incidence in Five Continents. Vol. III, I.A.R.C. Pub. No. 15, 1976.

[a]Adjusted to "World Population," Rates per 100,000 population.

Quebec. Among U.S. whites, the highest incidence rates were in the western states of New Mexico, California, and Utah and the lowest rates, in the eastern state of New York. In Europe, the lowest rates were found among the southeastern countries of Poland, Hungary, Romania, and Yugoslavia with the highest rates reported in the more northerly and western countries.

The distribution of incidence rates could be broadly categorized as follows: The highest rates occurred in the United States (particularly among blacks), Canada, and the northern European countries and Asia. Intermediate rates were found in the western European countries of Spain and the United Kingdom and the Latin American countries — Cuba, Jamaica, Brazil, and Colombia.

Within-Country Comparisons

Mortality. Lilienfeld (10) has presented an analysis by state of age–adjusted death rates for malignant neoplasms of the prostate for United States white males, 1959–1961, which showed that the highest rates occurred in the northern latitudes, particularly in the northeastern and western states. Rates in the highest quartile (13.7–15.6 per 100,000 population) were found in Maine, Vermont, New Hampshire, Washington, Oregon, Wyoming, Nevada, Utah, North Dakota, Nebraska, and Iowa, whereas rates in the lowest quartile (8.0–11.8 per 100,000 population) were found in Florida, Georgia, Texas, New Mexico, Colorado, Kansas, Arkansas, Kentucky, Virginia, West Virginia, and New York.

For nonwhite males high rates were found in the northern states with the exception of the Mountain states, which, along with the Pacific states, had the lowest rates. There was considerably greater variation among states for nonwhite rates than for white rates. For whites, the range in rates was from 11.7 to 13.1; whereas for nonwhites, rates ranged from 11.4 to 23.9.

For each geographic region, rates were higher for nonwhites than whites with the exception of the Mountain and Pacific divisions. This observation, plus the considerably lower rates in these divisions relative to the rest of the country for nonwhites, warrants further investigation.

The rank order of age-adjusted mortality rates for the several sites by geographic division was also presented by Lilienfeld (10). Prostatic cancer was the leading cause of cancer mortality among males in the New England division. It ranked as low as eighth for white males in the South Atlantic division and for nonwhite males in the Pacific division. For most areas of the United States, the rankings were similar for whites and nonwhites. The largest discrepancies occurred in the South Atlantic, West South Central, Mountain, and Pacific divisions where the rank varied by at least four. The widest disparity was in the Mountain division, where the rate for whites ranked first and for nonwhites, seventh.

An analysis of mortality data by large geographic areas such as states or divisions is of interest in looking for broad variations in rates which might indicate underlying etiologic factors. However, such an analysis is limited by the heterogeneity of a division and even a state and by numerous confounding factors such as availability, access to and utilization of medical care, diagnostic acumen and the quality and completeness of death certificates. For these reasons, smaller, more homogeneous areas are preferable.

An analysis of county cancer mortality rates for the period 1950–1969 was recently published by the National Cancer Institute (11–13). The highest prostatic cancer death rates for white males were found in counties in the upper midwestern states of Iowa, Minnesota, and North and South Dakota, and in counties in the northern New England area. Among nonwhites, the highest rates occurred in counties in the Northeast, Midwest, and Southeast.

Blair and Fraumeni (14) correlated these county rates with selected demographic, industrial and agricultural data. They found that mortality was higher in counties with a high percentage of residents of Scandinavian and German descent, in counties with metal and textile industries, and in counties with high consumption of fats.

Morbidity. The Third National Cancer Survey, conducted in nine areas of the United States, collected data on all newly diagnosed cancers during the period 1969–1971 (3). The average annual age–adjusted incidence rates per 100,000 population by race and area are presented in Table 2. For whites and blacks combined the lowest rate was in Iowa and the highest in Atlanta. For white males, the lowest rate was in Iowa and the highest ones were in Colorado and Minneapolis–St. Paul. Disregarding Iowa, Minneapolis–St. Paul, and Colorado, where the number of black males was less than 35,000 (3.2% of total male population), the lowest rate for blacks was in Birmingham and the highest was in Dallas–Fort Worth.

Despite the considerable variation among the nine areas, no clear geographic pattern was evident.

TABLE 2. Average Annual Age-Adjusted Incidence Rates for Prostatic Cancer Per 100,000 Population by Race and Area, 1969–1971[a]

Area	All races	White	Black
Dallas—Fort Worth, Texas	50.2	45.3	87.1
Birmingham, Alabama	52.6	44.8	70.5
Atlanta, Georgia	56.1	50.2	79.9
San Francisco—Oakland, California	50.0	49.3	81.9
Colorado	56.0	54.1	115.5
Pittsburg, Pennsylvania	43.9	41.9	70.7
Iowa	44.6	44.4	74.4
Detroit, Michigan	50.7	46.2	80.3
Minneapolis–St. Paul, Minnesota	54.6	54.1	63.1
All Areas	48.6	46.1	78.3

Source: Cutler, S.J., Young, J.L., Jr., The Third National Cancer Survey: Incidence Data, Biometry Branch, National Cancer Institute Monograph 41, DHEW Pub. No. (NIH) 75-787, 1975.

[a]Adjusted to 1950 U.S. population.

Urban-Rural Differences. Although cancer of the prostate was not analyzed separately, Gover (15) found a positive correlation between degree of urbanization and deaths from cancers of the genital organs for United States males for the period 1930–1932. Spiegleman (16) found the genital organ cancer mortality rates in 1940 for U.S. males aged 20–74, to be 27 and 41% lower for whites and nonwhites respectively in rural areas than in urban areas with populations over 100,000.

To eliminate confusion between legal residence and post office address, an analysis of prostatic cancer mortality data for the period 1949–1951 by metropolitan and nonmetropolitan counties (those with and without a central city of 50,000 population or more respectively) revealed, for white males, a higher age-adjusted rate for metropolitan counties than for nonmetropolitan counties for all areas of the country with the exception of the New England states (17). For nonwhites, there was a similar general pattern of higher rates in metropolitan counties; however, for many areas of the country, the small number of deaths among nonwhites precluded any definitive statement.

In Connecticut, the 1950 census definitions of residence were considered to be inapplicable and the term rural was applied to a group of 93 towns with a population density of less than 130 persons per square mile (18). The remaining 76 towns with a higher population density were classified as urban. A comparison of the age-adjusted prostatic cancer incidence rates resulted in urban-nonfarm ratio with an urban-farm ratio.

An identical ratio was found in an analysis of incidence rates for New York State (exclusive of New York City) for the period 1949–1951 (19). In this study, the U.S. Census Bureau definition of urban (all incorporated places with a population of 2500 or over) was used. The upstate New York data also permitted an analysis of the urban-rural ratio for metropolitan and nonmetropolitan counties. The urban-rural ratios of the age-adjusted incidence rates were 1.23 for metropolitan counties and 1.22 for nonmetropolitan counties. The authors felt that this analysis reflected a comparison of an urban-nonfarm ratio with an urban—farm ratio.

Haenszel et al. (20) in 1950 conducted a morbidity survey of cancer in the state of Iowa. The age-adjusted incidence rate of prostate cancer was similar in urban and rural areas (ratio = 1.11). Mortality data for the same period revealed an urban-rural ratio of 0.87. Age-specific incidence rates showed marked variation. For the 75–84 age group, the urban-rural ratio was 1.30 and for the age group 85 and over, 0.58. For those cases which were microscopically confirmed, perhaps a better method of comparison, the urban-rural ratio was 1.31.

Lilienfeld's (10) analysis of U.S. mortality data for the period 1959–1961 showed no difference between urban and rural death rates for either white or nonwhite males. A later analysis of essentially the same data showed increasing mortality rates with urbanization for nonwhite males (14). Based on the 1960 census data, 95 U.S. counties were listed as 100% rural and 13 counties as 100% urban. Comparing the age-adjusted prostatic cancer mortality rates for 1950–69 for these two sets of counties, an urban-rural ratio of 0.96 was found (21).

Analyses of urban and rural rates have been reported for several countries.

Data from the Danish registry for the period 1943–1962 showed a higher rate of prostatic cancer in the urban area of Copenhagen and its suburbs than in the rural areas (22, 23). The rates for provincial towns were intermediate between those for urban and rural areas. In both Norway and Poland, the incidence rate was higher in urban than in rural areas (9). The urban-rural ratio of the age-adjusted prostatic cancer mortality rate in Poland was 1.49 in 1967–1969, a decrease from a ratio of 3.62 in 1959–1961 (24).

Armenian et al. (25) found that a significantly higher proportion of prostate cancer patients resided in rural areas and smaller towns as compared to their matched controls. However, they have concluded that this was probably a reflection of referral patterns at the Roswell Park Memorial Institute rather than an actual difference in the urban-rural distribution of the disease.

A summary of these studies is presented in Table 3. There does appear to be a slightly higher rate of prostatic cancer in urban areas. The higher urban rate may merely reflect greater availability, utilization, and quality of medical care. These factors are especially significant for a disease like prostate cancer where the amount of latent carcinoma is high and detection is influenced by the amount of diagnostic intervention (26–28). On the other hand, real differences in risk related to environmental exposures may also be reflected in these findings.

LATENT CARCINOMA

A proper evaluation of the geographic variation in prostatic cancer rates should consider the frequency of latent carcinomas, i.e., cancer diagnosed through routine autopsy or biopsy examination of prostatic tissue from asymptomatic men. These tumors, which are indistinguishable histologically from clinically apparent cases, are usually discovered as incidental findings in patients who have undergone a rectal examination as part of a routine physical which leads to a biopsy, or who had a transuretheral resection for benign prostatic hypertrophy, or as an incidental finding at autopsy of patients who have died of unrelated causes (29–32).

It has been recognized for many years that carcinomas are found quite frequently when prostates from autopsies or surgery are examined. In fact, the earliest observation of this latent phenomenon was made in 1900 (33). However, the biological significance of these latent cancers is unclear (34). Including them in the count of incident cases would increase the rate of prostatic cancer by several hundred times. Additionally, it is not known whether these latent cancers are an early stage in the natural history of the disease and would in fact with time become clinically apparent, or whether they are a separate clinical entity. Several studies have shown that the survival rates for latent cancers are better than those for clinically apparent prostatic cancer (35–42).

The frequency of such tumors varies considerably among the many studies reporting such rates (see Table 4) and has been found to be as high as 100% in men over the age of 80 (43). The differences reported both among and within countries are due to variations in selection of case material, frequency of biopsies and autopsies, diagnostic acumen of the physician, amount of tissue

TABLE 3. Summary of Urban–Rural Comparisons of Age-Adjusted Prostate Cancer Mortality or Incidence Rates

Author, year published (reference)	Place	Years studied	Type of data[a]	Race	Rate per 100,000 population Urban	Rural	Urban: rural ratio[b]
King et al., 1963 (17)	United States	1949–1951	M	White	15.2	14.6	1.04
				Nonwhite	20.8	16.9	1.23
Lilienfeld et al., 1968 (10)	United States	1959–1961	M	White	12.3	12.5	0.98
				Nonwhite	21.6	20.2	1.07
Hoover et al., 1975 (21)	United States	1950–1969	M	White	Not published		0.96
Blair and Fraumeni, 1978 (14)	United States	1950–1969	M	Nonwhite	Not published		1.12
Griswold et al., 1956 (18)	Connecticut	1947–1951	I	All	27.8	23.3	1.19
Haenszel et al., 1956 (20)	Iowa	1950	I	White	37.8	34.2	1.11
			M	White			0.87
Levin et al., 1960 (19)	New York State	1949–1951	I	Not stated	28.7	24.1	1.19
Clemmesen et al., 1956 (22)	Denmark	1953	I	All	27.0	19.0	1.42
Clemmesen, 1969 (23)	Denmark	1953–1957	I	All	25.7	17.7	1.45
		1958–1962	I	All	26.0	20.3	1.28
Waterhouse, 1976 (9)	Norway	1968–1972	I	All	36.3	31.0	1.17
Waterhouse, 1976 (9)	Poland	1968–1972	I	All	15.6	9.4	1.66
Staszewski, 1976 (24)	Poland	1959–1961	M	All	Not published		3.62
		1967–1969	M	All	Not published		1.49

[a]Incidence (I); mortality (M).

[b]Ratio of highest urban category (75–100% of population living in urban areas) to lowest urban category (0–24% of population living in Urban areas).

examined, frequency of rectal examinations in older men and variation in histological and diagnostic criteria. Nevertheless, it is apparent that a large proportion of the prostates of older men do undergo malignant changes.

Because of these differences, it is difficult to compare frequencies of latent cancers among countries. Only two studies have examined the prevalence of latent cancers of the prostate among countries using a standardized protocol to collect and analyze prostatic tissue (44–46).

Prostates obtained from autopsy of 239 men in Japan and 158 Japanese migrants to Hawaii were examined using a standard protocol for evidence of cancer (44). All subjects were over the age of 50 and had no clinical evidence of a prostatic disorder. For both groups the age-specific prevalence rates of latent carcinoma increased with age. With the exception of men over 80, the age-specific rates were similar between Japanese men and Japanese migrants to Hawaii. The overall age-adjusted rates for the two groups were 20.5% and 26.7%, respectively. The comparable rates of latent prostatic cancer found in the two series and the marked disparity in clinically apparent incidence rates between Japan and the United States suggested to the authors that the cause(s) of prostatic cancer was equally frequent in the two populations, but that the factors which promoted its growth were more frequent in the United States.

Seven areas of the world known to vary considerably in their frequency and mortality rates of prostatic cancer were selected for a study of latent carcinoma (46). Prostates were obtained from men over age 45 at consecutive autopsies where no clinical evidence of cancer of the prostate existed. Sections of the prostate were examined by a pathologist from the area of origin and by a second randomly selected pathologist from one of the study areas. In both cases, a standard protocol was used.

With the exception of Singapore and Israel, there was a marked increase in the frequency of latent carcinoma of the prostate with age. Overall, latent cancers were found in about 20% of all the prostates examined. Frequencies ranged from a low of 13.2% in Singapore to a high of 31.6% in Sweden. There was a strong correlation between the frequency of latent cancer and both the clinical incidence and mortality rates for the seven countries. The epidemiologic implications of these results are noteworthy. Since latent cancers of the prostate are fairly common in older men throughout the world and since the variation among countries in the prevalence of such tumors is much less than the variation in clinical carcinoma, it becomes necessary to consider the prevalence of latent cancers when designing a case-control study. If, in fact, there is an etiologic relationship between latent and clinical cancers, then failure to eliminate individuals in the control group with latent cancers would diminish the magnitude of the difference between cases and control. However, because a valid screening test is not available, elimination of such individuals is not entirely possible.

An alternative procedure would be to restrict the study to younger cases and their age matched controls. Because the rate of latent cancers increases with age, restricting the study to younger men (under 60 years of age) would result in relatively few controls with latent cancer. There is, however, one disadvantage to this method of case selection. A large study area, or perhaps a multicentric collaborative approach, would be required to generate a sufficient number of younger cases in a reasonable period of time.

TABLE 4. Percent of Latent Cancers of the Prostate by Age From Various Studies

Author, reference	Study period	Number subjects	Country	Percent latent carcinomas by age 40–49	50–59	60–69	70–79	80–89	90+	All ages
Rich (47)	1931–1934	292	United States		8.5	11.2	30.5	20.0		14.0
Kahler (48)	1938	381	United States				Not published			13.9
Baron and Angrist (43)	1935–1939	364	United States		6.4	8.1	16.0	21.0		9.9
Baron and Angrist (43)	1935–1939	50	United States		42.0	38.0	66.0	100.0		46.0
Buchert et al. (49)	1938–1946	1038	United States				Not published			13.0
Bauer et al. (36)	1940–1953	847	United States				41.0	← 57.0 →		46.0
Mathé and Ardila (50)	1940–1946	337	United States				Not published			8.4
Hirst and Bergman (51)	1950–1951	39	United States					48.5	80.0	53.8
Hudson (52)	1951	686	United States	3.2	9.5	14.0	← 31.3 →			11.1
Hudson et al. (53)	1954	300	United States	4.2	12.9	16.1	16.9	0.0		13.0
Scott et al. (54)	1949–1963	158	United States				36.0	← 45.0 →		39.0
Halpert et al. (55)	1949–1962	4696	United States	3.8	6.4	12.5	17.4	← 26.1 →		8.8
Strahan (56)	1961–1962	85	United States		12.3	18.0	18.3	← 35.9 →		19.7
Berg et al. (57)	1952–1964	5636	United States	3.1	4.5	23.0	← 53.4 →			19.5
Butler et al. (58)	1958	220	United States				Not published			32.3
Jordon and Kraeger (59)	1966	100	United States				Not published			14.0
Suen et al. (60)	1960–1970	1842	United States			9.5	14.6	10.0		11.4

Akazaki and Stemmermann (44)	1969–1972	158	United States		10.7	20.8	22.9	←57.1→		29.1
Edwards et al. (61)	1948–1949	173	Canada	4.3	9.7	18.5	25.0	17.6		16.8
Andrews (62)	1948	142	England	4.5	5.3	17.9	31.8			12.0
Franks (63)	1954	220	England		29.0	30.2	40.0	66.7	100.0	37.6
Moore (64)	1931–1932	375	Austria	17.4	13.8	23.4	20.6	29.2		16.8
Gaynor (65)	1938	1040	Austria		10.4	17.8	28.3	38.7	40.0	20.7
Oota (66)	1955	259	Japan	5.0	6.6	13.6	35.8	45.0	50.0	18.1
Karube (67)	1956–1959	229	Japan	2.2	5.1	18.2	22.9	0.0		10.9
Sugihara (68)	1959	157	Japan	2.5	4.9	19.4	30.0	0.0		10.9
Imai (69)	1960	129	Japan	0.0	8.8	9.7	15.0	25.0		7.7
Akazaki and Stemmermann (44)	1969–1972	239	Japan		12.3	18.0	18.3	←35.9→		19.7
Cooray et al. (70)	1936–1952	605	Ceylon			Not published				14.0
Liavag et al. (71)	1964–1966	340	Norway	8.0	20.0	23.0	28.6	46.7	66.7	26.5
Viitanen and Hellens (72)	1957	100	Finland		14.0	21.0	38.0			22.0
Lundberg and Berge (73)	1967	308	Sweden	57.0	23.5	38.8	47.1	48.2		42.9
Luciak (74)	1967	500	Poland	4.4	7.2	14.3	17.2	44.4		9.0
Dham and Hohback (6)	1968–1971	1049	Germany	8.5	11.3	20.9	23.0	←22.9→		19.3

SECULAR TRENDS

Mortality

The analysis of mortality data over time poses a number of problems. Such factors as increased access to medical care, better diagnostic acumen, improvements in treatment which result in increases in survival, changes in procedures for assigning cause of death on the death certificate, rules for classifying and coding of death on the death certificate, and accuracy of the population census must be considered in evaluating variations in mortality over time. However, barring such artifacts in the data, real changes in incidence which may reflect underlying genetic or environmental effects can be ascertained. Age-adjusted mortality rates from cancer of the prostate for 1930–1970 have been presented in a number of reports (10, 75–80).

In the United States, for all races combined, an overall increase in mortality of about 150% has occurred between 1930 and 1974 (see Table 5). The increase for nonwhites (322.1%) has been much greater than for whites (33.6%). For white males under age 75, there was a marked increase in the death rates between 1930 and 1940 followed by a decrease through 1970 (see Table 6 and Figure 2). For those 75–84, the rates increased through 1955 before declining. However, between 1965 and 1970, there was an increase of 4.8%. For the oldest age group the rates increased continuously through 1965 before turning downward. The trend for nonwhites under 65 was similar to that noted for whites, except that the downward shift did not begin until after 1950. For those over 65, the rates have increased steadily through 1970 (see Table 6 and Figure 2).

The overall greater increase in mortality since 1930 among nonwhites may reflect, at least in part, improved medical care. Since a large percentage of prostatic cancer cases are asymptomatic and detected during routine rectal examinations, the frequency of use of medical care can increase the incidence of prostatic cancer. However, the higher rate among nonwhites is probably not entirely accounted for by this factor (81).

Twenty-three of the 24 countries in the report by Segi and Kurihara (77)

TABLE 5. Age-Adjusted Prostatic Cancer Death Rates by Race United States, 1930–1974[a]

	1930	1935	1940	1945	1950	1954–1956	1959–1961	1964–1966	1969–1971	1973–1974	Percent change 1930–1974
White	11.6	14.4	16.7	16.5	15.7	16.1	14.9	14.9	14.8	15.5	+33.6
Nonwhite	6.8	10.1	13.0	15.5	19.6	23.3	24.7	24.8	27.2	28.7	+322.1

Source: Devesa, S. S., Silverman, D. T., Cancer incidence and mortality trends in the United States: 1935–1974, J. Natl. Cancer Inst., 60, 545–571, 1978, Gordon T., Crittenden, M., Haenszel, W., Cancer Mortality Trends in the United States, 1930–1955, End Results and Mortality Trends in Cancer, NCI monograph No. 6, 1961.

[a]Average annual number of deaths per 100,000 population; age-adjusted to the 1950 United States population.

TABLE 6. Prostatic Cancer Death Rates Per 100,000 Population by Age and Race, United States, 1930–1970

Age group	1930	1935	1940	1945	1950	1955	1960	1965	1970
					Whites				
35–44	0.3	0.4	0.5	0.4	0.3	0.2	0.1	0.1	0.2
45–54	2.8	3.3	3.3	3.2	2.6	2.4	2.1	2.3	1.9
55–64	23.0	24.9	27.8	25.0	21.9	21.6	18.9	19.4	19.0
65–74	87.8	103.7	118.5	108.0	98.4	102.4	92.6	92.8	91.1
75–84	165.5	230.7	275.0	290.0	287.0	296.3	277.1	270.9	284.0
85+	174.2	238.1	295.7	397.7	434.5	463.3	480.4	499.7	431.5
					Nonwhites				
35–44	0.8	1.1	1.0	1.5	1.1	0.7	1.0	0.6	0.4
45–54	4.7	7.8	10.8	11.3	13.2	10.1	8.8	7.6	8.3
55–64	22.5	32.5	39.8	46.1	55.6	62.5	54.9	52.5	52.2
65–74	48.1	62.5	78.6	101.9	115.8	178.5	178.1	200.0	223.0
75–84	58.6	101.3	151.6	141.5	244.8	280.7	322.0	314.3	470.3
85+	53.6	109.5	113.1	293.3	300.0	256.3	412.4	373.2	447.8

Source: Gordon, T., Crittenden, M., Haenszel, W. Cancer Mortality Trends in the United States, 1930–1955. National Cancer Institute Monograph 6, 1961. 1960–1970 from U.S. Vital Statistics.

showed increases in mortality from cancer of the prostate between 1950 and 1967. The exception, Australia, showed a very slight decrease (0.6%) in rate during this time. In general, the percentage increase varied from 0.7% in Denmark to 378.9% in Japan. The rapidly increasing death rate in Japan has continued through 1974 (82). As a result of this increase, the difference between the rates for U.S. whites and Japanese diminished between 1950 and 1974 from a 30- to a sixfold disparity in the 65–69 year age group and from a 50- to a sixfold disparity in the 70–74 year age group. The increase in the Japanese rate may reflect an increase in exposure to an envirnomental factor and warrants further investigation. It is interesting to note that the increase in the Japanese consumption of dietary fat parallels their increase in the mortality rate (83).

Separate reports from Canada and Scotland show an increasing death rate of prostatic cancer (84, 85). A seven-fold increase was noted in the age-adjusted mortality rate in Scotland between 1911 and 1966 (85). Between 1931–1933 and 1970–1972 the age–standardized prostate cancer mortality rate in Canada increased by an average of 0.07 deaths per 100,000 population per year, a relatively modest rate of increase (84).

Morbidity

United States. Three national cancer surveys have been conducted in the United States by the National Cancer Institute (3, 86, 87). For various reasons, the Third National Cancer Survey was not conducted in the same areas cov-

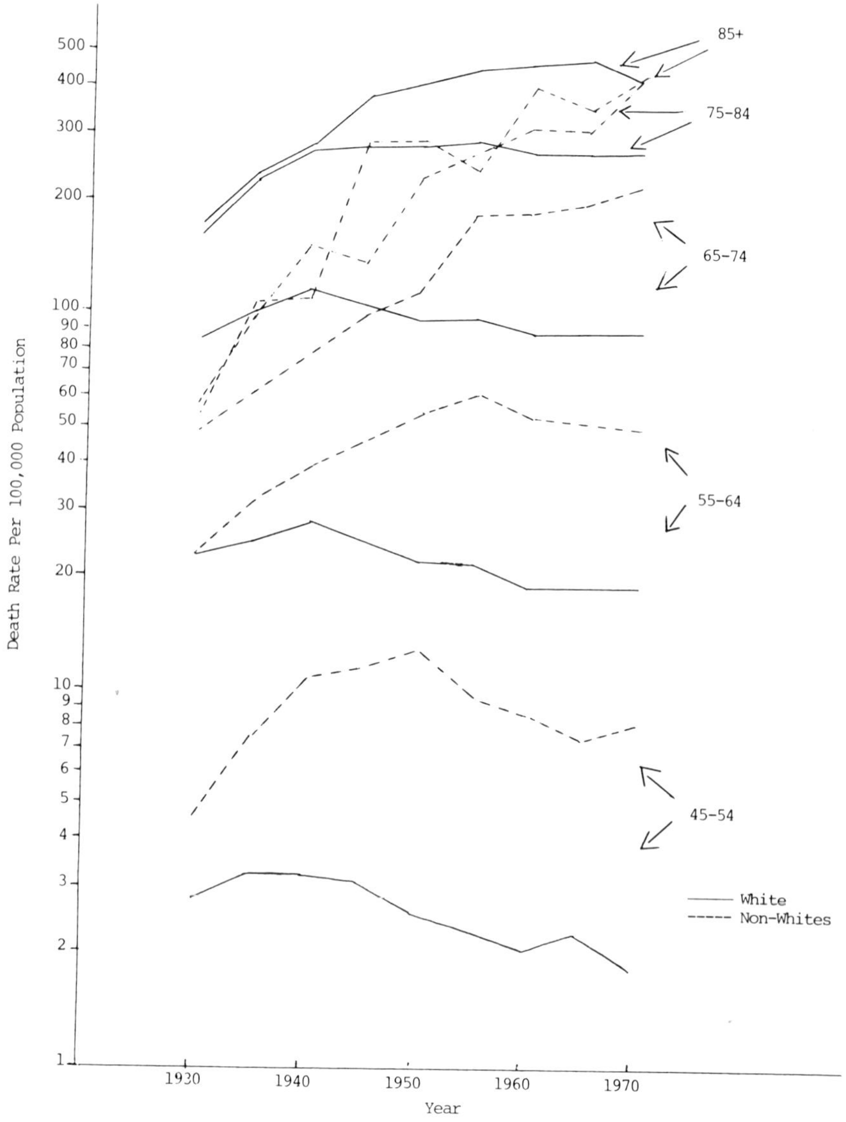

FIGURE 2. Prostatic Cancer Death Rates Per 100,000 Population by Age and Race, United States, 1930–1970.

ered in the first two surveys (80). Nevertheless, since seven of the nine areas covered in the Third National Cancer Survey were included in the first two surveys, comparisons can be made among the three surveys to provide data on the changing incidence of prostatic cancer.

Table 7 presents the age-specific and age-adjusted prostate cancer incidence rates from the three surveys. Overall, for all nine areas, the rates for whites and nonwhites increased 53.3% and 151.6%, respectively. This is probably slightly in excess of the true increase if the comparison was based only on the seven common areas included in all three surveys. When Devesa and Silverman (80) reanalyzed the Third National Cancer Survey data for the seven common areas, they found the age-adjusted rates to be 45.2 for whites and 68.6 for nonwhites per 100,000 population as compared to 46.1 and 78.3 for all nine areas.

For both races, the rates generally increased with age with a slight downward turn in the oldest age groups. The nonwhite–white ratio was smaller in the 1937–1939 survey (1.03) than in the 1969–1971 survey (1.70). This mainly reflects the more rapid increase in the nonwhite rate as compared to the white rate, particularly in the age groups 80–84 and 85+ where the nonwhite rates increased 372.2% and 541.5%, respectively.

For whites the rate of increase between the first and third surveys varied from 30.8% for the 50–54 age group to 115.8 percent for the 85+ group. For nonwhites the increase varied from 100 to 541.5% for the 50–54 and 85+ age groups, respectively.

Other studies have also examined the change in the rate of prostatic cancer over time. Griswold (88), using data from a ten-year survey of all hospitalized prostatic cancer cases in Connecticut, reviewed the number of cases between 1935 and 1945. Although there was an overall increase in incident cases, he

TABLE 7. Age-Adjusted and Age-Specific Prostate Cancer Incidence Rates by Race for Three United States National Cancer Surveys[a]

	1937–1939		1947–1948		1969–1971		Percent increase from 1937–1939 survey to 1969–1971 survey	
Age	W	NW	W	NW	W	NW	W	NW
50–54	13	18	13	40	17	36	30.8	100.0
55–59	34	46	33	81	52	118	52.9	156.5
60–64	86	111	90	189	127	270	47.7	143.2
65–69	171	205	175	310	255	465	49.1	126.8
70–74	317	336	334	535	431	785	36.0	133.6
75–79	417	390	506	523	658	926	57.8	137.4
80–84	408	270	670	460	829	1275	103.2	372.2
85+	412	135	771	379	889	866	115.8	541.5
All Ages	30	31	35	50	46	78	53.3	151.6

Source: Hutchison, G. B., Epidemiology of prostatic cancer, Sem. Oncol. 3, 151–159, 1976. Reprinted by permission of Grune & Stratton, Inc.

[a]Average annual rates per 100,000 population adjusted to 1950 U.S. population.

failed to compute rates and to take into account the parallel changes in population growth during this time period.

Sullivan et al. (90) analyzed incidence data from the Connecticut Tumor Registry for the period 1935–1965 for ten major primary sites of cancer including prostatic neoplasms. Sex- and age-specific incidence rates were computed for each site for each year and age-adjusted to the 1950 U.S. population. There was a substantial increase in the age-adjusted incidence of cancer of the prostate from 24.9 per 100,000 population in 1935–1938 to 37.7 per 100,000 population in 1962–1965. This increase (51.4%) was similar to that noted for white males between the First and Third National Cancer Surveys discussed earlier.

Between 1942 and 1955, New York State, exclusive of New York City, recorded a 27% increase in the incidence of prostatic cancer based on data from the state Cancer Registry (91). A more recent update of these data demonstrated an additional 37% increase from 1956 to 1972 (92). Overall, there was a 58% increase in the rate between 1942 and 1972.

In Alameda County, California, nonwhites have one of the highest rates among those in all the registries reported in the Five Continent Survey (9). Between 1960 and 1969 there was a statistically significant increase of 22.2% in the incidence of all prostatic cancer based on data from the Alameda County Cancer Registry (93). Unfortunately, no breakdown by race was provided, as the authors felt that data for nonwhites were unreliable due to the variability of the rates. Nevertheless, they did indicate that the increase was apparent for both races.

The authors compared these data for Alameda County with data covering the same time period derived from the Connecticut Tumor Registry. Data from Connecticut showed that the rates for prostatic cancer had actually decreased from 42.5 per 100,000 population in 1960 to 39.5 per 100,000 population in 1969. However, data for the same period from the New York State Registry are similar to those for Alameda County. For the period 1960–1969, New York had a 25.8% increase in the incidence of prostatic cancer.

Other Countries. Incidence data from the cancer registry of Denmark showed a marked increase in crude incidence rates for carcinoma of the prostate between 1943 and 1953 (22). Similar increases were noted for Copenhagen, provincial towns and rural areas, although the rates for any year were in general highest for Copenhagen and lowest for the rural areas. The authors speculated that at least some of this increase was due to more extensive application of histological examinations in the more recent time period.

Analyses of the data for 1953 through 1962 showed a continuation in the upward trend for prostatic cancer for all areas of Denmark (23). The increase in age-adjusted incidence rates during this period was more modest, ranging from 1.2% in the capital to 14.7% in the rural areas. A more recent report substantiated this marked increase (94). For the entire period between 1943 and 1972, the age-adjusted incidence rate for all areas doubled from 18.2 to 37.2 per 100,000 population.

The Finnish Cancer Registry provided the data for Saxen et al. (95) to examine the trend in the incidence of prostatic cancer between 1954 and 1963. Prostatic cancer, which accounts for about 6% of all male cancers in Finland has risen slightly (13%) in incidence from 12.6 per 100,000 population in 1954 to 14.2 in 1963. Teppo et al., using incidence data for 1957–1969 from the Finnish Cancer Registry, attempted to predict the incidence rates of cancer for various sites for the year 1980 (96). Applying linear regression analysis to the age-adjusted incidence rates he predicted an increase in the rate of prostatic cancer for the year 1980 based on an increasing trend in prostatic cancer between 1957 and 1968.

The recording of all cases of malignant neoplasms in the population of Warsaw, Poland, in 1963–1970, permitted Gadomska and Romejko (97) to compute the incidence of a number of cancer sites including cancer of the prostate. Prostatic cancer accounted for 5.1% of all male malignancies during this time period. The trend of changes in the incidence rates was elucidated by use of linear regression analysis. Because of the relatively few cases of prostatic carcinoma in men less than 60 years of age, the incidence of the tumors was analyzed only in two age groups, 60–69 years and 70 or more years. There was an overall decrease in the rate of incidence from 1963 to 1970 which was particularly conspicuous in the 60–69 year age group. The mean annual percent change showed a decline of 3.9% in this age group and 0.8% in the older age group. The percentage of histologically confirmed cases of prostatic carcinoma rose from 15.4% in 1963 to 33.3% in 1970.

In virtually all areas of the world for which data are available, an increase in the rate of prostatic cancer has been noted (9, 98). Exceptions to this increase were reported in Australia, Poland, Cali, Colombia, and Miyagi Prefecture of Japan, although the overall rate for Japan has increased steadily since World War II.

The reasons for this increase are not known. Undoubtedly, some contribution to the higher rates in more recent time periods may be due to an increased utilization of medical services, and in particular an increase in autopsy and biopsy examinations (22). However, it is unlikely that the total increase can be accounted for by this factor. It is reasonable to speculate that there has been a real increase in prostatic cancer and that it is probably attributable to an increased exposure to an environmental factor.

Cohort Analysis

Grouping mortality or morbidity data according to date of birth of the subjects permits an evaluation of common experiences or exposures. Three attempts have been made to ascertain a possible cohort effect for prostatic cancer (75, 99, 100). Neither Case (99), nor Gordon et al. (75) demonstrated such an effect using mortality data for England and Wales for the period 1911–1954 and mortality data for the United States for the period 1930–1955, respectively. Ernster et al. (100) analyzed prostatic cancer mortality rates among U.S. nonwhite males aged 45 to 84 for separate birth cohorts extending from 1846 to 1925. Rates for all age groups peaked in the birth cohort of 1896 to 1900 and declined thereafter. A continuation of this trend would result in an overall decline of the nonwhite prostatic cancer mortality rate. Furthermore, as pointed out by the authors, research into the early experiences of 1896 to 1900 and prior birth cohorts might provide etiologic clues.

AGE

Cancer of the prostate is a disease of older men. It rarely occurs in men under the age of 50; rates increase rapidly with advancing age (see Table 8 and Figure 3). In fact, Cook et al. (101) have shown that prostatic cancer increases in incidence with age more rapidly than any other cancer. A similar rate of increase for latent cancer of the prostate has also been demonstrated (102).

As shown in Table 8 and Figure 3, for both races, the rate of incidence of prostatic cancer increases with age, virtually doubling with each 5-year age interval between 55 and 74 years of age. The rate of increase after age 70–74 is markedly diminished. With the exception of the below-40- and above-85-year-olds, rates for the black males exceed those for white males. These differences are greatest in the age group 50–65 where the rate for blacks is 120% greater than that for whites.

Of interest is the difference in the percent distribution by age. For whites, 18.7% of all cases were among men less than 65 years of age, whereas for blacks 26.6% of cases were diagnosed in this age group. Almost one half (46.1%) of all cases among whites occurred in men over the age of 75, whereas for blacks less than one-third (30.4%) occurred in this age group. The median age of diagnosis was 73 for whites and 70 for blacks.

The age increase in the rate of prostatic cancer is apparent throughout the world. Every registry in the Five Continent Study generally demonstrated an increasing rate with age (9).

Mortality also increases with age (see Table 9). For each age group, rates for black males exceed those for white males. For all races combined, mortality rates virtually double from one age group to the next up to the age of 75 after which the rates of increase diminish. This rate of increase is greater for white than for black males. (see Figure 4).

RACE

U.S. Blacks

There are striking differences in the distribution of prostatic cancer by race. Noteworthy is the relatively high rate of the disease among blacks in the United States (3, 9, 10, 13, 81, 103–107). In fact, the Alameda County Cancer Registry and the San Francisco–Oakland Area Registry reported the highest rates of prostatic cancer in blacks of all registries covered in the Five Continent Study (9).

Data from the Third National Cancer Survey showed that blacks had a 70% higher age-adjusted incidence rate than whites (3). Similar excesses were found in both Alameda County (86%) and the San Francisco–Oakland (73%) area (9). Rates for blacks exceeded those for whites in each of the nine areas included in the Third National Cancer Survey, ranging from a low of a 17% excess in Minneapolis–St. Paul to a high of 113% in Colorado (see Table 2). Black-white ratios were greater in the lower age groups (under 65 years of age) where they were of the order of 2:1 (see Table 8). After age 65, the ratios decreased with age and by age 85+ the rate for whites was slightly greater than for blacks. Similar patterns existed for both San Francisco–Oakland and Alameda County although at each age group the ratios were slightly greater.

TABLE 8. Number and Percent Distribution of Incident Cases by Age and Average Annual Age-Specific Incidence Rates of Prostatic Cancer by Race, Third National Cancer Survey (All Areas Combined, 1969–1971)[a]

Age group	All races			White males			Black males		
	Number	Percent	Rate	Number	Percent	Rate	Number	Percent	Rate
<40	10	0.1	0.2	9	0.1	0.2	1	0.1	0.1
40–44	28	0.2	1.5	23	0.2	1.4	5	0.3	2.9
45–49	91	0.6	4.9	78	0.6	4.6	12	0.6	7.1
50–54	305	2.1	18.2	252	2.0	16.6	53	2.8	36.2
55–59	840	5.7	58.0	679	5.3	52.2	151	8.1	116.6
60–64	1640	11.0	139.5	1341	10.4	126.8	274	14.7	269.5
65–69	2408	16.2	273.6	1995	15.5	254.2	380	20.4	462.6
70–74	2990	20.1	457.8	2540	19.8	429.5	421	22.6	785.3
75–79	3035	20.4	673.3	2733	21.3	655.9	273	14.7	922.6
80–84	2152	14.5	847.6	1940	15.1	825.6	191	10.3	1274.6
85+	1359	9.1	871.8	1247	9.7	882.4	100	5.4	865.8
Total	14,858	100.0	48.6	12,837	100.0	47.7	1861	100.0	57.9

Source: Cutler, S. J., Young, J. L., Jr., Third National Cancer Survey: Incidence Data, Biometry Branch, National Cancer Institute, Monograph 41, DHEW Pub. No. (NIH) 75-787, 1975.

[a]Average annual rates per 100,000 population.

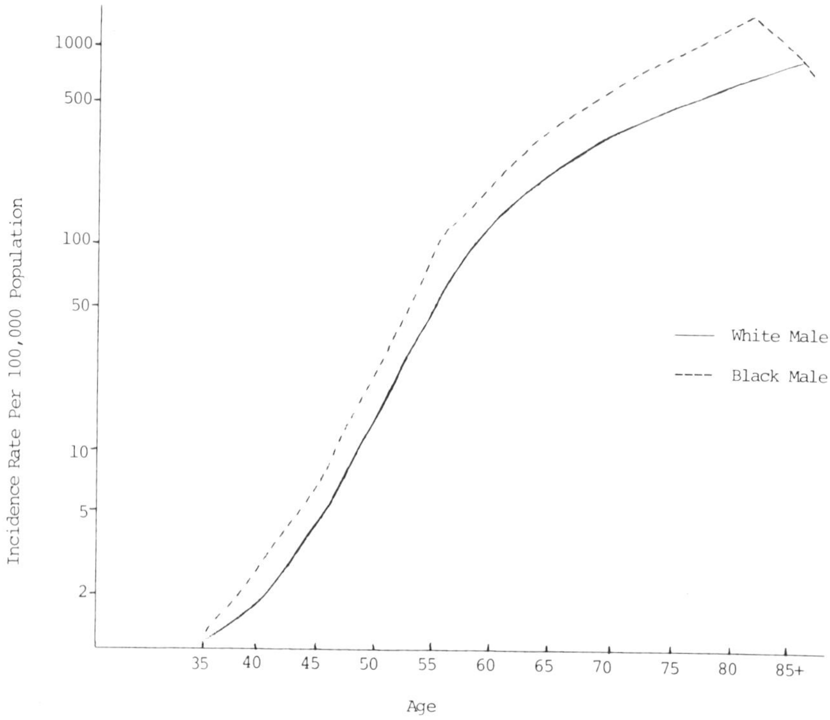

FIGURE 3. Age-Specific Incidence Rates For Prostatic Cancer by Race, Third National Cancer Survey, 1969–1971.

Source: S. J., Young, J. L., Jr. Third National Cancer Survey: Incidence Data, Biometry Branch, National Cancer Institute. Monograph 41. DHEW Pub. No. (NIH) 75–787, 1975.

TABLE 9. Age-Specific Mortality Rates for Prostatic Cancer by Race, United States, 1975[a]

Age group	All races	White males	Black males
40	—	—	—
40–44	0.2	0.2	0.9
45–49	1.0	0.8	2.4
50–54	3.7	2.9	12.0
55–59	12.6	10.9	32.5
60–64	33.2	28.9	81.5
65–69	72.0	64.2	154.7
70–74	149.4	133.8	352.9
75–79	253.6	236.5	499.1
80–84	400.6	390.6	564.0
85+	489.4	483.8	603.8
Total	18.7	18.1	26.0

Source: Vital Statistics of the United States, 1975, National Center for Health Statistics, D.H.E.W., 1979.

[a]Rates per 100,000 population.

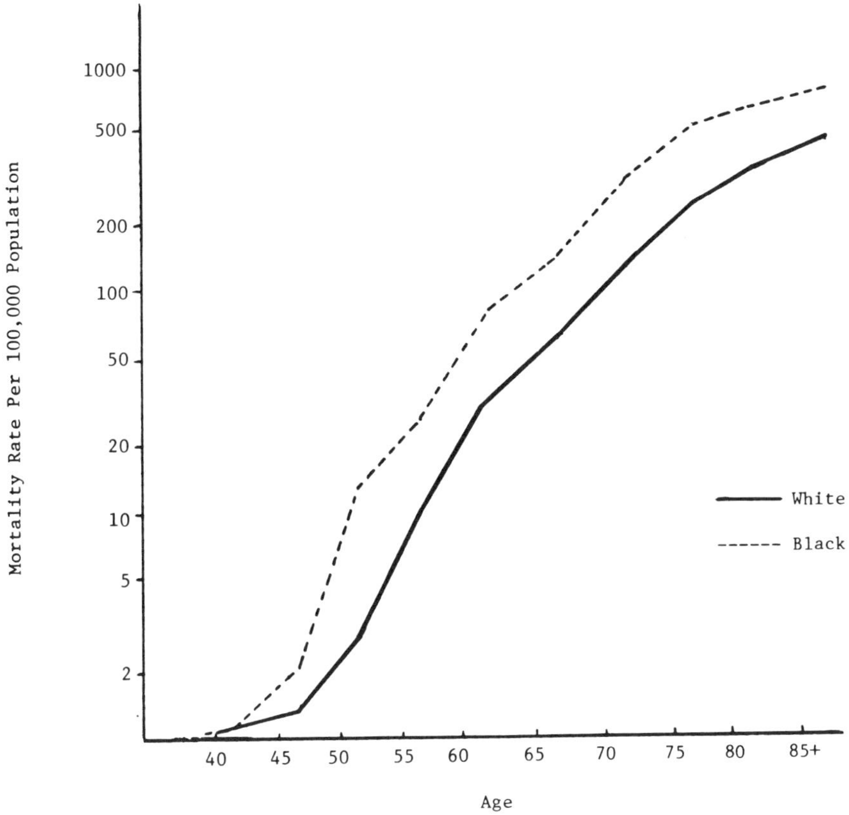

FIGURE 4. Age-Specific Mortality Rates For Prostatic Cancer by Race, United States 1971.

Source: Vital Statistics of the United States 1971. National Center for Health Statistics, DHEW, 1974.

Mortality rates were similarly distributed (see Table 9), that is, rates for blacks were 40% greater than those for whites. The largest differential between black and white rates occurred in the younger age groups where rates for blacks were 3 to 3.5 times greater than rates for whites. The higher rates in blacks were less pronounced after age 70, but beyond age 85, the rates were very similar (103).

Japanese

Incidence rates for Japanese men are considerably lower than for U.S. males (108, 109). In fact, the United States has an incidence rate about 15–20 times greater than that in Japan (9). Similar disparities exist between U.S. males and all oriental races (9, 108, 110). Japanese men from Hawaii and other parts of the United States were found to have a significantly lower mortality rate from cancer of the prostate than U.S. men (111). The standardized mortality ratios for Japanese compared to white and nonwhite U.S. males were 24 and 18, respectively.

Quisenberry (112) found that the incidence rate for prostatic cancer was nine times higher in Caucasian Hawaiians than in Japanese Hawaiians. The rate for Hawaiians and part-Hawaiians was approximately half that of Caucasians and was over four times as great as the rate for Japanese men. Smith (113), using data for the period 1949–1952, found standardized mortality ratios of 50 and 12 for Hawaiians and Filipinos, respectively, when compared to U.S. nonwhites. An analysis of cancer mortality among the various racial groups in Hawaii was made by Kagan (114). For the period 1957 through 1963, the rate for Caucasian men was about three times the rate of Japanese and Filipino men, twice that of Chinese men and three times that of Hawaiian men.

Recent cancer registry data reveal the following standardized prostatic cancer incidence rates per 100,000 population: Japan—2.73, Hawaiian- Japanese —24.6, U.S. whites—40.37, U.S. nonwhites—73.03 (109).

American Indians

An analysis of U.S. mortality data for the years 1950–1967 showed that American Indians had a significantly lower mortality rate from cancer of the prostate than white or black males (115). The standardized mortality ratios were 57.7 based on white rates and 36.7 based on black rates. These findings were consistent with previous observations (10, 116, 117). Although possible artifacts in the data, such as percentage of deaths attributed to senility and ill-defined causes, errors in the population census, death certification practices, completeness of reporting, and diagnostic acumen, might account for some of the deficit, available evidence suggests that the lower rates of prostatic cancer in American Indians is not entirely due to such artifacts but reflects real differences in risk (116, 117).

Tissue specimens from 693 histologically diagnosed cancers for U.S. Indians were available from Indian Health Facilities in 14 states (118). The examination of such specimens obviates in part the problem of relying on death certificates as the basic source of data. However, it cannot be assumed that the tissues submitted were in any way representative of prostatic cancer cases in the catchment area. The authors compared the "age-corrected frequency ratios" (proportional incidence ratios) among the Indian population with similar ratios for U.S. whites and found that the ratio among the Indian population was somewhat greater that that among U.S. whites (11.5% vs. 8.1%). This is contrary to the previous findings of lower rates among Indians. However, caution must be exercised in interpreting these results because of the probable selection bias in the data and the method of analysis. According to the Third National Cancer Survey, 15.8% of all male cancers were due to prostate cancer, which is similar to the percentage observed among the U.S. Indians.

Spanish Americans

Incidence data from the University of Southern California Cancer Surveillance Program in Los Angeles County were divided by the patients' surnames into Spanish and non-Spanish categories, using the detailed Spanish surname list from the 1970 U.S. Census (119). Lower incidence rates of prostatic cancer were found in male Spanish-surnamed residents of Los Angeles County when compared to other whites. Further classification of the Spanish-surnamed males by dichotomizing into immigrant Mexican-Americans and indigenous Mexican-Americans resulted in greater disparities in rates. Immigrant Mexican-Americans had incidence rates from prostatic cancer much lower than other whites whereas indigenous Mexican-Americans had rates that were intermediate between the other two groups. These findings were similar to those reported by Creagan and Fraumeni (115) for the American Indians.

Alaskan Natives

Alaskan natives (Eskimos, Indians, and Aleuts) were found to have a significantly lower than expected incidence of prostatic cancer (120). The lower risk was particularly striking among Eskimos.

A summary of the data on race is presented in Table 10. The high rates in U.S. blacks and low rates in Orientals are particularly noteworthy. It also appears that American Indians, Mexican-Americans and Alaskan natives have lower rates than U.S. whites. However, further work on these latter racial groups is necessary before their rates and relative position could be considered to be firmly established.

MIGRANTS

The study of migrants provides a unique opportunity to determine if the etiology of a disease is due to genetic or environmental factors (121,122). Steiner referred to migrants as providing an opportunity to observe natural experiments on the etiology of cancer in humans (123). A comparison of the mortality experience of migrants with that in their country of origin and in their country of adoption can provide valuable insight as to the relative contribution of exogenous or endogenous factors in disease. If migrants have a mortality rate similar to that in their country of adoption and quite dissimilar to the rate prevailing in their country of origin, then it is more likely that an environmental factor is responsible for the migrants' assumption of the new rate in their country of adoption. On the other hand, a genetic factor would more likely explain the situation where the migrants retained the mortality rate prevailing in their country of origin despite emigrating to a country with a markedly different rate.

Naturally, there can be exceptions to these outcomes. A number of factors must be considered in the analysis and interpretation of migrant data. These include artifacts in the data such as the accuracy and completeness of death certification, the etiological importance of the premigration environment, and the characteristics, particularly the health status, of migrants relative to those from their country who do not migrate. Data on these factors, however, are not always available. Nevertheless, awareness of the potential sources of bias in migrant studies does suggest caution in their interpretation.

Lombard and Doering (124) were perhaps the first to provide a systematic review of a number of site specific cancer mortality rates for the foreign–born living in Boston. However, little attention was devoted to migrant studies un-

TABLE 10. Summary of Results of Studies on the Relationship Between Cancer of the Prostate and Race

Author, date (Reference)	Source of data	Time period	Racial group	Racial group/white ratio
Cutler and Young, 1975 (3)	Third National Cancer Survey	1969–1971	U.S. blacks	1.70
Five Continent Study, 1976 (9)	Alameda County Cancer Registry	1969–1973	U.S. blacks	1.86
Dunn, 1975 (108)	Bay Area Cancer Registry	1969–1973	U.S. blacks	1.74
Ernster 1977 (105)	Alameda County Cancer Registry	1960–1969	U.S. blacks	1.20
Burbank, 1972 (103)	U.S. Mortality Data	1950–1967	U.S. blacks	1.69
Ernster, 1977 (105)	Alameda County Mortality Data	1968–1972	U.S. blacks	1.20
Smith, 1956 (116)	U.S. Mortality Data	1948–1952	American Indians	0.13
Smith, 1957 (117)	U.S. Mortality Data	1949–1952	American Indians	0.58
Creagan, 1972 (115)	U.S. Mortality Data	1950–1967	American Indians	0.46
Menck, 1975 (119)	U.S.C. Cancer Survellance Program	1972–1973	Mexican Americans	0.69
Lanier, 1976 (120)	Hospital and Registry Data	1969–1973	Alaska natives	0.60
Smith, 1956 (111)	U.S. Mortality Data	1949–1952	Japanese Americans	0.24
Quisenberry, 1960 (112)	Hospital Records, Hawaii	1944–1954	Japanese Americans	0.11
Dunn, 1975 (108)	Bay Area Cancer Registry	1969–1973	Japanese Americans	0.40
Kagan, 1971 (114)	Mortality Data, Hawaii	1957–1963	Japanese Americans	0.38
Quisenberry, 1960 (112)	Hospital Records, Hawaii	1944–1954	Chinese Americans	0.17
Kagan, 1971 (114)	Mortality Data, Hawaii	1957–1963	Chinese Americans	0.55
Fraumeni, 1974 (110)	U.S. Mortality Data	1950–1969	Chinese Americans	0.30
Dunn, 1975 (108)	Bay Area Cancer Registry	1969–1973	Chinese Americans	0.40
Smith, 1957 (113)	Mortality Data, Hawaii	1949–1952	Hawaiians	0.50[a]
Quisenberry, 1960 (112)	Hospital Records, Hawaii	1944–1954	Hawaiians	0.48
Kagan, 1971 (114)	Mortality Data, Hawaii	1957–1963	Hawaiians	0.33
Smith, 1976 (113)	Mortality Data, Hawaii	1944–1952	Filipinos	0.12[a]
Kagan, 1971 (116)	Mortality Data, Hawaii	1957–1963	Filipinos	0.33

[a]Compared to U.S. nonwhite rates.

til Haenszel's (125) extensive analysis of over 34,000 cancer deaths in 1950 among foreign-born whites in 35 U.S. states. Perhaps this neglect was due to the pessimistic conclusion of Lombard and Doering, who stated that "the differences we have found in the cancer death rates by site and nativity groups are subject to speculation. Nothing can be definitely established."

Haenszel (125) experienced greater success. He found that in general the mortality ratio for prostatic cancer for the foreign-born whites was lower than for the native-born U.S. whites. However, this was not true for every country. The migrants from Ireland, Norway, Canada, and Sweden had a prostatic cancer mortality rate greater than the native-born. Migrants from Poland, Austria, Russia, and Italy had lower rates than the native-born. The most noteworthy result was for the foreign-born from Ireland. Although the prevailing prostatic cancer mortality rate in Ireland at that time was lower than for U.S. whites, the Irish migrants had a rate almost two and one-half times greater than that in Ireland. For the other countries, the rates among the foreign-born were not significantly different from those in their countries of origin. Haenszel concluded from this analysis that prostatic cancer was more likely due to an endogenous factor, a position supported by Kmet (126).

Lilienfeld et al. (10) analyzed mortality data for 1959–1961 for U.S. native-born whites, migrants to the United States from selected countries, and residents of these countries of origin. A summary of these findings is presented in Table 11. Migrants from countries with rates significantly lower than U.S. rates (Czechoslovakia, Germany, Hungary, Ireland, Italy, Mexico, Poland, United Kingdom, and Yugoslavia) had higher rates than those prevailing in their country of origin, that is, the migrants assumed the rates of their country of adoption. There were only two countries with rates significantly greater than the U.S. native white rate—Norway and Sweden. Migrants from Sweden had a rate intermediate between the rate in Sweden and the rate in the United States. Norwegian migrants had a rate slightly higher than that prevailing in their country of origin. Migrants from Ireland had a significantly higher rate than that among residents of Ireland or United States native whites. The same disparity was found in Haenszel's earlier analysis [125]. No explanation was offered in either study to explain this result. It appears that either only migrants who are at a high risk from cancer of the prostate migrated to the United States or that this group underwent a drastic change in an environmental factor (perhaps dietary) so as to significantly elevate their rate. This latter explanation assumes an exogenous rather than endogenous etiologic factor. The analysis by Lilienfeld et al. (10) is suggestive of an environmental influence since the migrants, particularly from countries with lower rates than those for U.S. native-born whites, assumed the prevailing rates of their country of adoption.

Haenszel (127) analyzed three sources of data on Jewish migrants to the United States. Using data from his earlier study on U.S.S.R. migrants and from both MacMahon's (128) and Seidman's (129) studies of New York Jews, Haenszel reviewed the internal consistency of these sources of information on prostatic cancer mortality among U.S. Jews (125). All three sources of data demonstrated the lower prostatic cancer mortality among foreign and U.S.-born Jews.

TABLE 11. Age-Adjusted Prostatic Cancer Death Rates[a] for United States Native Whites, for Migrants To the United States From Selected Countries, 1959–1961 and For Residents of These Countries of Origin, 1960

United States Native Whites = 12.9

Country	Mortality rate among residents	Mortality rate among migrants
Austria	13.0	13.7
Canada	12.2	15.3
Czechoslovakia	7.4	11.0
Finland	11.8	11.8
Germany	11.4	13.4
Hungary	10.6	11.5
Ireland	9.3	19.3
Italy	8.1	9.5
Mexico	4.1	7.7
Norway	15.4	16.4
Poland	3.5	10.9
Sweden	16.5	14.1
United Kingdom	11.5	12.7
Yugoslavia	5.2	12.0

Source: Lilienfeld, A. M., Levin, M. L., Kessler, I. I., Cancer in the United States, APHA Monograph, Harvard University Press, 1972.

[a]Rates per 100,000 population.

Greenwald (130) analyzed mortality data on Russian-born residents of New York State (exclusive of New York City) who died during the years 1969–1971. The distinction between Jewish and non-Jewish segments of the Russian-born population was based, as in previous studies, on the religious affiliation of the cemetery of burial or the funeral home listed on the death certificate. Overall the prostatic cancer mortality rate of all Russian-born residents was similar to that expected (SMR=97). Because no population data by country of birth and religion were available, a proportional mortality comparison was made for the Jewish and non-Jewish segments of the study population. The cause-specific proportionate cancer mortality of all residents of New York State (exclusive of New York City) for the years 1969–1971 was used to derive expected values. There was no significant difference between the observed and expected values of prostatic cancer among the Jewish or non-Jewish Russian-born populations, although the latter group had a much greater disparity between observed and expected values.

Because baseline mortality data were not available for Poland at the time Haenszel conducted his study, Staszewski (131) later presented an analysis of cancer mortality data for Poland and Polish migrants to the United States for the year 1950 using the same method as Haenszel. The results were similar to those of Lilienfeld et al. (10). Poland had one of the lowest prostatic cancer mortality rates in the world. Migrants from Poland to the United States were found to have rates intermediate between those for native Poles and U.S. native whites. This was particulary apparent for migrants who died at ages 65 and over. For deaths at an earlier age, the rate for migrants was somewhat greater than those for both native-born Poles and native-born Americans. However, the small numbers of deaths in the younger age groups made it impossible to draw any firm conclusions from the data.

Both China and Japan have low rates of prostatic cancer (9). Migrants from both these countries have been studied and found to have rates intermediate between those in their country of origin and those in the United States (132–134). For the Japanese, comparisons between Issei and Nisei were not possible because of the scarcity of Nisei males over the age of 65. For the Chinese, comparisons between foreign-born and native-born U.S. Chinese (referred to as Idai and Eidai by King and Haenszel) were possible. The standardized mortality ratio (SMR) for the Eidai (35) was somewhat higher than the SMR for the Idai (29). However, the difference was modest and was based on small numbers. The most recent published analysis of foreign and native-born Chinese and Japanese was based on data from 1959–1962 (132–134). Because the 1970 census data are available, it is now possible to update this analysis for the period around 1970.

The State of Israel provides a unique opportunity to study disease rates among the various migrant groups. Israel's unrestricted immigration policy grants every Jew the right to make Israel his or her home and to receive citizenship. As a result, large groups of people migrated to Israel from Europe, Asia, Africa, and America, especially in the period between 1948 and 1953. An analysis of the cancer incidence and mortality rates for Israeli, African, Asian, European, and American-born Jews was conducted using incidence data for 1960–1966 from the Central Cancer Registry in Israel and mortality data for 1950–1967 (135). The patterns of the age-specific incidence rates varied greatly. For the youngest age group, 45–54, African- and Asian-born Jews had a rate almost twice as high as that for European- and American-born Jews. No data were available for this age group for Israeli-born Jews. For the age group 55–64, Israeli-born Jews had the highest rate, European- and American-born Jews the lowest, and African- and Asian-born Jews were intermediate between the two. Just the opposite was found for the age group 65 and over where the European and American Jews had the highest rate and Israeli-born Jews the lowest.

An analysis of the mortality data revealed that the age-adjusted rates for European- and American-born Jews were greater than for African- and Asian-born Jews for the period 1950–1965; after that time the rates were reversed.

Steinitz and Costin (136) analyzed the cancer incidence registry data by specific country of origin. The age-adjusted prostatic cancer death rates were highest for Jews born in Greece and Bulgaria (22.80) followed by Egyptian-born Jews (20.78), Northwest African-born Jews (18.09), and Iranian-born Jews (15.53). In all, there was considerable variation among the countries. The lowest rates were found for Yemenite Jews.

Overall, the data on migrating populations tend to favor an environmental hypothesis. However, there is as yet only a small body of data on this subject.

RELIGION

Religion can be a useful classificatory variable in epidemiologic studies because it can help to identify a group of individuals whose culture, behavioral and ethnic practices make them fairly homogenous. There is undoubtedly considerable variability in the degree of homogeneity between religious groups. However, certain customs, habits, practices, or behaviors are common to virtually all members of a particular religious group. Circumcision, abstinence from tobacco and alcohol, and a vegetarian diet characterize Jews, Mormons, and Seventh Day Adventists, respectively. Therefore, the ascertainment of disparities in disease rates among religious groups could suggest factors of possible etiologic significance for further study.

MacMahon (128) examined cancer mortality among the white ethnic subgroups of New York City. Deaths of residents of New York City in 1955 were divided into three religious groups, Catholic, Protestant, and Jewish, on the basis of the cemetery of burial. (Ascertaining religion on the basis of cemetery of burial was previously used in a study on mortality among Jews in New York City conducted in 1931 (137).) Data on religious distribution in the general population were obtained from a sample survey undertaken by the Health Insurance Plan of New York. The highest mortality rate for prostatic cancer was found for Protestants and the lowest for Jews.

Newill (138) extended the New York study by including 6 years of mortality data, 1953–1958, to ascertain if the differences noted in MacMahon's study were still evident in a larger series of deaths. The results were similar to those found in MacMahon's study. The death rate from prostatic cancer among Protestants was 57% higher than that among Jews and 28% higher than among Catholics. These compare with excesses of 66% and 19% in the previous study.

King (139) attempted to determine religious preference of decedents more directly than by using cemetery of burial as recorded on the death certificate. In a study conducted in 1959 in Baltimore City and Baltimore County, King used the funeral home where the funeral service was held to obtain information on the religious preference of 1754 decedents. The information was obtained by a mailed questionnaire sent to 152 undertakers in Maryland requesting religious identification of decedents. The findings for prostatic cancer varied slightly from those of both MacMahon and Newill (128, 138). The highest rate was among Catholics and the lowest among Jews, although the rates for Protestants and Catholics were virtually identical.

Seidman (129) analyzed mortality data for New York City for the period 1949–1951 to examine the relationship between cancer mortality and both religion and socioeconomic status. As in MacMahon's study, religious denomination was ascertained from the cemetery of burial listed on the death certificate. For all socioeconomic classes combined, Jews were found to have the lowest age-adjusted death rate from prostatic cancer, Catholics the highest, and Protestants were intermediate between the two. The low rate among Jews was not evident in the lowest socioeconomic class where the Protestant rate was lower than that for Jews.

Three of these four studies ascertained religion from the religious affiliation of the cemetery of burial. MacMahon and Koller (140) compared religion as stated on hospital records with religion designated by cemetery of burial on death certificates for a group of leukemia deaths. They found that persons buried in Catholic and Jewish cemeteries were almost exclusively Catholic and Jewish respectively. Of those individuals buried in Protestant and nonsectarian cemeteries, and of those cremated, 63% were Protestant, 22% Catholic, 8% Jewish, and 7% of other religious affiliation. Therefore, information on cemetery of burial does classify Jews and Catholics accurately, but does not provide for a satisfactory ascertainment of Protestants. However, in allocating deaths to the three religious groups, both MacMahon (128) and Newill (138) adjusted the distribution to the Protestant category in accordance with the data from the MacMahon and Koller study. Seidman (129) included as Protestant those individuals buried in Protestant and nonsectarian cemeteries plus a "proportional allocation" of all others.

The three studies by MacMahon, Newill, and Seidman were conducted in New York City utilizing death certificates from about the same time period. Although all three studies found a lower rate of prostatic cancer among Jews (considering all socioeconomic groups combined in Seidman's study), there was some disagreement as to the religious group with the highest rate. The differences could be due to two aspects of the studies: (1) both MacMahon and Newill considered white males age 45 and over, whereas Seidman used white males age 25–64 (2) both MacMahon and Newill estimated Protestants in the same manner whereas Seidman's method differed.

The significantly lower rate of prostatic cancer among Jews found in the four previous studies that analyzed mortality data was also found in case-control studies by Wynder (141) and Krain (142, 143). Although Krain concluded in his two papers that no statistically significant differences were found in the religion of the patients versus the controls, there were almost twice as many Jews among controls as compared to cases. Wynder showed that among white males over the age of 60 the prostatic cancer group contained a smaller percentage of Jews than the control group. Under the age of 60, there was no difference between cases and controls in the percentage of Jews.

Data from the Five Continent Study lend further support to the consistent finding of a lower rate of prostatic cancer among Jews (9). The age-adjusted incidence rate for Jews in Israel for the period 1967–1971 was among the lowest rates for the registries that reported data.

In a study of 3914 clergymen of the United Lutheran Church of America, King and Bailar (144) found that the mortality rate from prostatic cancer was no different from that expected among U.S. white males. A later study of ministers of the Protestant Episcopal Church in the United States and of clergymen of the Church in England, reported a lower than expected prostatic cancer mortality rate (SMRs = 85 and 78, respectively) (145).

Versluys (146), analyzing mortality data for the Netherlands for the period 1931–1935, found six prostatic cancer deaths among Roman Catholic priests, whereas 4.5 would have been expected. A preliminary study of Catholic priests was conducted in Minnesota (147). Three hundred and seven deaths among priests from six dioceses in Minnesota occurred between 1960 and

1975. Death certificates obtained on 300 of them revealed four deaths from cancer of the prostate. A proportional mortality analysis using the age-comparable Minnesota male population to derive expected values yielded no significant difference between the four observed and seven expected deaths. The continued interest in the relationship between sexual behavior and prostatic cancer does suggest the need, for a larger, perhaps collaborative study, of Catholic priests.

The unique lifestyles of both the Mormons and the Seventh-Day Adventists have made them the subject of a number of epidemiologic studies (148–157). The Mormon religion advocates abstention from the use of alcohol, tobacco, coffee, and tea and proscribes all extramarital sexual activity. Seventh-day Adventists, a religious group with about 500,000 U.S. members, advocate abstention from the use of tobacco and alcohol and, to a lesser extent, from coffee, tea, fish, and meat. Both groups have been found to have a lower mortality rate from most causes of death.

Mormons

Cancer of the prostate is one of the few cancers for which Mormons appear to have a higher mortality rate than expected (153, 154). In a comparison of average annual age-adjusted cancer death rates among U.S. white males and both Utah county and Utah State males, Enstrom (153) found only two male cancer sites which were greater among Mormons than among U.S. whites: cancers of the prostate and of the nervous system. Utah county, whose population is 85% Mormon, had the highest prostatic cancer rate (20.0 per 100,000), followed by the State of Utah, which is 70% Mormon (19.71 per 100,000). United States whites, with a population which is only 0.5% Mormon, had the lowest rate (17.84 per 100,000).

An analysis of observed and expected cancer mortality among Mormons in California during 1970–1972 was conducted by Enstrom (153) using annual ward reports from the Church Historical Department. Prostatic cancer mortality was not found to be in excess among this group, in fact, the observed-to-expected ratio ranged from 0.30 to 0.51, depending upon which of three standard populations were used. However, data resulting from this study must be interpreted with caution for several reasons: estimates had to be derived for the age distribution of the California Mormon population; reporting of deaths was incomplete; out-of-state deaths were not completely ascertained; inactive members who moved out of the ward or died were probably removed from the ward membership lists; and errors or omissions occurred in the California mortality records.

Incidence data from the Utah Cancer Registry for the years 1966–1970 provided an opportunity to analyze the cancer morbidity experience of Utah Mormons (154). Standardized incidence ratios were derived from age-, sex-, and race-specific incidence rates of the Third National Cancer Survey. The results were similar to those from Enstrom's (153) mortality analysis of Utah Mormons; namely, two sites had higher incidence rates for Mormon males—prostate with an 11% excess of the rate expected from the Third National Cancer Survey and brain and nervous system neoplasms, with a 12% excess. Non-Mormon males in Utah had fewer cases than expected at both sites.

A later study compared incidence data from the Utah Cancer Registry for 1966–1970 with incidence data from the Third National Cancer Survey and mortality data for the same period in Utah with U.S. mortality data for 1968 (155). For prostatic cancer, both the incidence and mortality rates in Utah were greater than the rates in the comparison groups. The standardized mortality ratio, 113.9, was significant at the $P < 0.01$ level. The standardized incidence ratio, although greater than 100 (103.4), did not approach statistical significance.

In a recent study, Enstrom (157) examined the cancer mortality among active Mormon males in California and Utah and contrasted these results with his earlier study of all Mormon males. The active Mormons were identified as the High Priests (local church leaders and members of the various councils) and the Seventies (adult missionaries who attempt to convert nonmembers to the Mormon faith). These groups were selected for separate analysis, as they were more likely to adhere to the Church-advocated lifestyle. Based on a comparison with the 1970 age-specific cancer mortality rates for U.S. white males 35 years of age and older, active California Mormons had a prostatic cancer standardized mortality ratio of 79. For active Utah Mormons, the SMR was 107. Thus the previously noted higher prostate cancer rates among all Mormons do not hold for active Mormons, who are believed to abstain almost completely from tobacco, alcohol, coffee, and tea.

Differences in cancer mortality or morbidity among all Mormons could be the result, at least in part, of underreporting (157). The reliance on ward clerks or "home teachers" to maintain membership rosters and the lack of a systematic followup procedure for inactive members could result in an underascertainment of deaths. Nevertheless, it is unlikely that this underreporting would be site-specific and therefore, the excess rate of prostatic cancer noted in both studies probably is a minimum estimate of the true difference.

Seventh Day Adventists

In a study based on admissions to eight hospitals, under the direction of the Seventh-Day Adventist Church, virtually no difference was found between the number of men admitted with prostatic cancer and the number expected (148).

Analyzing mortality data for the Seventh-Day Adventists, Phillips (152) found that the standardized mortality ratio (SMR) for prostatic cancer, although not statistically significant, was 19% lower than expected in the general population. When comparisons were made to a population "more similar to Adventists and more particular to Adventists who choose to enroll in a prospective study," the SMRs were reduced. By use of the general California population the SMR was 68 and of the nonsmoking population from Hammond's American Cancer Society prospective study the SMR was 65.

Hutterites

The Hutterite Brethren, a Christian sect, comprise a genetic isolate with a unique lifestyle of communal living and diversified farming. Cancer incidence data on a large colony of Hutterites living in Alberta, Canada, were analyzed to determine if their cancer rates were different from an age and sex comparable population of Alberta (158). Data for 1953–1974 were ascertained from the Alberta Cancer Registry. Hutterites were identified by both computer and manual search of the registry data for 195 contemporary Hutterite surnames. The other sources, the Patient Index System, death certificates, and nonreporting pathology laboratories, were also searched for possible names. Because these surnames were not exclusive to the Hutterites, all persons with street addresses were excluded and information such as ethnic origin, religion, place of birth, and colony address was used to identify study subjects. The observed number (6) of prostatic cancer cases was somewhat higher than expected (4.5) but was not statistically significant.

Parsi

Cancer of the prostate is the most common site of cancer in Parsimen (159,160). The incidence rate is 50% greater than in the total male population of Bombay. The Parsi have several unique customs, habits, and religious beliefs. Generally, they do not smoke or chew tobacco, they marry at the relatively late age, they are highly inbread, they are literate and prosperous, and they consume a Westernized diet.

There are consistent and noteworthy findings among the studies on religious groups—the low rate among Jews and Seventh Day Adventists and the slightly elevated risk among Mormons as well as the higher one among Parsis. The significance of thise findings is not readily apparent. However, the unique dietary patterns of these groups warrant attention.

SOCIOECONOMIC STATUS

Socioeconomic status, often used interchangeably with social class, is a widely used concept in the epidemiologic literature. It encompasses a number of variables, such as education, income, occupation, social prestige, area of residence, and general living conditions or lifestyle. Studies differ in their definition of socioeconomic status ranging from a single variable such as median family income or occupation to a complex index constructed from a combination of some of the variables mentioned above. As an example of the latter, Hollingshead and Redlich (161) in their study of mental illness used, as an index of socioeconomic status, a combination of occupation, education and residence. However, because of this diversity of definitions of socioeconomic status, caution must be exercised in comparing studies on social class.

The census tract, which is a small (population = 3000–6000) relatively homogeneous administrative unit of a city, can be classified according to some measures of socioeconomic status. Thus, census tracts are classified according to the percentage of population in certain occupational categories, median income of the population, population density, housing conditions, and so on. Disease rates can be calculated and compared for residents of these census tracts. Gordis et al. (162) demonstrated the utility of such an approach in a study of the association between the incidence of rheumatic fever and socioeconomic status. As a measure of socioeconomic status, they grouped 168 census tracts in Baltimore City into five socioeconomic categories according to the median rental value of the houses in each tract.

Occupation is often used as a measure of socioeconomic status because of its availability and comparability. Great Britain has presented mortality data by occupation since 1855 and has developed a classification which divides occupations into five broad classes—Professional (I), Intermediate (II), Skilled (III), Semiskilled (IV), and Unskilled (V) (163, 164).

A considerable amount has been written on the various measures of socioeconomic status and their relationship to disease (165–167). Regardless of the specific measure of socioeconomic status, its relationship to disease can be characterized as shown in Table 12. As can be seen, socioeconomic status itself is not an etiological factor of disease but, as an indicator or measure of variables, such as diet, crowding, availability and utilization of medical care, or stress, it can provide valuable clues as to factors of possible etiological significance.

A number of attempts have been made to correlate prostatic cancer and social class using a number of different measures of social class. The variability in the methods used to classify socioeconomic status must be considered in the interpretation of the results of the various studies.

Most of the studies which have examined the association between prostatic cancer and socioeconomic status have concluded that "generally no regular socioeconomic gradient is apparent" (17); or "there is no clear relationship between prostatic cancer and socieconomic status" (168); or "sociocconomic circumstances are not consistently related" (169); or "investigations of the variation of incidence of prostatic cancer with various measures of socioeconomic status have generally shown weak or nonsignificant associations" (88); or ". . . the results reveal no concensus" (105); or "there seems to be no consistent correlation between the incidence of prostatic cancer and socioeconomic status" (141). Thus there is agreement in the literature that socioeconomic status is of little or no importance in prostatic cancer. These conclusions are probably accurate since gradients of mortality/morbidity with some measure of social class (usually divided into four or five classes) are non-existent and in the relatively few instances where such patterns emerge, differences are usually small and comparisons between studies yield conflicting results.

A summary of the studies on social class is presented in Table 13. Comparing just the highest and lowest social classes, the studies reviewed

TABLE 12. Possible Relationship Between Selected Population Variables and Specific Components Influenced by Social Class

	Population variable	Components	Physiological or cellular	End result
Social Class	Medical Care Diet Working Conditions Psychosocial Stress Other	Specific Therapy Occupational Exposures Other Components	Biochemical Mechanism	Specific Disease or Cause of Death

Source: Lilienfeld, A. M., Foundations of Epidemiology, Oxford University Press, New York, 1976.

TABLE 13. Summary of Studies on the Relationship Between Prostatic Cancer and Socioeconomic Status

Author, year (reference)	Source of prostatic cancer data[a]	Source of data on socioeconomic class	Ages	Rate in high socioeconomic class[a]	Rate in low socioeconomic class[a]
Young, 1926 (170)	Mortality data, England and Wales, 1910–1912	Occupation from death certificate	25+	69	36
Registrar-General, 1938 (17)	Mortality data, England and Wales, 1921–1923	Occupation from death certificate	20–64	110	86
Registrar-General, 1954 (17)	Mortality data, England and Wales, 1930–32	Occupation from death certificate	35–65	111	106
Registrar-General, 1957 (17)	Mortality data, England and Wales, 1949–1953	Occupation from death certificate	20–64	128	102
			65+	129	84
Buell, 1960 (171)	Mortality data, California, 1949–1951	Occupation from death certificate	20–64	135	52
Guralnick, 1963 (172)	Mortality data, United States, 1950	Occupation from death certificate	20–64	116	94
Richardson, 1965 (173)	Mortality data, Scotland, 1963	Occupation from death certificate	50–64	12	10
			65–74	95	79
			75+	278	227
	Hospital and nursing home records, Scotland, 1961–1902	Area of residence	50–59	33	35
			60–69	153	108
			70–79	263	200
			80+	631	232

Hoover, 1975 (21)	Mortality data by County, United States, 1950–1969	Counties classified on basis of median number of school years completed	All	1.09	1.00
Clemmesen, 1951 (174)	Danish Cancer Registry, Copenhagen, 1943–1947	22 administrative subdistricts divided into five social classes on basis of rental value of homes	All	78	114
Dorn, 1959 (87)	National Cancer Survey, United States 1947–1948	Median family income of census tract of residence	All	88	112
Graham, 1960 (175)	Erie County Cancer Registry, 1948–1952	Median rental value of census tract	All	27.6	28.2
Seidman, 1970 (129)	Mortality data, New York City, 1949–1951	Index based on median family income, percentage of dwellings with adequate plumbing, percentage of labor force employed, and percentage of professionals	25–64	4.9	5.4
Ernster, 1977 (105)	Mortality data, Alameda County, 1968–1972	Percentage of individuals in census tract with some college education	50–59	2.8	6.3
			60–64	6.8	30.2
			65–69	36.7	41.0
			70–74	79.8	101.8
			75+	363.3	308.2
	Alameda County, Cancer Registry, 1960–1969	As above	50–59	37.0	49.9
			60–64	63.3	131.2
			65–69	254.1	310.0
			70–74	402.0	527.4
			75+	582.0	689.4

[a]Rates are expressed as standardized mortality ratios, age-specific and age-adjusted mortality ratio, ratios of age-adjusted rates.

can be divided almost equally between those suggesting a positive association of prostatic cancer with social class and those showing a negative association. However, virtually all of the studies in which a higher prostatic cancer rate was found in the higher socioeconomic class, used the occupation recorded on the death certificate as an index of socioeconomic status. On the other hand, the studies in which a negative association was found—that is, a higher rate in the lowest socioeconomic class—used residence as an index of socioeconomic status. Usually, this involved selecting a proxy variable such as median income or median rental value for the census tract in which the subject last resided.

It appears then that the lack of any consistent findings on the relationship between social class and the rate of prostatic cancer may be due, at least in part, to a lack of consistency in the measure of social class. Clearly, further work is needed in this area to delineate the association with social class.

Education is often used as a parameter of social class. However, there are relatively few data on the relationship between prostatic cancer and educational attainment. United States mortality data for white males age 25 or over and age 65 or over showed a positive relation between cancer of the prostate and education (10). College-educated males (one or more years) had twice the death rate of males with a high school or lower education.

Wynder et al. (141) found no significant differences in education levels between prostatic cancer cases and controls, although slightly more cases than controls had a college education. For men, under 60, 31% of the cases and 23% of the controls had a college education.

Both mortality and incidence data were analyzed for Alameda County, California, using education and income of the census tract in which the case resided at the time of diagnosis as a measure of socioeconomic status (105). Although no consistent pattern was evident, white male mortality data revealed a slightly higher rate for the census tracts in which over 45% of its population had some college education compared to those census tracts where less than 14% were college educated. The opposite trend was noted for black males and for the analysis of the incidence data for both races.

Among prostate cancers cases in the Philippines a greater than expected number had completed high school and college (176).

OCCUPATION

In addition to being used as a measure of socioeconomic status, occupation can be used to identify specific disease risks associated with specific exposures. There have been a number of such studies for prostatic cancer.

In a clinical study of a small group of men exposed for at least 10 years to cadmium oxide in the manufacture of alkaline batteries, three of the five cancer deaths were due to cancer of the prostate (177). Although there was no comparison made with expected deaths, the high proportionate mortality rate was suggestive.

Following up on these findings, Kipling and Waterhouse (178) studied 248 workers who were exposed for at least one year to cadmium oxide. Comparing the observed incidence rates with expected rates derived from the

Birmingham Regional Cancer Registry, a statistically significant excess rate of prostatic cancer was found ($P < 0.003$).

Holden (179), in a letter to the editor of Lancet, disputed the earlier findings, by reporting that only one prostatic cancer death occurred among 42 men exposed from 2 to 40 years to cadmium oxide. No mention is made of the total number of deaths. However, assuming that all 42 men died, the proportionate mortality rate from cancer of the prostate would be 0.024, a rate which exceeds that for U.S. white males age 65 or over.

A nonconcurrent cohort mortality study was conducted on 292 white males with at least 2 years of employment at a smelter which produced cadmium metal and cadmium compounds (180). As in the previous studies, an excess of prostatic cancer deaths was found (4 observed vs. 1.15 expected). This excess was not statistically significant. A further analysis by time interval since onset of exposure did reveal a significantly ($P < .05$) increased risk of prostatic cancer for men who had worked at least 20 years.

Although the numbers involved in all three studies are small, the consistency in the results do warrant further study. Kolonel (181) conducted a case-control study of white males aged 50–79 referred to Roswell Park Memorial Hospital in Buffalo, New York. Using the occupational history obtained from each individual on admission to hospital to elicit cadmium exposure, he found no excess of such exposure among prostatic cancer cases. In two other studies, one of 58 male alkaline battery workers and one following eight cases of chronic cadmium poisoning, no deaths from cancer of the prostate were found (182, 183). However, the small numbers involved in both studies preclude any definitive conclusion. An attempt to find cases of prostatic cancer among groups of cadmium workers in Sweden, France, the United States, Germany, and the Eastern European countries revealed but one case in a man from Germany employed in making nickel–cadmium batteries (184).

The rubber industry has been the subject of a number of epidemiologic studies primarily because of the many hazardous chemicals used therein (185, 186). In a nonconcurrent cohort study of 6678 male rubber workers in Akron, Ohio, McMichael et al. (187) observed an excess of prostatic cancer deaths. The standardized mortality ratios were 147 and 142 for the age groups 40–64 and 40–84, respectively with the latter achieving statistical significance at the 0.05 level. A proportional mortality analysis of five other plants from throughout the United States found an excess of prostatic cancer deaths for the age group 40–64; however, for the 40–84 age group, only two of five plants had an excess. Undoubtedly, the relatively small numbers of deaths in this latter analysis may have compromised the results. Following a second phase analysis of employment histories, McMichael et al. suggested that the higher than expected prostatic cancer rates may be the result of exposure to cadmium compounds used as vulcanization (curing) accelerators (188). However, this hypothesis proved to be unwarranted when company officials stated that exposure to cadmium compounds was nil (189).

Pursuing an alternative hypothesis that the excess prostatic cancer deaths in the rubber industry resulted from exposure to heavy metals and organic compounds used as accelerators and antioxidants, Goldsmith (189) conducted a case-control study on 88 prostatic cancer deaths and 258 matched controls.

The highest odds ratio for both black and white males was found in batch preparation where exposure to heavy metal oxides and organic compounds was considered to be greatest.

Monson (191) in a study of 13,571 employees of the six major United States rubber companies found a higher than expected number of prostatic cancer deaths among white males employed in the "miscellaneous tire" work area (190). No information was provided on possible exposures in this area although Monson did suggest that chemicals used in the rubber industry might, in general, be responsible for the higher than expected cancer rates.

A study of over 8,000 employees from a single rubber manufacturing plant in Ohio yielded a significant excess of deaths from cancer of the prostate (192, 193). When the data were analyzed by specific work experience, the excess of prostatic cancer deaths was found primarily in the General Service area which represents all operations associated with power plant, quality control, trucking, janitorial, and clerical services, in general, a diversified category representing a variety of exposures.

Roswell Park Memorial Institute, a cancer diagnostic, treatment, and research facility located in Buffalo, New York, routinely collected, between 1956 and 1965, detailed information from all admitted patients, including a lifetime occupational history. This information was obtained prior to the diagnostic examination. Utilizing these data, the relative frequency of a given occupation among patients with a specific form of cancer was compared with the relative frequency among persons with nonneoplastic disease (194). For cancer of the prostate significant relative risks were found for blacksmiths, farmers, managers of dairy farms, foremen of all industries, mechanics, repairmen, and operatives in miscellaneous manufacturing industries. Although not statistically significant, age-specific relative risks exceeding 3.0 were found for bakers (age 60+), operatives in rubber and plastics industry (less than 60), shoemakers and repairers, except factory (60+), stationary engineers (less than 60), and operatives in the textile mill industry (60+). Further analysis of occupations involving exposure by inhalation of chemicals or combustion products revealed a significant relative risk for mechanics and repairmen, particularly, to those men over the age of 60 (195).

A study of 58,828 steelworkers employed in seven Allegheny County Steel plants who were followed through 1966 showed a statistically significant relative risk for nonwhite males employed as janitors in the plants (196–198).

A followup evaluation was conducted of the cancer risk among coke oven workers (199). An elevated, but insignificant prostatic cancer mortality rate was found for long-term coke oven workers employed for five or more years at the time of entry to the study. A similar study in a single steel mill showed no excess in prostatic cancer deaths (200). However, differences in the processes and chemical exposures in the plants between the two studies and the incomplete followup in this latter study, could account for the different results.

A significantly higher than expected prostatic cancer mortality rate was found among men employed in the wood and pulp industry in Washington State (201).

Henry et al. (202) analyzed prostatic and bladder cancer mortality data for England and Wales for the period 1921 to 1928. The most disparate observed-to-expected ratios (SMR) were found for the following occupations: gas work managers (333), laborers at patent fuel works (250), gas stokers (229), brick kiln and oven men (222), gas fitters (210), cellarmen (200), barmen (61), chimney sweeps (61), plumbers (56), gas work inspectors (45), and hairdressers (26).

A similar analysis was conducted on mortality data from the Netherlands during the years 1931 to 1935 (203). The most striking disparities between observed and expected prostatic cancer deaths occurred in the following occupations (SMR): Masters—secondary and grammar school (268); university men—physicians, clergymen, engineers, lawyers (242); tailors and tailor journeymen (181); soldiers—land and naval forces (164); grocers (50); commercial travelers (45); and navvies (33). A later analysis of the changes in cancer frequency during the period 1930 to 1957 in the male population of the Netherlands in a few selected occupations revealed nothing noteworthy (204).

The British have analyzed occupational data from death certificates since 1851 (163). A recent analysis of such data revealed significant higher prostatic cancer death rates for men employed as farmers, foresters, and fisherman; sales workers, administrators, and managers; and professionals, technical workers, and artists (205).

Guralnick (206) analyzed United States mortality data for males 20 to 64 for 1950 and 26 groups of occupation classes. The groupings into classes were based on the Bureau of Census Intermediate Occupational Classification. As in previous studies, occupation was ascertained from death certificates. For 13 of 26 occupational classes the standardized mortality ratio did not deviate by more than ± 10% from 100. Some of the more extreme values for all males age 20 to 64 were (SMR): mine operators and laborers (200), laborers in metal manufacturing (175), laborers in other manufacturing (192), laborers in other nonmanufacturing industries (157), laborers except those on the farm (148), foremen (71), drivers and deliverymen (70), clerical and kindred workers (65), and mechanics and repairmen, except radio (60).

A random 10% sample of all incident invasive tumors occurring in 3 years in eight areas surveyed by the Third National Cancer Survey was selected for a detailed personal interview which included an employment history (207, 208). A comparison was made between the proportions of specific main lifetime industries and occupations among patients with cancer of a particular site and patients with cancers of all other sites. For major industrial groups, the transportation industry experienced a relative odds ratio of 0.54 ($P < 0.05$). Specific industries showing significant relative odds ratios were coal mining (1.47), rubber products (1.60), wholesale and retail trade–apparel and shoes (4.03), and charitable and religious services (1.76). Among the major occupational groups that were examined, significant relative odds ratios were found for managers and administrators except farmers (0.75), craftsmen and related workers (1.31), and farmers and farm laborers (1.52). For specific occupations, clergymen (6.71), plumbers and pipefitters (7.35), farm laborers (3.22), food service workers (4.12), and truck drivers (0.35) all showed significant relative odds ratios.

Milham (209) analyzed the occupational and cause of death information on about 30,000 Washington State white male death certificates for the years 1950–1971. Using an age-standardized proportionate mortality ratio (PMR) method of analysis, he found statistically significant ($P < 0.05$) PMRs for the following occupation (PMR) dentists (177); optometrists (273); physicians (186); surveyors (226); ranchers (142); railroad conductors (188); stock clerks, storekeepers, and warehousemen (160); insurance agents, brokers, underwriters, and appraisers (169); oil drillers and welldrillers (281); meatcutters and butchers (36); mine operatives and laborers (68); painters (144); brewery workers (246); farm laborers (53); produce, seed, feed, and grain company workers (236); loggers (114); and laborers (71).

Because age-specific death data were also provided, it was possible to examine the proportion of prostatic cancer deaths which occurred among those under the age of 65. For U.S. white males about 12% of all prostatic cancer deaths occur in this age group (106). The highest proportions of this age group among the Washington State deaths occurred for officers and enlisted men of the navy, coast guard, army, air force, and marine corps (36%); Boeing workers (45%); Atomic Energy workers (43%); bus drivers (36%); deliverymen (33%); and taxi drivers and chauffeurs (57%). In a study of 111 age- and race-matched prostatic cancer cases and controls, significantly more cases than controls were exposed to fertilizers or auto exhaust fumes (210).

Occupational data derived from death certificates are of questionable value. These data are usually provided by the funeral director based on information supplied by an informant. Gurnalnick reviewed one month's shipment of death certificates from each state for 1950 and found them to be grossly inadequate for a mortality study (211). Of a group of questionnaires sent to state registrars for additional information, only 55% were returned. Only 81.5% of all death certificates contained data on both occupation and industry (83.5% and 70.2% for white and nonwhite males, respectively). For prostatic cancer, the average age at death is beyond retirement and occupation is often reported as "retired." Furthermore, when occupation is recorded, it is often the last known occupation and not the usual occupation.

Studies of specific occupational groups, particularly rubber workers and those with cadmium exposure (mining and battery workers) warrant consideration. The cadium studies, unfortunately, are based on small series and need further confirmation. However, the findings from the studies of rubber workers are quite consistent. Further confirmation of this association is provided by the interview data collected during the Third National Cancer Survey (TNCS) [207,208].

Galvanized pipe, commonly used in the United States, contains high concentrations of cadmium. Thus, the high relative odds ratio found for plumbers and pipefitters (7.35) in the TNCS analysis could lend some support to the cadmium exposure studies.

The lack of consistency for other occupations among the many studies is difficult to interpret.

TRACE METALS

Zinc

Although zinc is found in all tissues of the body, the concentration is especially high in the human prostate gland (212–215). The prostate gland is, in fact, the richest repository of zinc in the body (216). This is also true in at least two other species of animals, the rat and the rabbit, which also show unusually high concentrations of zinc in the prostate, particularly in the lateral as opposed to the dorsal prostate (217, 218). The zinc concentrations vary markedly within the prostate gland (219). Studies of human prostates have shown that relative to normal, nondiseased prostates, cancerous prostates have significantly lower concentrations of zinc, whereas hyperplastic prostates have significantly elevated levels of zinc (220–226).

The effect of castration and hormones on zinc concentrations in the prostates has also been studied (222, 227, 228). Studies of both rats and dogs have shown that castration results in a marked decrease in the size and total zinc uptake of the prostate. In these studies, the administration of testosterone to the castrated animal prevented the reduction of zinc and resulted in far less diminution in the size of the prostate. Testosterone administered to the intact animal decreased the efficiency of the prostate to concentrate zinc.

Estradiol administered to the castrated animal was effective in preventing the marked decrease in the efficiency of zinc uptake which resulted from castration alone. It was also somewhat effective in maintaining the weight of the prostate. The intact animal, when administered relatively small doses of estradiol ($< 10\ \mu g$), showed a decrease in the size and total zinc uptake of the prostate. At doses between 10 and 100 μg, the efficiency of the prostate to concentrate zinc was not depressed. It was also shown that the capacity of the prostate to concentrate zinc increased as the age of the rat increased. Further evidence of the effect of hormones on zinc concentration has been provided in a study that showed that plasma zinc concentrations decrease in normal women following menopause (229).

The above findings are particularly relevant in evaluating the significance of zinc levels in human prostates. Studies of zinc levels in cancerous prostates must take into account that these prostates probably have been compromised by castration, in a few instances, or, more commonly, by estrogenic therapy. Both of these procedures will result in markedly diminished concentrations of zinc.

Cadmium

Cadmium has a strong affinity for dithiols and thus may interfere with lipoic acid coenzymes and alter the growth rates of tissues (215). Although mesenchymal tissue appears particularly vulnerable to cadmium, animal studies have shown other tissues also to be susceptible to carcinogenic changes following cadmium exposure (230). In fact, several cadmium compounds have been reported to be carcinogenic. Injection of cadmium metal powder and various cadmium compounds such as oxides of cadmium, cadmium sulfate, cadmium sulfite and cadmium chloride, have produced tumors in animals (231–238).

Cadmium depressed the capability of the dorsolateral prostate to take up administered $zinc^{65}$ (239). $Zinc^{65}$ uptake in the ventral prostate, which is not under androgen control, was not altered in the presence of cadmium. Gunn et al. (240) demonstrated in animals that cadmium-induced tumors could be prevented by the simultaneous injection of a zinc solution. As demonstrated in animals, the relationship between cadmium and zinc with respect to hypertension, might also be of etiologic importance in prostatic cancer (241). There were no neoplastic changes in the prostates of rats injected subcutaneously over a 2-year period with cadmium sulfate (242). Similar experiments administering cadmium sulfate, either by gastric instillation or in aqueous solution by stomach tube, failed to produce any macroscopic or microscopic changes in the prostate glands of the experimental animals (243, 244).

Cadmium is used in industry in the manufacture of pigments and in electroplating parts used in switches and switch gear (245). As discussed in the previous section, studies of men occupationally exposed to cadmium have shown that they are at increased risk of prostatic cancer (177, 178, 180, 246).

Other Metals

Other trace metals that have been studied in prostatic cancer patients are copper and magnesium. Wiederanders and Evans (247) found no significant difference between the copper concentration of hyperplastic prostatic tissue and carcinomatous prostatic tissue. Tissues from normal prostates were not analyzed. No difference was found in magnesium concentrations between normal and cancerous prostates (225). However, the concentrations were almost twice as high in hyperplastic prostates as in either normal or cancerous prostates.

AIR QUALITY

Two studies have shown a positive association between air pollution and prostate cancer mortality (248, 249). In the Nashville Air Pollution Study, the highest prostatic cancer mortality rates were found in the areas with the highest levels of SO_3, soiling, and dustfall (248). No differences were found with SO_2. The Erie County Study found the highest prostatic cancer mortality rates in areas with the highest suspended particulate levels (249). The authors hypothesized that cadmium, which is a component of air pollution in some urban areas, might be the factor of etiological significance. Unfortunately, levels of cadmium were not measured in Erie County.

WATER HARDNESS

In an analysis of 80 county boroughs of England and Wales for the years 1958–1967, a higher than expected prostatic cancer proportionate mortality ratio was found in hard water areas where water was obtained mainly by boreholes in chalk (250). In all, the associations were weak and unimpressive.

RADIATION

Little attention has been placed on the possible affects of radiation on the development of prostatic cancer. The few animal studies that have been done are inconclusive.

Upton et al. (251) suggested that there was no increase in prostatic carcinoma as a result of radiation exposure. Other studies have shown weak, but significant, effects of radiant energy on the development of prostatic adenocarcinoma in rats (252, 253). The Japanese National Institute of Health—Atomic Bomb Casualty Commission Life Span Study provided some data on the effects of varying doses of radiation exposure on humans. Results from routine autopsies performed during 1961–1969 on 1,357 men from Hiroshima and Nagasaki and on three age–matched groups of 71 autopsied men with little or no radiation exposure showed no association between radiation exposure based on the distance from the hypocenter of the bomb and cancer of the prostate (254). A similar study conducted with fewer cases also failed to reveal any association (255). Watanabe (256) also reported on the Hiroshima survivors. He found no increase in prostatic cancer.

SMOKING

Dorn found an unexplainable excess of prostatic cancer deaths among cigarette smokers as compared to nonsmokers in his follow–up study of U.S. Government life insurance policyholders (257). Among British physicians, no significant difference was found between smokers and nonsmokers (258). Wynder (141), who examined this association in a case-control study, found no difference in the proportion of smokers or in the amount smoked between prostatic cancer cases and hospital controls.

ALCOHOL

Three mortality followup studies, one of a group of alcoholics undergoing treatment at the Toronto Clinic of the Addiction Research Foundation, a second of a group of patients treated for alcoholism and discharged from a Norwegian Psychiatric Hospital, and the third of a group of alcoholics ascertained through a survey of a large U.S. company, all showed that alcoholics had a higher than expected number of prostatic cancer deaths (259–261). However, the observed number of prostatic cancer deaths in all three series was extremely small (6, 10, and 3, respectively). A cohort study of patients admitted to a Massachusetts mental hospital with a diagnosis of alcoholism revealed fewer prostatic cancer deaths than expected (262). As in the previous studies, the numbers were very small (3 observed versus 7.5 expected).

In a case-control study, no significant difference in alcohol consumption was found between prostatic cancer cases and hospital controls (141). Data collected by personal interview from a sample of cases ascertained in the Third National Cancer Survey revealed a significant odds ratio (prostatic cancer cases compared to all other cancer cases) for wine consumption (263). The odds ratios for beer and hard liquor were less than 1.0 but were not significant. There were at least two major problems with this study. The response rate among prostatic cancer cases was only 53% (207). Furthermore, for 27% of all patients who agreed to the interview, the responses to the alcohol questions were "unknown." An additional problem may have resulted from the use of "intercancer" controls, that is, comparing responses from patients with cancer at a single site with responses of patients with cancer at other sites could result in spurious associations.

Negative but nonsignificant correlations were found between the prostatic cancer mortality among white males in 41 states of the United States and per capita consumption of distilled spirits and wine (264). Correlations between age-specific prostatic cancer incidence rates for 24 countries and per capita consumption of alcohol were positive but not significant.

Other available data that could shed light on the relationship between prostatic cancer and alcohol consumption can be derived from the studies on Seventh Day Adventists and Mormons, two groups who consume very little alcohol. Seventh Day Adventists and active Mormons have a lower than expected prostatic cancer rate; however, all Mormons have just the opposite, a higher than expected rate (149–157).

Although definitive evidence is not yet available, from the available data it would appear that alcohol may not be of direct etiologic importance in prostatic cancer. Nevertheless, its effect on sex-hormone metabolism and on liver disease, which is negatively associated with prostatic cancer, makes it worthy of further consideration and study.

Effect of Alcohol on Hormones

It has been demonstrated that alcohol fed to rats and mice results in a reduction of plasma testosterone concentration and, in rats, prostatic and seminal vesicle atrophy (255, 266). Studies of men have shown that alcohol depressed plasma testosterone concentrations, decreased testosterone production rates, reduced the frequency and dampened the episodic bursts of testosterone secretion by the testes, increased metabolic clearance of testoterone in men ingesting alcohol over a short period of time, and decreased plasma leutenizing hormones in chronically exposed men (267–271). Alcoholism has also been shown to increase protein binding of the sex steroids abnormally (272).

The decreased plasma concentration and production rates of testosterone associated with alcohol consumption are similar to those found in cirrhosis of the liver (273, 274). However, one study has shown that the metabolic clearance rate of testosterone, rather than increasing as with alcohol consumption, decreases with cirrhosis of the liver (274).

Cirrhosis of the Liver

Early studies of both animals and man indicated that the liver was the chief, and perhaps only organ involved in the inactivation of estrogens (275–281). Cirrhotic patients are known to suffer from gynecomastia, testicular atrophy, and an increased urinary excretion of estrogens (279, 282–288).

A functioning liver is necessary for the proper removal or inactivation of endogenous estrogen (289). Therefore, hyperestrogenism, which often accompanies advanced hepatic cirrhosis, could result from the inability of the damaged liver to metabolize estrogen (290). Since estrogen has been used in the treatment of prostatic cancer, consideration has been given to the possibility of decreased frequency of the disease in men with cirrhosis of the liver. A number of studies have been undertaken to examine this relationship (See Table 14).

A review of all autopsies performed during 1939 to 1946 at the Los Angeles County Hospital yielded 316 cases of cirrhosis of the liver and 174 cases of prostatic cancer in males over the age of 50 (290). Prostatic cancer was somewhat less frequent among patients with cirrhosis of the liver (2.8%) than it was among patients without cirrhosis (3.1%). Furthermore, the frequency of cirrhosis of the liver was lower among prostatic cancer patients (5.2%) than among patients without prostatic cancer (5.5%). Three other similarly conducted studies using autopsy material found essentially the same results (291–294).

Robson (293) reported on the relationship of severity of cirrhosis and clinical signs of hyperestrogenism to the incidence of prostatic cancer. Data for this study were collected from the hospital records of the cirrhotics ascertained from the autopsy series. The five signs used for severity were jaundice, ascites, esophageal varices, hepatic coma, and liver enlargement. Clinical signs of estrogen activity were gynecomastia, testicular atrophy, female hair distribution, palmar erythema and spider angiomata. Forty-nine cases of cirrhosis were classified as severe on the basis of having three of five severity signs. Among these severe cirrhosis cases, there were no cases of prostatic cancer whereas 10 prostatic cancer cases were found among the nonsevere group (100 cases), a difference that was significant at the 5% level. Thirty-seven cases, having 2 or more physical signs of hyperestrogen activity, were considered hyperestrogenic. Of these cases, 2.7% had prostatic cancer compared to 8.0% of the controls. This difference was not statistically significant.

A lower frequency of benign prostatic hypertrophy has also been found among cirrhotics when compared with noncirrhotics (285, 291, 293, 295).

Wynder (141), in a case-control study, found no difference for a history of hepatitis or liver cirrhosis between prostatic cancer cases and controls.

FAMILIAL AGGREGATION

Although there have not been many studies on familial aggregation of prostatic cancer, the few studies that have been done all demonstrate a higher frequency of prostatic cancer among male relatives of cases than among male relatives of controls. The first study to demonstrate this relationship was conducted among 183 prostatic cancer cases admitted to the urology clinic of the University of Milan between 1939 and 1954 (296). The number of pro-

TABLE 14. Summary of Autopsy Studies on Cirrhosis of the Liver and Cancer of the Prostate

Author, date (reference)	Years autopsies performed	Age group	Percentage with prostatic cancer: Cirrhotics	Percentage with prostatic cancer: Controls
Johns and Hirst, 1950 (290)	1939–1946	50+	2.8	3.1
Stumpf and Wilens, 1953 (291)	1953–1961	50+	5.0	7.0
Glantz, 1964 (292)	1920–1962	45+	3.3	9.1
Robson, 1964 (293)	1946–1960	50+	8.3	11.7

static cancer deaths among male relatives of cases was 11 times greater than the number of such deaths among the male relatives of 183 age matched controls.

Woolf (277) selected propositi from death certificates for the state of Utah for the years 1942 to 1958. The selection was restricted to 228 white males who died from cancer of the prostate and were born in Utah or resided there most of their life. Deaths among parents and siblings were ascertained by tracing names of survivors listed in the propositi's obiturary column and through the archival records of the Geneological Society of the Mormon Church in Utah. This latter procedure may have introduced a bias in favor of ascertaining Mormons in the study group. A control group was selected consisting of white individuals who matched the deceased relatives of the propositi on sex, age (−3 and +5 years), year, and county of death. By use of the double dichotomy method of analysis, a statistically significant excess number of prostatic cancer deaths were found among fathers and brothers of propositi compared to fathers and brothers of controls. Although not statistically significant, an excess was also observed for all other cancer deaths among relatives of propositi. The author suggested that a higher prostatic cancer rate among Mormons could account for the results in view of the selection bias of propositi. In fact, as indicated earlier, Mormons, as a total group, do have a higher than expected prostatic cancer rate, although a study of *active* Mormons did not show such an increase (153, 154, 157).

Lynch et al. (298) reported on a single family in which four of seven members of a sibship had histologically confirmed carcinoma of the prostate. A 10-year survey of 109 histologically confirmed prostatic cancer cases revealed five first-degree relatives with prostatic cancer, a number considered to be in excess of that expected.

The Michigan Cancer Foundation collected data on cancers in families of 2411 white proband women participating in a study on the relationship of virus–like particles in human milk to family history of cancer (299). Information was obtained on 4635 lineages containing 31,945 people. The observed to expected ratio of prostate cancer, although greater than one (1.23), was not statistically significant.

In two case-control studies, significantly more prostatic cancer cases than matched controls reported a family history of prostatic cancer (142, 143, 300, 301).

BLOOD GROUP

In 1962, Bourke and Griffin, in a letter to *Lancet*, reported a significant association between blood group A and cancer of the prostate (302). Two subsequent studies failed to demonstrate any such relationship (141, 303).

BENIGN PROSTATIC HYPERTROPHY (BPH)

For many years it was thought that the prostate increased in size through early life and adolescence and reached a plateau at about age 20, and that after age 20 it remained constant in size until about age 50, when it began to increase again (304). However, more recently, examination of prostates from accident victims has indicated that hyperplasia can be found in the periuretheral region of the gland of men in their twenties (305). Regardless of the age when the hypertrophic process begins, it is generally agreed that by age 80, most prostates, perhaps as many as 75%, contain demonstrable hyperplastic spheroids (306).

Despite the prevalence of BPH, relatively little epidemiologic data are available. Consideration of certain characteristics of this disease would be helpful in speculating on its relationship to prostatic cancer. The data which are available do indicate that the distribution of BPH in terms of age, race, and international variation is very similar to prostatic cancer. BPH is relatively rare before age 40 and is estimated to be detectable at autopsy in approximately 75% of all males over the age of 80 (307, 308). Mortality rates are highest in Iceland, Germany, Austria, Norway, and Denmark and lowest in Japan, China, and the Philippines. In the United States, rates for black males are higher than those for white males. Also of interest is the correlation ($r = 0.73$ $P < 0.001$) found between mortality from BPH and mortality from prostatic cancer (309).

Several authors have suggested that prostatic cancer and benign prostatic hypertrophy may co-exist in the same patient and perhaps share a common etiology (310, 311). In fact, Sommers et al. (310) found that 80% of the prostatic cancer cases also showed evidence of benign hypertrophy. Edwards et al. suggested that latent cancer of the prostate was often found among the larger glands in which hypertrophy was also present. In their study, they found that 27.8% of 173 cases of hypertrophy showed malignant changes while only 10.8% of individuals without hypertrophy showed such changes.

A more direct approach to study of the relationship between BPH and prostatic cancer has been attempted in two studies (312, 313). Armenian et al. (312) conducted a mortality followup of 338 patients with a primary diagnosis of benign prostatic hyperplasia, discharged between 1945 and 1967 from Roswell Memorial Institute in Buffalo, New York. For each case a matched (age and year of admission) control was selected from among patients with nonneoplastic diagnoses discharged during the same time period. Cases and controls with a prostatic malignancy ascertained by a rectal examination at the time of admission were not included. The death rate from prostatic cancer was found to be 3.7 times greater among the BPH cases than among the controls.

A case-control study of 290 prostatic cancer cases and an equal number of matched controls was also conducted. Using the resources of Roswell Park, with their detailed questionnaire which was administered to all incoming patients prior to a diagnostic evaluation, Armenian et al. (312) found a significant relative risk of 5.1 for the antecedent hospital admissions for possible BPH.

Greenwald's (313) study of patients from the Lahey Clinic Foundation in Boston included 838 benign prostatic hyperplasia patients with no evidence of malignancy who were less than 80 years of age at the time of resection, and 802 age-matched controls who had surgery for some other condition and no known prostatic disease or malignancy. Eigty-eight percent of the cases and

91% of the controls selected from records between 1940 and 1959 were followed until death or December 31, 1970. No significant difference was noted in the rate of prostatic cancer between cases and controls (2.9% vs. 3.2%). Further analysis of the data using a modified life-table method yielded essentially the same result. For BPH patients there was no significant association between the development of cancer and the amount of tissue removed.

The results of these two studies are clearly contradictory. Armenian and his colleagues (312) found a significant relationship between BPH and cancer of the prostate using both a retrospective–cohort and case-control study design. Greenwald using a retrospective–cohort design found no such relationship. However, both studies contain potential sources of bias and these have been addressed by a number of authors (169, 314–317).

Armenian et al. relied on a clinical diagnosis for 48% of the cases; 27% were biopsied and 26% underwent surgery. The authors were aware of the possibility that microscopical cancer of the prostate may have been present and missed at the time of diagnosis. Suggestive of this possibility is the fact that the death rate from prostate cancer was lower (5.1 per 1,000 person-years) among the men who had had prostatectomies as compared to men who had had no prostatectomies (11.3 per 1,000 person-years).

Another potential source of bias is the fact that patients with hypertrophy may have undergone more frequent prostatic evaluation and hence may be at an increased risk of having a cancer diagnosed. Indicative of this is the significantly higher frequency of hospital admissions for noncancerous prostatic conditions among prostate cancer cases as compared to matched controls.

Greenwald's (313) study has been criticized on the basis that the BPH cases selected for study had all undergone a subtotal prostatectomy and hence the removal of prostate tissue diminished their chance of developing cancer. However, as pointed out by Franks (314), subtotal prostatectomy does not remove the outer area of the prostate where most prostatic cancer begins. A further potential source of bias may have been introduced by the selective histological examination of prostates from benign hypertrophy cases and not from controls. As stated by Higgins (169), "by eliminating latent disease from their case group but not from their controls, it seems possible that a twofold increase in risk of clinical cancer might have also been eliminated."

The relationship between benign prostatic hypertrophy and prostatic cancer is unresolved. On the basis of the available evidence, it is premature to conduct a randomized clinical trial of prostatectomy in symptom-free patients with hypertrophy as suggested by Armenian et al. (312). Additional epidemiologic studies are required to clarify the relationship between these diseases.

SOMATIC CHARACTERISTICS

Ogawa (318, 319), intrigued by the early reports that described benign prostatic hypertrophy patients as obese males with scanty hair growth and female-like pelvis, compared the constitutional characteristics of 30 patients with cancer of the prostate and 40 normal controls in Japan. He found that the prostatic cancer patients were more slender and had broader shoulders; none was obese.

Wynder et al. (141) found that more prostatic cancer patients than controls had heavy beards, chest, and leg hair; however, the differences were not statistically significant. They found no significant differences in height and weight of the cases and controls.

Greenwald et al. (320) examined a number of anthropometric indices and ratings among cases of prostatic cancer and controls. He found that somatotype, gynandromorphy (morphologic femininity in the male physique), androgyny (degree of femininity of build in the male), degree of baldness, pilosity, height, and weight were similar in cases and controls.

Rotkin (210) found that cases of prostate cancer had a somewhat retarded development of secondary sexual characteristics—voice pitch; development of pubic, axillary, and chest hair; and enlargement of pubertal genitalia. The differences, however, between cases and controls were not statistically significant.

Sex hormones influence the development and function of the prostate gland and, at least in part, determine physical characteristics. If differences between cases and controls in early physical characteristics existed, an etiologic role for sex hormones in prostate cancer could be postulated.

MARITAL STATUS

Both mortality and morbidity data show a higher rate of prostatic cancer among ever-married than never-married men (see Tables 15 and 16).

King et al. (17) in a review of mortality data for 1940 found that widowed and divorced males had higher mortality rates from cancer of the genital organs than single or married men regardless of race, age group, or residence. The only exception was divorced nonwhites in rural areas. United States mortality data for the years 1949–1951 showed a similar pattern, that is, higher rates from cancers of the genital organs for widowed and divorced men than for single or married men (321).

TABLE 15. Death Rates[a] for Cancer of the Prostate by Age, Race and Marital Status. United States, 1959–1961

	White				Nonwhite			
Age	Single	Married	Widowed	Divorced	Single	Married	Widowed	Divorced
45–49	0.8	0.7	0.6	0.9	2.9	3.3	5.6	4.9
50–54	2.9	3.5	3.2	6.5	13.6	12.1	50.8	21.4
55–59	8.8	10.3	17.0	17.3	26.1	32.4	54.2	41.6
60–64	29.3	27.4	37.7	40.2	63.5	74.0	132.9	105.3
65–69	59.2	64.5	72.5	90.6	122.1	132.2	216.5	208.5
70–74	113.9	129.5	149.6	157.2	180.7	208.4	253.1	269.8
75–79	217.4	227.1	256.2	271.5	254.2	269.4	351.1	368.5
80–84	319.0	389.8	405.7	524.6	245.0	382.3	437.3	354.2
85 and over	438.6	518.0	529.5	579.4	344.2	380.4	475.5	962.4

Source: Lilienfeld, A. M., Levin, M. L., Kessler, I. I., Cancer in the United States, Cambridge, Mass., Harvard University Press, 1972.

[a]Rates per 100,000 population.

TABLE 16. Incidence Rates[a] for Cancer of the Prostate by Age, Race, and Marital Status, Denmark, 1953–1957

Age	Marital status: Ever married	Marital status: Unmarried
45–49	1.2	1.4
50–54	4.7	6.6
55–59	22.2	12.4
60–64	52.6	35.1
65–69	110.7	99.6
70–74	206.5	171.8
75–79	313.7	216.0
80+	409.6	275.8

Source: Clemmesen, J., Statistical studies in malignant neoplasms, Acta Pathol. Microbiol. Scand., Suppl. 174, 348, 1965.

[a]Rates per 100,000 population.

Mortality data from New York City for the years 1939–1941 revealed that married men had a less favorable mortality from prostatic cancer than single men, particularly at ages 55–74 (322). In Canada in 1970–1972, the highest prostatic cancer mortality rates occurred among widowed and divorced men (84). Single men had the lowest rates.

An analysis of 1959–1961 mortality data for the United States showed that, for white males aged 55 and over, death rates from prostatic cancer were greatest for divorced men, followed respectively by widowed men, married men, and single men (10). Essentially, the same pattern was apparent for nonwhites, with a reversal in position of divorced and widowed rates for ages 55–69 and 80–84. This trend may be due to random variation because of small numbers or, as suggested by King et al. (17), there may be greater error in reporting of marital status among nonwhites. In Australia, Lancaster (323) found a higher than expected mortality rate from cancers of the male genital organs among married men with children than among those never married and those married without children.

Data on marital status have been ascertained in a number of case-control studies. Steele et al. (300) found a higher proportion of single men among controls than among prostatic cancer cases. In separate studies, Wynder (141) and Krain (143) found essentially no differences in marital status between cases and controls.

Greenwald et al. (320) in a followup study of a cohort of Harvard University students on whom demographic, physical, and anthropometric measurements were obtained, ascertained 268 deaths from prostatic cancer and 536 matched controls. The proportion ever married, age at first marriage, age at first child, and total number of children were the same for both cases and controls. Within the married group, 14.7% of the prostate cancer cases and 21.5% of the controls had no children, suggesting the possibility of increased fertility among the cases. Wynder et al. (141) found a similar pattern. Although not statistically significant, more cases than controls had children.

The hypothesis of increased fertility gained further credence with the results of Armenian's study (25). Using prostate cancer cases and age-matched controls ascertained from the records of the Roswell Park Memorial Institute in Buffalo, New York, Armenian found that, although there were no significant differences between cases and controls on marital status, number of times married, and age of first marriage, prostate cancer cases were married longer, had significantly more children, and their wives had more miscarriages and stillbirths. The total pregnancy experience (children + miscarriages + stillbirths), used as an indicator of fertility, suggested to the authors that certain constitutional patterns could predispose to both high fertility and prostatic cancer.

It is unlikely that either marriage or children cause prostatic cancer; however, as indicators of sexual behavior or fertility, they can provide etiologic insights. The general consistency in the relationship between prostate cancer and marital status and number of children warrants further investigation.

SEXUAL FACTORS

Case-Control Studies

The first case-control study of the relationship between prostatic cancer and sexual behavior was conducted by Steele et al. (300, 301). Thirty-nine histologically confirmed cases, 39 age-matched controls with no genitourinary or cancerous condition, and 35 patients with benign hyperplasia of the prostate were selected for study. All subjects were interviewed in hospital by a physician from the Department of Urology. Since prostatic cancer cases and controls were matched, there was no age difference between these two groups; however, the hyperplasia cases were not matched and were found to be somewhat older than the other two groups. More of the cancer group had been married and had more marital partners than the control groups. Prostatic cancer cases were found to have more premarital and extramarital sexual partners than controls (34.2% of the cases and 10.5% of the controls had six or more partners).

In response to the question "What was the maximum number of coital events ever in a single week?" 53.9% of the cases and 71.8% of the controls stated that they had more than 3 coital experiences during this time of peak sexual activity. This question is particularly revealing since Martin (324, 325) considers it to be an indicator of total ejaculatory performance during an individual's lifetime. If this is indeed the case, then one would conclude on the basis of this variable that prostatic cancer cases had fewer sexual experiences than controls.

Data, however, indicated that the general pattern of coital frequency throughout life was similar between cases and controls; 53.9% of the cases and 56.4% of the controls indicated coital frequencies of one or more times per week. More detailed breakdown of frequencies greater than one might have been more informative and resulted in a different conclusion.

Cases of prostatic cancer indicated slightly greater sexual activity in the 5-year period preceding the illness that necessitated hospital admission (33.3% vs. 28.2% one or more times per week). Interest in more coitus than occurred was expressed by significantly more prostatic cancer cases than controls which suggested a greater sexual drive among the cases. A higher frequency of cases than controls reported a previous history of venereal disease which was consistent with the finding on multiple partners. More cases than controls reported using condoms.

In general, these findings suggest that prostatic cancer cases experienced a greater sexual drive throughout their life than controls. They had more sexual partners and, perhaps as a result, more venereal disease. However, it does not appear that they experienced greater sexual activity except for the few years preceding hospitalization.

Krain (142, 143) conducted two studies similar to the one by Steele (300, 301). The first included all cases ($N = 136$) of histologically confirmed prostatic cancer from seven Los Angeles area hospitals from January 1, 1971, to June 1, 1972. The second study included cases ($n = 211$) through December 31, 1972. In both studies age and race-matched controls with no genitourinary or cancerous condition were selected. However, in the second study, all controls had prostatic acid phosphatase determinations and rectal examinations to eliminate cases with latent cancer of the prostate. Despite these efforts, it is unlikely that these would ensure the elimination of latent cases (326–328). The results of both studies were similar and confirmed the earlier findings of Steele—cases reported a great number of pre- and extramarital partners, greater coital frequency in the 10-year period preceding hospitalization, higher frequency of venereal disease, and greater use of condoms.

Rotkin (210) presented a preliminary analysis of data obtained from 111 age- and race-matched prostatic cancer cases and controls from two participating institutions, one in Los Angeles, and one in Chicago. Despite the apparent matching, it appeared that the controls were slightly older than the cases for white males and slightly younger than the cases for nonwhite males. Unfortunately, some of the conclusions presented by the author were not supported by the data presented in the paper. The data showed that more cases than controls masturbated during adolescence, had their first ejaculation between ages 12 and 17, experienced nocturnal emissions, had their first coital experience between ages 18 and 23 and had more unfulfilled erections prior to age 20. A similar number of cases and controls experienced two or more sexual partners in their life, although slightly more cases than controls were married more than once.

Cases over 50 years of age experienced fewer sexual acts than controls. However, no data were presented on sexual activity between ages 20 and 50. Comparisons of men over the age of 50 may not be as informative in terms of etiology because of the probable effect of symptoms of the disease on sexual activity. More cases than controls experienced a voice change, development of pubic, axillary and chest hair, and enlargement of pubertal genitalia beyond the age of 15. The author considered this retarded development of secondary sexual characteristics to reinforce further the hypothesis of an endogenous influence upon the initiation of prostatic cancer. However, these differences were not significant. Furthermore, a similar number of cases and controls began to shave during adolescence and there were no differences in physical growth rates between the ages 12 to 17. Although a similar number of cases and controls were circumcised, significantly more cases than controls were circumcised at birth.

The validity of data on age at first masturbatory experience, nocturnal emission, pubic hair development and voice change is questionable. Unfortunately, there is no way to verify these data. The results from this study may have been biased at the outset by fully disclosing the purpose of the study to the subjects.

In a very preliminary analysis of 21 matched cases and controls, Jackson et al. (324) reported that the cases experienced a later age of puberty and a later age of first coitus. Another preliminary analysis of 53 prostatic cancer cases, 52 age and race matched hospital controls and 44 age- and race-matched neighborhood controls revealed that prostate cancer cases reported an earlier median age at first intercourse, a greater number of sexual partners and lower sexual activity than controls (330). A greater proportion of cases than controls reported a history of venereal diseases and experience with prostitutes.

How then does data on sexual behavior facilitate an understanding of the etiology of prostatic cancer? It is unlikely that too much or too little sexual activity is the cause of the disease. Sexual activity is probably related to a factor that is closely linked to the disease in the causal chain. Hormonal or viral factors in particular deserve consideration.

Hypotheses

Hormonal. A hormonal hypothesis would suggest that sexual activity is merely an indicator or indirect measure of hormonal status. Thus, the differences in sexual frequency between prostatic cancer cases and controls is simply a reflection of differences in one or more hormonal levels between these two groups. A similar hypothesis referred to by Armenian et al. (25) as the constitutional hormonal model, assumed an underlying genetic susceptibility which predisposed to both higher fertility and prostate cancer. In this way, the findings of a significant familial history of the disease could also be related. However, endocrine status could be influenced by external factors such as diet, thus modifying an individual's "inherited susceptibility" to the disease.

Viral. *Herpesvirus.* A second hypothesis deals with the venereal transmission of a virus. The association of viruses with diseases of the urogenital tract were derived initially from observations in the female (331–335). Although early electron microscopic examination of human prostatic carcinoma yielded findings suggestive of a tumor-associated virus (336, 337), the first suggestion of the etiologic importance of herpesvirus in prostate disease was presented by Morrisseau et al. (338) who found evidence of herpes infection in two men with prostatitis. No virus was recovered from 10 men with no prostatic symptoms. Two years later, using indirect immunofluorescence staining, Centifanto et al. (339) isolated herpesvirus from prostate tissue from 15% of a randomly selected population of 190 males without a history of herpes infection. These results suggested to the authors that the prostate may serve as a reservoir for the venereal transmission of the virus. Prompted by this finding, a search was made for herpesvirus particles in cells derived from a cancerous prostate (340). Indirect immunofluorescence staining and electron microscopy demonstrated the presence of herpes viral antigen in prostate tumor cells. Later evidence showed the in vitro transformation of hamster embryo cells by tumor associated herpesvirus type 2 from a human prostatic carcinoma (341).

Herpesvirus has been recovered from the male reproductive tract in subjects both with and without a history of herpes 2 infection (342–344). The frequency of such infection in subjects without a positive history ranged from 7.6% to 40%. Sabin and Tarro (345) found antibodies against a presumed herpesvirus antigen in the sera of all eight prostatic cancer patients studied. An attempt to culture the virus from semen obtained from 20 male student volunteers with a history of recurrent herpes 2 infection failed to demonstrate the virus in any of the specimens (346).

A seroepidemiologic study on 28 prostatic cancer patients and 20 benign prostatic hypertrophy patients did not show any difference in the geometric mean titer of antibodies of either herpesvirus type 1 or herpesvirus type 2 (347). Overall, 71% of the cancer cases and 66% of the hypertrophy cases had antibodies to herpesvirus type 2. Unfortunately, similar data were not obtained on a healthy control group.

Simian Virus 40. Experimentally, neonatal hamster prostate cells, transformed in vitro with simian virus 40 (SV40), a deoxyribonucleic acid oncogenic virus, and transplanted into adult hamsters, produced estrogenic and androgenic dependent prostatic tumors which morphologically resembled human prostatic carcinoma (348–352).

Neutralizing antibodies to SV40 were detected in the sera of 8.3% (2 of 24) patients with cancer of the prostate at the Roswell Park Memorial Institute. This was not considered statistically significant (353). A second study also failed to reveal a significant association between SV40 and prostatic cancer (354).

A serological comparison of patients with bladder cancer, patients with prostate cancer, and normal controls for SV40 neutralizing antibodies showed no differences among the 3 groups (355). Four of 68 prostatic cancer patients and 1 of 32 controls had a low titer of SV40 neutralizing antibodies. A single isolate of cytomegalovirus was recovered from the supernatant of a bladder cancer culture.

Cytomegalovirus. Cytomegalovirus (CMV) which has certain properties resembling herpesvirus, is known to persist in the human genital tract, particularly in semen (356, 357). Furthermore, there is evidence that CMV can induce oncogenic transformation of hamster embryo fibroblasts (358).

Sanford et al. (359) found significant titers of CMV antibodies in the sera of prostatic cancer patients. A greater percentage (95%) of these patients had titers greater than 1:4 against CMV than non–urogenital controls (61% and 78%). In addition, a strain of CMV (CMV-M_j) isolated from a prepubertal prostate at autopsy has been shown to transform normal human prostatic tissue into cells with malignant characteristics. This CMV isolate also established a long-term persistent infection of human embryo lung cells in vitro which resulted in the development of two CMV transformed human cell lines (360). These transformed cells were oncogenic in weaning mice.

A number of other studies have demonstrated the presence of virus-like particles in tissue removed from patients with prostatic cancer or have shown increased antibody titers in such patients (361–368). However, the presence of viral particles in a few selected samples of prostatic tissue does not confirm the etiologic role of the virus in the oncogenic process. Nevertheless, available evidence does suggest that further work, both epidemiologically and virologically, is required. Sanford et al. (369) suggest that the circumstantial evidence connecting viruses with prostatic cancer cannot be ignored. On reviewing the status of the viral etiology in prostatic cancer, Zeigel et al. (370) suggested that the lack of long term cell cultures of normal and pathological prostate epithelium from males of all ages presents a fundamental barrier to more sophisticated virologic studies.

Circumcision. In 1942, Ravich (371) reported that in a series of 843 cases operated on for prostatic obstruction, a 20% incidence of carcinoma was found among non-Jewish males (assumed to be uncircumcised) as compared to 1.7% among Jewish males (assumed to be circumcised). A later series of cases yielded essentially the same results (372). In both series, cases were selected from a few hospitals in New York City. The cases, reflecting the admission patterns of the hospitals involved, were 90.6% Jewish. Neither age nor race was considered in making the comparison between Jews and non-Jews. The authors, nevertheless, on the basis of these two reports, attributed the lower rate of cancer among Jews to the practice of circumcision and recommended it as a routine prophylactic against prostatic cancer. The evidence presented did not support this measure.

Gibson (373), expressing skepticism about these previous studies, attempted to test this hypothesis in London. All cases of prostatic neoplasia for the years 1940 to 1953, which occurred in a general hospital in suburban London, were reviewed for race. The frequency of malignant disease among Jews and Gentiles was 13.2% and 18.2%, respectively.

All hospital records at the Chicago Wesley Memorial Hospital from January 1958 through December 1964 with a tissue diagnosis of prostatic cancer or hypertrophy were reviewed to ascertain religion and a notation of the presence or absence of the prepuce (374). The frequency of prostate cancer was 8.8% among the Jewish patients and 23.9% among the non-Jewish patients. Of these non-Jewish patients, 35.9% were thought to be circumcised, but the authors noted that their method of ascertaining circumcision status was inappropriate. Unfortunately, these studies did little to clarify the relationship between circumcision and cancer of the prostate.

Apt (375) recognized the deficiencies in the earlier studies and attempted a more definitive study. However, the data he presented provided only more indirect evidence. First, he compared Scandinavian Jews, (virtually all males are circumcised), with the remaining Scandinavian male population (virtually all males are uncircumcised). For all cancer, the death rates were the same between the two groups, however, prostate cancer accounted for only 0.78% of all deaths among Scandinavian Jews and 1.9% among Swedish males. A further comparison was made between Sweden and Israel, two countries considered by the author to have comparable medical standards but differing in the proportions of circumcised males. The prostatic cancer incidence rate was considerably lower in Israel.

Wynder et al. (141) found no significant difference in circumcision status between non-Jewish prostatic cancer patients and controls. On the other hand, Rotkin (210) did find that significantly more cases (73%) than controls (48%) had been circumcised at birth.

Despite the lack of conclusive evidence, in 1971 Ravich (376) concluded: "it is now generally recognized that smegma, venereal infection, and sexual promiscuity, synergistically play essential etiologic roles in cancer of the prostate and cervix . . . complete circumcision at birth seems the most effective available preventive against genitourinary cancers."

These conclusions are unwarranted, based on the available evidence regarding circumcision. Additional properly designed case-control studies are required to determine whether an association exists between circumcision and cancer of the prostate. Consideration should be given to the problem of accurately ascertaining circumcision status (377).

Other Evidence. Assuming a viral etiology in prostatic cancer, Feminella and Lattimer (378) studied the frequency of cervical cancer in 101 wives of prostatic cancer patients, and 101 wives of a matched control group consisting of patients with benign prostatic hypertrophy. Although more wives of prostatic cancer cases had a history of cervical cancer than wives of hypertrophy cases, the difference was not statistically significant. However, compared to the general population, the cervical cancer rate among the wives of cases was highly significant. The small numbers of subjects involved in this study and the lack of a nongenitourinary disease control group precludes any substantive conclusion. Perhaps, a larger followup study which would also include the husbands of cervical cancer patients would shed more light on the question.

Greenwald et al. (379) in a case-control study of widowered men who died from prostate cancer and a case–control study of married men with prostate cancer found no significant relationhip in the occurrence of cancer in their wives.

NUTRITION

For the past several years there has been an increasing interest in the role of diet in the etiology of cancer. This has resulted from an accumulation of evidence associating dietary consumption patterns with cancer of a number of sites. Initial interests were in the gastrointestinal tract tumors; however, more recently, data have been generated which indicate that nutrition may effect the development of the endocrine-related organs, such as breast, ovaries, endometrium, and prostate (380–385).

Although the evidence is far from definitive and the precise mechanism has not yet been elucidated, speculation has evolved on the possible pathways through which diet could produce cancer (386). Nutritional influences may occur in the following ways:

1. Food additives, contaminants or specific elements could act as carcinogens or as initiators, promoters, or accelerators.

2. A dietary deficiency could initiate a neoplastic process through some biochemical malfunction.
3. A dietary excess could result in a cancer through a variety of metabolic abnormalties.

If diet is of etiologic importance in cancer of the prostate, a possible explanation of its action would be through some effect, probably as a modifier or promoter, on hormonal status. As pointed out by Lipsett (384), diet can affect endocrine levels by stimulating or inhibiting secretion, by altering rates and routes of metabolism and by changing receptor mechanisms. The paucity of dietary data for prostate cancer prevents any secure statement on which, if any, of the suggested pathways most aptly explains a nutritional influence on prostate cancer.

One hypothesis currently under consideration regarding the influence of diet deals with animal protein and/or fat, through a modification of endocrine status. Such an hypothesis has been proposed for breast cancer and may be of similar significance for prostatic cancer (383, 387–391).

Causal mechanisms are often ascertained through experimental studies with animals. The role of diet in the etiology of both colon and breast cancer has been studied in animals and a number of hypotheses developed. Unfortunately, there is no appropriate animal model for prostate cancer (392, 393). Nevertheless, a brief review of some of the experimental evidence linking dietary fat to cancer, namely breast cancer, an endocrime related tumor is presented. Following this, the epidemiologic evidence suggesting an association between dietary fat and prostate cancer is reviewed.

Fat

The role of dietary fat in tumorgenesis may be either as a cocarcinogen or as a carcinogen. There is little evidence for the latter, although lipid soluble compounds such as polycyclic hydrocarbons do have carcinogenic properties (394). Also, some evidence does exist from animal studies that carcinogens may result from the oxidation or polymerization of fats through heating or other processing in food preparation (395, 396). However, there is more support for a cocarcinogenic rather than a carcinogenic effect of dietary fat.

A number of animal studies have shown that skin cancer incidence is greater in rats fed a high fat diet and exposed to a carcinogen such as coal tar, benzypyrene, or ultraviolet light than in rats not fed a high fat diet and exposed to the same carcinogens (397–400). The tumor enhancing effect of fat seems to occur with all types of fat tested—butter, Crisco™, coconut oil, and cottonseed oil. The development of hepatomas, lung adenocarcinomas and mammary carcinomas was also greatly augmented in mice and rats fed a high fat diet (389, 400–403). Tumors appeared earlier and in greater numbers.

The type of fat may be important in mammary tumors. One study with rats found that 20% corn oil gave a higher tumor incidence than 20% coconut oil (389). Further studies by the same authors using different fats and oils fed as 20% of the rats' diet found that the animals on unsaturated fats had a higher tumor incidence than animals on saturated fats.

In general, mammary tumor incidence appears to increase with increasing levels of dietary fat, plateauing at about 16% fat (401). However, the tumor increase has not been arithmetically proportional to the fat content of the diet. Increasing the fat content from 2 to 8% resulted in the same tumor enhancement as increasing fat from 8 to 26%.

Weisburger et al. (383) suggested that diet and nutrition act as modifiers, either directly or indirectly, rather than as initiators of tumor development. This modifying effect acts directly through specific alterations in cell-membrane structure and functions or indirectly through a change in ongoing physiological processes.

Both estrogen and prolactin seem to play a role in the development of mammary tumors (404–408). Chan and Cohen (409–411) have suggested that a high fat diet may increase synthesis and/or secretion of prolactin by the pituitary gland, and that the increased growth of breast tumors in animals when fed diets high in fat, particularly unsaturated fat, may be due to a fat induced increase in the plasma prolactin to estrogen ratio. Hill et al. (391) demonstrated that prolactin levels were increased in rats fed a high fat diet. Hormonal assays on nurses transferred from a regular American diet to a meat-free diet for 2 months revealed decreased plasma testosterone and prolactin levels, a shortened menstrual cycle by 1–2 days, a shift in the luteinizing hormone peak from approximately the eight to the fifteenth day of the cycle, and a shift in the estrogen peak from approximately the sixth to the twelfth day.

The development of mammary tumors may, in fact, be related to a high prolactin to estrogen ratio which can be influenced by the fat content of the diet (399, 400). A similar mechanism could be of importance in the development of prostatic tumors.

Epidemiologic Evidence

A significant correlation coefficient of 0.89 was found between prostatic cancer mortality and per capita consumption of dietary fat based on data from 40 countries (389). An analysis of essentially the same data, but subdivided by specific food items, showed substantial correlation coefficients between the prostatic cancer mortality rate and per capita consumption of meat ($r = 0.74$), milk ($r = 0.70$), and fats ($r = 0.73$) (412, 413).

Lea, (414), analyzing data from Segi's 24 country mortality study, and from the United Nation's Food Production Yearbook, found a significant correlation between cancer of the prostate and per capita consumption of milk, animal protein, eggs, fats, and oils. Armstrong and Doll (380) analyzed prostatic cancer incidence data from 23 countries and mortality data from 32 countries and correlated these with per capita consumption dietary data. Mortality was highly correlated with the consumption of meats ($r = 0.60$), fats and oils ($r = 0.70$), animal protein ($r = 0.67$), sugar ($r = 0.63$) and total fats ($r = 0.74$); prostatic cancer incidence was not. The authors considered the mortality data more reliable since the "ascertainment of true incidence of prostatic cancer is likely to be deficient, varying from country to country according to diagnostic practices." In fact, the correlation between the incidence and mortality rates was only 5.7, among the lowest for the sites included in this study. The previously reported positive correlation between per capita consumption of coffee and mortality from cancer of the prostate (415) was attributed by Armstrong and Doll to an association between total fat and coffee consumption.

Age-adjusted prostatic cancer mortality rates for U.S. counties, 1950–1969, were highest in the areas of the United States with the highest consumption of beef, milk products, fats and oils, pork, and eggs (14).

Further support for a dietary-fat hypothesis comes from the earlier discussed findings of the lower rate of prostatic cancer among Seventh Day Adventists. Many Adventists follow a lacto-ovo-vegetarian diet that is free of any meat, poultry, or fish but does contain milk products and eggs (152). Virtually all Adventists abstain from pork products and other biblically defined unclean meats. This of course is also true of Jews, who were also found to have relatively low rates of the disease.

The low rate of prostatic cancer in Japanese men relative to U.S. males, may be related to their lower consumption of fats and oils (416). The marked postwar increase in Japan in the consumption of milk, meat, and eggs parallels the increased rate of prostatic cancer in Japan (417). A similar increase between prostate cancer and fat consumption has also been noticed in Poland (24).

Hirayama (417) speculated that the increase in prostatic cancer in Japan is related to the change to a westernized diet. In a census-population based prospective study, prostatic cancer was found to occur significantly less frequently in vegetarians. Furthermore, the dietary changes which have occurred between 1949 and 1973 have resulted in the following consumption increases: milk and milk products—23-fold, meat—13.7, eggs—12.9, and oil—7.8. Very little change occurred during this time in the consumption of fish, vegetables and rice.

In an 8-year followup of 265,118 people in Japan, a significantly lower rate (SMR = 0.33) of prostatic cancer was found for men who ate yellow-green vegetables daily (418). Daily consumption of meat, milk, and alcohol resulted in a slightly increased risk of disease that was not statistically significant. Issei (born in Japan and living in Hawaii), who have lower rates of prostatic cancer than the Nisei (Japanese born in Hawaii), have diets significantly lower in total and saturated fats (419).

The Chinese in Singapore have a low incidence rate of prostatic cancer (9). Shanmugaratnam and Wee (420) found that, among the Chinese in Singapore, the prostatic cancer rate was highest among the Cantonese as compared to the Hokkiens and Teochews. Although there are a number of differences in lifestyle among the three dialect groups, one notable difference is the variety of cooking methods used. Cantonese use deep fat frying more frequently than Hokkien or Teochew and have a preference for peanut oil.

The incidence of prostatic cancer has been found to be lower in Puerto Rico than in the United States (421). This finding is consistent with the relatively low consumption of fats in Puerto Rico in the past (422). More recently, Puerto Rico has experienced a marked increase in per capita consumption of beef, pork, milk, eggs, fats, and oils (422). This increase has been paralleled by a substantial increase in the incidence of prostatic cancer (9, 98).

In the only case-control study reported to date which examined the role of diet, the prostatic cancer cases reported a greater consumption of meats, eggs, cheeses, and creams than their matched controls (210).

Many epidemiologic studies have shown a strong correlation between the consumption of fat and the occurrence of both colon and breast cancer (389, 413, 423–429). The evidence linking dietary fat to prostatic cancer, although less convincing than for colon or breast cancer, is mounting. Countries with high rates of colon and breast cancer have high rates of prostatic cancer suggesting the possibility of a common etiology (9, 309, 412, 414, 430). Furthermore, there appears to be a familial association between breast cancer in women and prostatic cancer in men (431).

More work is needed to clarify the role diet may play in the etiology of cancer of the prostate. Needless to say, dietary studies are difficult to execute. Better methods for obtaining valid dietary data in a retrospective or case-control study need to be developed.

CONCLUSIONS

Because knowledge of the epidemiologic characteristics of prostate cancer is minimal, a formulation of specific hypotheses may be somewhat premature. Nevertheless, it does appear from this review that certain characteristics of the distribution of the disease are fairly well established (see Table 17)—increasing rate with age, high rate in blacks, low rate in Orientals, low rate in ever–married compared to never–married. men. In addition, there appears to be some association of the disease with an increased number of sexual partners, a history of venereal disease and a diet high in fat content. The interrelationships among these disparate facts and their significance in the etiology of prostate cancer are unclear.

The general influence of hormones on the disease is well documented. Androgenic levels, particularly testosterone, increase the rate of growth of prostate cancer and treatment of the disease is through the administration of estrogens. Thus, a hormonal etiological hypothesis seems intuitively obvious. However, data on the premorbid hormonal status of men are not available and, indeed, would be costly to obtain through a prospective or cohort study. Case-control studies of endocrine status may be biased in that the disease state may alter the serum hormone levels. Furthermore, the advisability of single specimen blood samplings for such determinations must be questioned, in view of an increasing amount of evidence that demonstrates the inappropriateness of such sampling (432). Multiple sampling to obtain circadian, ultradian, and circannual hormonal patterns may be required to ascertain differences of etiologic importance. Such "chronoepidemiological" studies might be conducted in selected groups of high- and low-risk men such as Japanese and Americans. A similar study of females was done for breast cancer (432).

A dietary hypothesis remains viable. Perhaps, the influencing of hormonal levels by dietary fat is of etiologic importance. Here again methodological problems are extant, particularly with regard to dietary questionnaires (433–436). Until a better methodological approach is developed to elicit valid dietary information, such studies may be of questionable value.

TABLE 17. Summary of the Epidemiologic Characteristics of Cancer of the Prostate

International Variations	Mortality	—Hi:	Northern Europe, New Zealand, Australia, United States
		—Lo:	South and Southeast Asia, Latin America
	Incidence	—Hi:	United States (Blacks), Canada, Northern European
		—Lo:	Southeast Europe, Eastern Asia
Within Country Variations	U.S. mortality	—Hi:	Northern United States
		—Lo:	Southeastern United States
Urban–Rural	Urban rates slightly higher		
Latent Cancers	Occur in about 20% of all men over the age of 40 Rate increases with age		
Secular Trend	Mortality—rate increased 150% since 1930 (33.6% for white males, 322.1% for nonwhite males)		
	Increases noted in virtually all countries, particularly striking in Japan		
	Incidence—rate increased 53.3% for white males and 151.6% for nonwhite males since 1937		
Age	Increases with age. Average age at diagnosis, 73		
	Rare prior to age 60		
Race	High in U.S. blacks (about 1.5 white rate)		
	Low in Japanese, Chinese, American Indians		
Migrants	Rates increased in Japanese, Chinese, Polish, and Irish migrants to the United States		
Religion	Rates higher in Protestants than in Catholics, who have higher rates than Jews		
	Slightly elevated in Mormons (except active Mormons), Parsis		
	Lower than expected in Seventh-Day Adventists		
Socioeconomic status	Results of studies inconclusive—slightly higher among men with some college education and professionals		
Occupation	Possible relationship with cadmium exposures—rubber workers, plumbers, and pipefitters		

(continued)

TABLE 17. Summary of the Epidemiologic Characteristics of Cancer of the Prostate (*continued*)

Trace Metals	Decreased zinc levels found in cancerous prostates
Air Quality	Positive association between SO_3, soiling, dustfall, particulates, and prostate cancer
Radiation	Probably no association
Alcohol	No consistency in the data
Cirrhosis of the liver	Prostate cancer decreased in cirrhotics
Familial aggragation	Positive relationship
Benign Prostatic Hypertrophy	Relationship questionable
Marital status	Rates higher in ever married than never married men Rates higher in widowed and divorced men than in married men who have higher rates than single men Rates higher in married men with children than married men without children
Sexual Factors	More pre- and extramarital partners Greater sexual drive Greater coital frequency in 10-year period preceeding diagnosis Possible later age at first coitus
Venereal Disease	Positive association
Circumcision	Relationship questionable
Viral	Possible association with herpesvirus 2, simian virus 40, or cytomegalovirus. Further research needed
Diet	Positive association with dietary fat

The importance of sexual behavior in the development of prostate cancer requires further study. The few studies that have been done are provocative, and more work in this area is indicated.

Although the evidence for a viral hypothesis is far from overwhelming, few adequately designed studies have been conducted. Whether or not circumcision is associated with the development of prostatic cancer also remains to be resolved.

In evaluating the rather meager and contradictory data, a specific etiologic hypothesis is difficult to develop. Perhaps the wisps of evidence suggest a common thread, such as a hormonal hypothesis. Could differences in sexual behavior between cases and controls merely be a reflection of differences in endogenous endocrine status between these groups? Could differences in fertility between these groups also reflect endocrine status? If dietary fat is, in fact, related to the development of prostatic cancer, could it act through some alteration of hormonal status? Similarly, differences among countries and between racial and ethnic groups might also be explained on the basis of differences in endocrine status. Such conclusions are tempting, particularly in view of the fact that cancer of the prostate is considered an endocrine dependent tumor. However, in view of the paucity of data, it is premature to cast the die. Nevertheless, a synthesis of the evidence to date might explain the apparently unrelated findings and direct future research endeavors.

REFERENCES

1. Bush, R. B., Bush, I. M. (1977) Early Developments in the History of Prostatic Disorders In: Urologic Pathology. Tannenbaum, M. (ed.). Philadelphia: Lea and Febiger, pp. 7–22.
2. Murphy, L. J. T. (1972) The Prostate. In: The History of Urology. Springfield, Illinois: Charles C. Thomas, pp. 378–452.
3. Cutler, S. J., Young, J. L., Jr., (1975) Third National Cancer Survey: Incidence Data. National Cancer Institute Monograph 41, DHEW Pub. No. (NIH) 75–787.
4. American Cancer Society (1980) 1980 Cancer Facts and Figures. New York.
5. Dunham, L. J., Bailar, J. C. (1968) World maps of cancer mortality rates and frequency ratios. J. Natl. Cancer Inst. 41, 155–203.
6. Dhom, G., Hohbach, M. (1972) Mortality and morbidity of prostatic carcinoma. Rec. Results Cancer Res. 39, 139–147.
7. World Health Organization (1973) Epidemiology and Vital Statistics Report, Geneva.
8. Segi, M. (1978) Age-Adjusted Death Rates for Cancer for Selected Sites (A Classification) in 52 Countries in 1973. Segi Institute of Cancer Epidemiology, Japan.
9. Waterhouse, J., Muir, C. Correa, P., Powell, J. (1976) Cancer Incidence in Five Continents, Vol. III, International Agency for Research on Cancer Pub. No. 15.
10. Lilienfeld, A. M., Levin, M. L., Kessler, I. I. (1972) Cancer in the United States. Cambridge, Mass; Harvard University Press, APHA Monograph.
11. Mason, T. J., McKay, F. W. (1974) U.S. Cancer Mortality By County: 1950–1969. Washington: National Cancer Institute, U. S. Department of Health, Education and Welfare.
12. Mason, T. J., McKay, F. W., Hoover, R., Blot, W. J., Fraumeni, J. F., Jr. (1976) Atlas of Cancer Mortality for U. S. Counties, 1950–1969. Washington: National Cancer Institute, U. S. Department of Health, Education and Welfare.
13. Mason, T. J., McKay, F. W., Hoover, R., Blot, W. J., Fraumeni, J. F., Jr. (1976) Atlas of Cancer Mortality Among U.S. Nonwhites, 1950–1969. Washington: National Cancer Institute, U. S. Department of Health, Education and Welfare.
14. Blair, A., Fraumeni, J. F. Jr. (1978) Geographic Patterns of prostate cancer in the United States. J. Natl. Cancer Inst. 61, 1379–1384.
15. Gover, M. (1940) Cancer mortality in the United States. III. Geographic variation in recorded cancer mortality for detailed sites for an average of the years 1930–1932. Pub. Health Bull. No. 257.
16. Spiegleman, M. (1952) Demographic differentials in cancer mortality in urban and rural areas of the U. S., 1940. Vital Statistics Special Report 33, No. 14.
17. King, H., Diamond, E., Lilienfeld, A. M. (1963) Some epidemiological aspects of cancer of the prostate. J. Chron. Dis. 16, 117–153.
18. Griswold, M. H., Wilder, S. S., Cutler, S. J., Pollach, E. (1956) Cancer in Connecticut, 1935–1951. Connecticut State Health Department.
19. Levin, M. L., Haenszel, W., Carroll, B. E., Gerhardt, P. R., Handy, V. H., Ingraham,

S. C. (1960) Cancer incidence in urban and rural areas of New York State. J. Natl. Cancer Inst. 24, 1243–1257.
20. Haenszel, W., Marcus, S. C., Zimmerer, E. G. (1956) Cancer Morbidity in Urban and Rural Iowa. Public Health Monograph No. 37.
21. Hoover, R., Mason, T. J., McKay, F. W., Fraumeni, J. F. (1975) Geographic patterns of cancer mortality in the United States. *In*: Persons at High Risk of Cancer. Fraumeni, J. F. (ed.) New York: Academic Press.
22. Clemmesen, J., Nielson, A. (1956) Cancer incidence in Denmark 1943–1953. Danish Med. Bull. 3, 36–43.
23. Clemmesen, J. (1969) Statistical studies in the aetiology of malignant neoplasms. Acta. Path. Microbiol. Scand. Suppl. 209.
24. Staszewski, J. (1976) Epidemiology of Cancer of Selected Sites in Poland and Polish Migrants. Cambridge, Mass: Ballinger Publishing Co.
25. Armenian, H. K., Lilienfeld, A. M., Diamond, E. L., Bross, I. D. J. (1975) Epidemiologic characteristics of patients with prostatic neoplasms. Am. J. Epidemiol. 102, 47–54.
26. Liavag, I., Harbitz, T. B., Haugen, O. A. (1972) Latent carcinoma of the prostate. Rec. Results Cancer Res. 39, 131–137.
27. Lefer, L. G., Rosier, R. P. (1977) Increased prevalence of prostatic carcinomas due to more thorough microscopical examination. N. Engl. J. Med. 296, 109.
28. Medart, W. S. (1977) "Prevalence" of prostatic cancer. N. Engl. J. Med. 296, 759.
29. Franks, L. M. (1956) The natural history of prostatic cancer. Lancet 271, ii, 1037–1039.
30. Liavag, I. (1967) Carcinoma of the Prostate. Oslo: Universitetsforlaget.
31. Franks, L. M. (1972) The incidence of carcinoma of prostate: An epidemiological survey. Rec. Results Cancer Res. 39, 149–155.
32. Mears, E. M. (1972) Current concepts in the management of carcinoma of the prostate gland. Calif. Med. 117, 27–34.
33. Albarran, J., Hallé, N. (1900) Hypertrophie et néoplasies épithéliales de la prostate. Ann. Mal. Org. Gen. Urin. 18, 113–147.
34. Editorial (1973) Carcinoma of the prostate. Br. Med. J., 566–567.
35. Hinman, F., Jr., Hinman, F. (1949) Occult prostatic carcinoma diagnosed upon transurethral resection. J. Urol. 62, 723–729.
36. Bauer, W. C., McGravran, M. H., Garlin, M. R. (1960) Unsuspected carcinoma of the prostate in suprapubic prostatectomy specimens. Cancer 13, 370–378.
37. Mellinger, G. T., Gleason, D., Bailar, J. (1967) The histology and prognosis of prostatic cancer. M. Urol. 97, 331–337.
38. Cook, G. B., Watson, F. R. (1968) A comparison by age of death rates due to prostate cancer alone. J. Urol. 100, 669–671.
39. Veterans Administration Cooperative Urologic Research Group (1968) Factors in the prognosis of carcinoma of the prostate. A cooperative study. J. Urol. 100, 59–65.
40. Corriere, J. N., Carnog, J. L., Murphy, J. J. (1970) Prognosis in patients with carcinoma of the prostate. Cancer 25, 911–918.
41. Gilbertsen, V. A. (1970) Improved prognosis for survival following earlier detection of cancer. Geriatrics 25, 149–154.
42. Hanash, K. A., Utz, D. C., Cook, E. N., Taylor, W. F., Titus, J. L. (1972) Carcinoma of the prostate. A 15-year follow up. J. Urol. 107, 450–453.
43. Baron, E., Angrist, A. (1964) Incidence of occult adenocarcinomas of the prostate after 50 years of age. Arch. Pathol. 32. 787–793.
44. Akazaki, K., Stemmermann, G. N. (1973) Comparative study of latent carcinoma of the prostate among Japanese in Japan and Hawaii. J. Natl. Cancer Inst. 50, 1137–1144.

45. Akazaki, K. (1973) Comparative histological studies on the latent carcinoma of the prostate under different environmental circumstances. *In*: Host Environmental Interactions in the Etiology of Cancer in Man. Lyon, France: International Agency for Research on Cancer.
46. Breslow, N., Chan, C. W., Dhom, G., Drury, R. A. B., Franks, L. M., Gellei, B., Lee, Y. S., Lundberg, S., Sparke, B., Sternby, N. H., Tulinius, H. (1977) Latent carcinoma of prostate at autopsy in seven areas. Int. J. Cancer 20 680–688.
47. Rich, A. R. (1935) On frequency of occurrence of occult carcinoma of prostate. J. Urol. 33, 215–223.
48. Kahler, J. E. (1939) Carcinoma of prostate gland: A pathologic study. J. Urol. 41, 557–573.
49. Buchert, W. L., Culp, D. A., Jones, C. H. (1947) An analysis of 135 cases of carcinoma of the prostate gland. Pa. Med. 51, 165–173.
50. Mathé, C. P., Ardile, C. E. (1947) Review of 130 cases of carcinoma of the prostate. Surg. Gynecol. Obstet. 84, 276–282.
51. Hirst, A. E., Bergman, R. T. (1954) Carcinoma of the prostate in men 80 or more years old. Cancer 7, 136–141.
52. Hudson, P. B. (1957) Prostatic cancer, XIV. Its incidence and extent and behavior in 686 men studied by prostatic biopsy. Am. Geriatr. Soc. J. 5, 338–350.
53. Hudson, P. B., Finkle, A. L., Hopkins, J. A., Sproul, E. E., Stout, A. P. (1954) Prostatic cancer: XI. Early prostatic cancer diagnosed by arbitrary open perineal biopsy among 300 unselected patients. Cancer 7, 690–703.
54. Scott, R., Jr., Mutchnik, D. L., Laskowski, T. Z., Schmalhorst, W. R. (1969) Carcinoma of the prostate in elderly men: Incidence, growth characteristics and clinical significance. J. Urol. 101, 602–607.
55. Halpert, B., Sheehan, E. E., Schmalhorst, W. R., Scott, R. (1963) Carcinoma of the prostate. A survey of 5000 autopsies. Cancer 16, 737–742.
56. Strahan, R. W. (1963) Carcinoma of the prostate: Incidence, origin, pathology. J. Urol. 89, 875–880.
57. Berg, J. W., Hajdu, S. I., Foote, F. W. (1971) The prevalence of latent cancers in cancer patients. Arch. Pathol. 91, 183–186.
58. Butler, J., Braunstein, H., Freeman, D. G., Gall, E. A. (1959) Incidence, distribution and enzymatic activity of carcinoma of the prostate gland. Arch. Pathol. 68, 243–251.
59. Jordon, W. P., Kreager, J. A. (1967) Incidentally discovered microscopic carcinoma of the prostate. J. Urol. 97, 751–754.
60. Suen, K. C., Lau, L. L., Yermakov, V. (1974) Cancer and old age (An autopsy study of 3, 535 patients over 65). Cancer 33, 1164–1168.
61. Edwards, C. N., Steinthorsson, E., Nicholson, D. (1953) Autopsy study of latent prostatic cancer. Cancer 6, 531–554.
62. Andrews, G. S. (1949) Latent carcinoma of the prostate. J. Clin. Pathol. 2, 197–208.
63. Franks, L. M. (1954) Latent carcinoma of prostate. J. Pathol. Bacteriol. 68, 603–616.
64. Moore, R. A. (1935) The morphology of small prostatic carcinoma. J. Urol. 33, 224–234.
65. Gaynor, E. P. (1938) Zur Frage des Prostatakrebses. Virchows Arch. Pathol. Anat. 301, 602–652.
66. Oota, K. (1961) Latent carcinoma of the prostate among the Japanese. Acta Un. Int. Cancer 17, 952–957.
67. Karube, K. (1960) Study of latent carcinoma of the prostate in the Japanese based on necropsy material. Tohoku J. Exp. Med. 73, 265–285.
68. Sugihara, K. (1959) A study on latent carcinoma of the prostate in Japanese. Gann. 50, Suppl. 163–164.
69. Imai, T. (1961) *In*: Oota, K., Latent carcinoma of the prostate among the Japanese, Acta Un. Int. Cancer 17, 952–957.

70. Cooray, G. H., Panabokke, R. G., Wijesekera, S. V. J. (1954) Some observations on prostatic carcinoma in Ceylon. Ceylon J. Med. Sci. 8, 191–197.
71. Liavag, I. (1968) The localization of prostatic carcinoma. An autopsy study. Scand. J. Urol. Nephrol. 2, 65–71.
72. Viitanen, I., Hellens, A. V. Latent carcinoma of the prostate in Finland. Acta. Pathol. Microbiol. Scand. 44, 64–67.
73. Lundberg, S., Berg, T. (1970) Prostatic carcinoma. An autopsy study. Scand. J. Urol. Nephrol. 4, 93–97.
74. Luciak, M. (1969) Problem of the occult prostatic cancer. Slaska Akademia Medyczna, Poland.
75. Gordon, T., Crittenden, M., Haenszel, W. (1961) Cancer Mortality Trends in the United States, 1930–1955. End Results and Mortality Trends in Cancer, National Cancer Institute Monograph No. 6.
76. Burbank, F. (1971) Patterns in Cancer Mortality in the United States, 1950–1967. National Cancer Institute Monograph 33.
77. Segi, M., Kurihara M. (1972) Cancer Mortality for Selected Sites in 24 Countries, No. 6, 1966–1967. Japan Cancer Society.
78. Silverberg, E., Holleb, A. I. Cancer Statistics. CA 22, 2–7.
79. Tulinius, H. (1977) Epidemiology of prostate carcinoma. Rec. Results Cancer Res. 60, 3–13.
80. Devesa, S. S., Silverman, D. T. (1978) Cancer incidence and mortality trends in the United States: 1935–1974. J. Natl. Cancer Inst. 60, 545–571.
81. Henschke, U. K., Leffall, L. D. Jr., Mason, C. H., Reinhold, A. W., Schneider, R. L., White, J. E. (1973) Alarming increase of the cancer mortality in the U.S. black population. Cancer 31, 763–768.
82. Hirayama, T. (1978) Comparative Epidemiology of Cancer in the U.S. and Japan–Mortality. U.S.–Japan Cooperative Cancer Research Program.
83. Hirayama, T. (1975) Epidemiology of cancer of the stomach with special reference to its recent decrease in Japan. Can. Research 35, 3460–3463.
84. Wigle, D. T. (1978) Cancer patterns in Canada. Can. J. Pub. Health, 69, 113–120.
85. Haddow, A. J. (1968) Cancer as a Scottish problem. Scot. Med. J. 13, 338–348.
86. Dorn, H. F. (1944) Illness from cancer in the United States. Pub. Health Rep. 59.
87. Dorn, H. F., Cutler, S. J. (1958) Morbidity from Cancer in the United States. U. S. Pub. Health Service Monograph No. 56. Washington, D. C.: Government Printing Office.
88. Hutchinson, G. B. (1976) Epidemiology of prostatic cancer. Semin. Oncol. 3, 151–159.
89. Griswold, M. (1946) Cancer of the prostate in Connecticut. Conn. State Med. J. 10:2, 106–109.
90. Sullivan, P. D., Christine, B., Connelly, R., Barrett, H. (1972) Analysis of trends in age-adjusted incidence rates for 10 major sites of cancer. Am. J. Pub. Health 62, 1065–1071.
91. Gerhardt, P. R., Handy, V. H., Ferber, B. (1957) Trends in cancer incidence, mortality and probability in the state of New York. N. Y. State J. Med. 57, 1387–1390.
92. Greenwald, P., Burnett, W. S., Kirms, V., Brennan, K., Nasca, P. C. (1976) Cancer Incidence and Mortality in New York State. Bureau of Cancer Control, N. Y. State Department of Health.
93. Arellano, M. G., Linden, G., Dunn, J. E. (1972) Cancer patterns in Alameda County, California. Br. J. Cancer 26, 473–482.
94. Clemmesen, J. (1977) Correlation of sites, *In:* Hiatt, H. H., Watson, J. D., Winsten, J. A., (eds.). Origins of Human Cancer. Book A. Cold Spring Harbor Laboratory.

95. Saxen, E., Hakama, M., Lehtonen, M. (1969) Cancer in Finland 1954–1963. Ann. Clin. Res. 1, 291–300.
96. Teppo, L., Hakulinen, T., Saxen, E. (1974) The prediction of cancer incidence in Finland for the year 1980 by means of cancer registry material. Ann. Clin. Res. 6, 122–125.
97. Gadomska, H., Romejko, A. (1973) Incidence of malignant neoplasms in five most frequently involved organs in the population of the city of Warsaw. 1963–1970. Polish Med. Sci. History Bull. Abstr. 1, 13–23.
98. Doll, R., Payne, P., Waterhouse, J. (1966) Cancer Incidence in Five Continents. Lyon, France: International Union Against Cancer.
99. Case, R. A. M. (1956) Cohort analysis of cancer mortality in England and Wales, 1911–1954, by site and sex. Br. J. Prev. Soc. Med. 10, 172–199.
100. Ernster, V., Selvin, S., Winkelstein, W. (1978) Cohort mortality for prostatic cancer among United States nonwhites. Science 200, 1165–1166.
101. Cook, P. J., Doll, R., Fellingham, S. A. (1969) A mathematical model for the age distribution of cancer in man. Int. J. Cancer 4, 93–112.
102. Ashley, D. J. B. (1965) On the incidence of carcinoma of the prostate. J. Pathol. Bacteriol. 90, 217–224.
103. Vital Statistics of the United States, 1975. National Center for Health Statistics, DHEW, 1979.
104. Young, J. L., Jr., Devesa, S. S., Cutler, S. J. (1975) Incidence of cancer in United States blacks. Cancer Res. 35, 3523–3536.
105. Ernster, V. L., Winkelstein, W., Selvin, S., Brown, S., et al. (1977) Race, socioeconomic status and prostatic cancer. Cancer Treat. Rep. 61, 187–191.
106. National Center for Health Statistics (1977) Vital Statistics of the United States, 1975. Volume II. Mortality. Washington: U. S. Department of Health, Education and Welfare. (PHS) 78–1102.
107. Jackson, M. A., Ahluwalia, B. S., Herson, J., Heshmat, M. Y., Jackson, A. G., Jones, G. W., et al. (1977) Characterization of prostatic carcinoma among blacks: A continuation report. Cancer Treat. Rep. 61, 167–172.
108. Dunn, J. E., Jr. (1975) Cancer epidemiology in populations of the United States—with emphasis on Hawaii and California—and Japan. Cancer Res. 35, 3240–3245.
109. Hirayama, T. (1978) Comparative Epidemiology of Cancer in the U.S. and Japan—Morbidity. U. S.–Japan Cooperative Cancer Research Program.
110. Fraumeni, J. F., Mason, T. J. (1974) Cancer mortality among Chinese Americans, 1950–1969. J. Natl. Cancer Inst. 52, 639–665.
111. Smith, R. L. (1956) Recorded and expected mortality among the Japanese of the United States and Hawaii, with special reference to cancer. J. Natl. Cancer Inst. 17, 459–473.
112. Quisenberry, W. B. (1960) Sociocultural factors in cancer in Hawaii. Ann. N. Y. Acad. Sci. 84, 795–806.
113. Smith, R. L. (1957) Mortality attributed to cancer among Hawaiians and Filipinos and other racial groups of the United States and Hawaii. J. Natl. Cancer Inst. 18, 397–405.
114. Kagan, A. (1971) Cancer mortality among ethnic groups in Hawaii. Israel J. Med. Sci. 7, 1451–1454.
115. Creagan, E. T., Fraumeni, J. F., Jr. (1972) Cancer mortality among American Indians, 1950–67. J. Natl. Cancer Inst. 49, 959–967.
116. Smith, R. L., Salisbury, C. G., Gilliam, A. G. (1956) Recorded and expected mortality among the Navajo, with special reference to cancer. J. Natl. Cancer Inst. 17, 77–89.

117. Smith, R. L. (1957) Recorded and expected mortality among the Indians of the United States with special reference to cancer. J. Natl. Cancer Inst. 18, 385–396.
118. Dunham, L. J. Bailar, J. C., III, Laqueuer, G. L. (1973) Histologically diagnosed cancers in 693 Indians of the United States, 1950–65. J. Natl. Cancer Inst. 50, 1119–1127.
119. Menck, H. R., Henderson, E. E., Pike, M. C., Mack, T., Martin, S. P. (1975) Cancer incidence in the Mexican-American. J. Natl. Cancer Inst. 55, 531–536.
120. Lanier, A. P., Bender, T. R., Blot, W. J., Fraumeni, J. Fl, Hurlburt, W. B. (1976) Cancer incidence in Alaska natives. Int. J. Cancer 18, 409–412.
121. Lilienfeld, A. M. (1976) Foundations of Epidemiology. New York: Oxford University Press.
122. Haenszel, W. (1970) Studies of migrant populations. J. Chron. Dis. 23, 289–291.
123. Steiner, P. E. (1954) Cancer: Race and Geography. Baltimore: The Williams Wilkins Co.
124. Lombard, H. L., Doering, C. R. (1929) Cancer studies in Massachusetts. Cancer mortality in nativity groups. J. Prev. Med. 3, 343–361.
125. Haenszel, W. (1961) Cancer mortality among foreign-born in the United States. J. Natl. Cancer Inst. 26, 37–132.
126. Kmet, J. (1970) The role of migrant population in studies of selected cancer sites: A reveiw. J. Chron. Dis. 23, 305–324.
127. Haenszel, W. (1971) Cancer mortality among U. S. Jews. Israel J. Med. Sci. 7, 1437–1450.
128. MacMahon, B. (1960) Ethnic distribution of cancer mortality in New York City, 1955. Acta. Un. Int. Cancer 16, 1716–1724.
129. Seidman, H. (1970) Cancer death rates by site and sex for religious and socioeconomic groups in New York City. Environ. Res. 3, 235–250.
130. Greenwald, P., Korns, R. F., Nasca, P. C., Wolfgang, P. E. (1975) Cancer in United States Jews. Cancer Res. 35, 3507–3512.
131. Staszewski, J., Haenszel, W. (1965) Cancer mortality among the Polish born in the United States. J. Natl. Cancer Inst. 35, 291–297.
132. Buell, P., Dunn, J. E. (1965) Cancer mortality among Japanese Issei and Nisei of California. Cancer 18, 656–664.
133. Haenszel, W., Kurihara M. (1968) Studies of Japanese migrants. 1. Mortality from cancer and other diseases. J. Natl. Cancer Inst. 40, 43–68.
134. King, H., Haenszel, W. (1973) Cancer mortality among foreign and native-born Chinese in the United States. J. Chron. Dis. 26, 623–646.
135. Halevi, H. S., Dreyfuss, F., Pertiz, E., Schmelz, U. O. (1971) Cancer mortality and immigration to Israel. Israel J. Med. Sci. 7, 1386–1404.
136. Steinitz, R., Costin, C. (1971) Cancer in Jewish immigrants. Israel J. Med. Sci. 7, 1413–1435.
137. Bolduan, C., Weiner, L. (1933) Causes of death among Jews in New York City. N. Engl. J. Med. 208, 407–416.
138. Newill, V. A. (1961) Distribution of cancer mortality among ethnic subgroups of the white population of New York City, 1953–58. J. Natl. Cancer Inst. 26, 405–417.
139. King, H., Diamond, E., Bailar, J. C. III (1965) Cancer mortality and religious preference. Milbank Mem. Fund. Quart. 43, 349–358.
140. McMahon, B., Koller, E. K. (1957) Ethnic differences in the incidence of leukemia. Blood 12, 1–10.
141. Wynder, E. L., Mabuchi, K., Whitmore, W. F. (1971) Epidemiology of cancer of the prostate. Cancer 28, 344–360.
142. Krain, L. S. (1973) Epidemiologic variables in prostatic cancer. Geriatrics 28, 93–98.

143. Krain, L. S. (1974) Some epidemiologic variables in prostatic carcinoma in Califronia. Prev. Med. 3, 154–159.
144. King, H., Bailar, J. C. (1968) Mortality among Lutheran clergymen. Mill. Mem. Fund. Quart. 46, 527–548.
145. King, H. (1971) Clerical mortality patterns of the Anglican communion. Sociol. Biol. 18, 164–177.
146. Versluys, J. J. (1949) Cancer and occupation in the Netherlands. Br. J. Cancer 3, 161–185.
147. Mandel, J. S., Hollingsworth, C., Murray, S. Mortality from cancer of the prostate among Catholic priests. Unpublished report.
148. Wynder, E. L., Lemon, F. R., Bross. I. J. (1959) Cancer and coronary artery disease among Seventh-Day Adventists. Cancer 12, 1016–1028.
149. Lemon, F. R., Walden, R. T., Woods, R. W. (1964) Cancer of the lung and mouth in Seventh-Day Adventists. Cancer 17, 486–497.
150. Lemon, F. R., Walden, R. T. (1966) Death from respiratory system disease among Seventh-day Adventist men. J.A.M.A. 198, 117–126.
151. Phillips, R. L. (1974) Cancer and Adventists. Science 183, 471.
152. Phillips, R. L. (1975) Role of lifestyle and dietary habits in risk of cancer among Seventh-Day Adventists. Cancer Res. 35, 3513–3522.
153. Enstrom, J. E. (1975) Cancer mortality among Mormons. Cancer 36, 825–841.
154. Lyon, J. L., Klauber, M. R., Gardner, J. W., Smart, C. R. (1976) Cancer incidence in Mormons and non-Mormons in Utah, 1966–1970. N. Engl. J. Med. 294, 129–133.
155. Lyon, J. L., Gardner, J. W., Klauber, M. R. (1977) Low cancer incidence and mortality in Utah. Cancer 39, 2608–2618.
156. Phillips, R. L., Kuzma, J. W. (1977) Rationale and methods for an epidemiologic study of cancer among Seventh-Day Adventists. Epidemiology and Cancer Registries in the Pacific Basin. National Cancer Institute Monograph 47.
157. Enstrom, J. E. (1978) Cancer and total mortality among active Mormons. Cancer 42, 1943–1951.
158. Gaudette, L. A., Holmes, T. J., Laing, L. M., Morgan, L., Grace, M. G. A. (1978) Cancer incidence in a religious isolate of Alberta, Canada, 1953–74. J. Natl. Cancer Inst. 60, 1233–1238.
159. Jussawalla, D. J., Deshpande, V. A., Haenszel, W., Natekar, M. V. (1970) Differences observed in the site incidence of cancer between the Parsi community and the total population of greater Bombay: A critical appraisal. Br. J. Cancer 24, 56–66.
160. Gangadharan, P., Jussawalla, D. J., Rao, D. N., Paymaster, J. C. (1974) Multiple study approaches (for cancer) to a well defined population of Parsis. *In*: Bucalossi, P., Vernesi, U., Cascinelli, N. (ed.). Cancer Epidemiology. Environmental Factors. Florence: Proceedings of the International Cancer Congress. American Elsevier Pub. Co.
161. Hollingshead, A. B., Redlich, F. C. (1958) Social Class and Mental Illness. A Community Study. New York: John Wiley Sons.
162. Gordis, L., Lilienfeld, Al, Rodriguez, R. (1969) Studies in the epidemiology and preventability of rheumatic fever—II. Socioeconomic factors and the incidence of acute attacks. J. Chron. Dis. 21, 655–666.
163. Registrar General for England and Wales (1855) Fourteenth Annual Report, England and Wales, 1851. London: Her Majesty's Stationery Office.
164. Registrar General for England and Wales (1954) Occupational mortality, England and Wales, 1951. The Registrar General's Decennial Supplement, Part II, Vol. I and II. London: Her Majesty's Stationery Office.
165. Petras, J. W., Curtis, J. E. (1968) The current literature on social class and mental disease in America: critique and bibliography. Behav. Sci. 13, 382–398.

166. Green, L. W. (1970) Manual for scoring socioeconomic status for research on health behavior. Pub. Health Rep. 85, 815–827.

167. Susser, M. W., Watson, W. (1970) Sociology in Medicine. London: Oxford University Press.

168. Owen, W. L. (1976) Cancer of the prostate: A literature review. J. Chron. Dis. 29, 89–114.

169. Higgins, I. T. T. (1975) The epidemiology of cancer of the prostate. J. Chron. Dis. 28, 343–348.

170. Young, M. (1926) Variations in mortality from cancer of different parts of the body in groups of men of different social status. J. Hyg. 25, 109–271.

171. Buell, P., Dunn, J. E., Brewlow L. (1960) The occupational social class risks of cancer mortality in men. J. Chron. Dis. 12, 600–621.

172. Richardson, I. M. (1965) Prostatic cancer and social class. Br. J. Prev. Soc. Med. 19, 140–142.

173. Guralnick, K. (1963) Mortality by Occupational Level and Cause of Death Among Men 20 to 64 Years of Age: United States, 1950, Vital Statistics—Special Reports, 53, no. 3. United States Department of HEW. Washington, C. C.: U. S. Gov. Printing Office.

174. Clemmesen, J., Nielsen, A. (1951) The social distribution of cancer in Copenhagen, 1943–1947. Br. J. Cancer 5, 159–171.

175. Graham S., Levin, M., Lilienfeld, A.M. (1960) The socioeconomic distribution of cancer of various sites in Buffalo, N.Y., 1948–52. Cancer 13, 180–191.

176. Basa, G.F. Hirayama, T., Cruz-Basa, A.G. (1977) Cancer epidemiology in the Philippines. Epidemiology and Cancer Registries in the Pacific Basin. National Cancer Institute Monograph 47.

177. Potts, C.L. (1965) Cadmium proteinuria—the health of battery workers exposed to dust. Ann. Occup. Hyg. 8, 55–61.

178. Kipling, M.D., Waterhouse, J. A. H. (1967) Cadmium and prostatic carcinoma. Lancet i, 730–731.

179. Holden, J. (1969) Cadmium toxicology. Lancet ii, 57.

180. Lemen, R. A., Lee, J. S., Wagoner, J. K., Blejer, H. P. (1976) Cancer mortality among cadmium production workers. Ann. N. Y. Acad. Sci. 271, 273–279.

181. Kolonel, L. N. (1972) An epidemiological investigation of cadmium carcinogenesis. Ph.D. thesis. University of California, Berkeley; 109 pp.

182. Friberg, L. (1948) Proteinura and kidney injury among workmen exposed to cadmium and nickel dust. J. Indust. Hyg. 30, 33–36.

183. Humperdink, K. (1968). Kadmium and Lungenkrebs. Med. Klin. 63, 948–950.

184. Malcolm, D. (1972) Potential carcinogenic effects of cadmium in animals and man—effects of cadmium on the genito-urinary tracts of animals. Ann. Occup. Hyg. 15, 33–36.

185. Wilson, R. H. (1944) Health hazards encountered in the manufacture of synthetic rubber. J.A.M.A. 124, 701–703.

186. Wilson, R. H., Hough, G. V., McCormick, W. E. (1948) Medical problems encountered in the manufacture of American-made rubber. Ind. Med. Surg. 17, 199–207.

187. McMichael, A. J., Spirtas, R., Kupper, L. L. (1974) An epidemiologic study of mortality within a cohort of rubber workers. J. Occup. Med. 16, 458–464.

188. McMichael, A. J., Spirtas, R., Gamble, J. F., Tousey, P. M. (1976) Mortality among rubber workers: Relationship to specific jobs. J. Occup. Med. 18, 178–185.

189. Goldsmith, D. F., Smith, A. H., McMichael, A. J. (1977) Prostate cancer among a cohort of rubber workers. Paper presented at American Public Health Association meeting, Washington, D. C.

190. Monson, R. J., Nakano, K. K. (1976) Mortality among rubber workers. I. White male union employees in Akron, Ohio. Am. J. Epidemiol. 103, 284–296.

191. Monson, R. J., Nakano, K. K. (1976) Mortality among rubber workers. II. Other employees. Am. J. Epidemiol. 103, 297–303.

192. Andjelkovic, D., Taulbee, J., Symons, M. (1976) Mortality experience of a cohort of rubber workers, 1964–73. J. Occup. Med. 18, 387–394.

193. Andjelkovic, D., Taulbee, J., Symons, M., Williams, T. (1977) Mortality of rubber works with reference to work experience. J. Occup. Med. 19, 397–405.

194. Decoufle, P., Stanislawczyk, K., Houten, L., Bross, I. D., Viadana, E. (1977) A retrospective survey of cancer in relation to occupation. Department of Health, Education and Welfare. NIOSH, Publ. No. 77–178.

195. Viadana, E., Bross, I. D., Houten, L. (1976) Cancer experience of men exposed to inhalation of chemicals or to combustion products. J. Occup. Med. 18, 787–792.

196. Lloyd, J. W., Ciocco, A. (1969) Long-term mortality study of steelworkers. I. Methodology. J. Occup. Med. 11, 299–310.

197. Lloyd, J. W, Lundin, F. E. Jr., Redmond, C. K. (1970) Longterm mortality study of steelworkers, IV. Mortality by work area. J. Occup. Med. 12, 151–157.

198. Redmond, C. K. (1975) Comparative Cause-Specific Mortality Patterns by Work Area Within the Steel Industry. Washington: U.S. Department of Health, Education and Welfare, National Institute of Occupational Health and Safety.

199. Redmond, C. K., Ciocco, A., Lloyd, W., Rush, H. W. (1972) Long-term mortality study of steelworkers VI. Mortality from malignant neoplasms among coke oven workers. J. Occup. Med. 14, 621–629.

200. Radford, E. P. (1976) Cancer mortality in the steel industry. Ann. N. Y. Acad. Sci. 271, 228–238.

201. Milham, S., Jr. (1976) Neoplasia in the wood and pulp industry. Ann. N. Y. Acad. Sci. 271, 294–300.

202. Henry, S. A., Kennaway, M. N., Kennaway, E. L. (1931) The incidence of cancer of the bladder and prostate in certain occupations. J. Hygiene 31, No. 2, 125–137.

203. Versluys, J. J. (1949) Cancer and occupation in the Netherlands. Br. J. Cancer 3, 161–185.

204. Versluys, J. J. (1960) Study on the changes in cancer frequency in the total male population and in various branches of occupation during the period 1930–1957. Acta. Un. Int. Cancer 16, 1771–1775.

205. Adelstein, A. M. (1972) Occupational mortality: Cancer Ann. Occup. Hyg. 15, 53–57.

206. Guralnick, L. (1963) Mortality by occupation level and cause of death among men 20 to 64 years of age: United States, 1950. Washington: U. S. Department of Health, Education and Welfare, Vital Statistics—Special Reports, Vol. 53, No. 5.

207. Williams, R. R., Stegens, N. L. Horm, J. W. (1977). Patient interview study from the Third National Cancer Survey: Overview of problems and potentials of these data. J. Natl. Cancer Inst. 58, 519–524.

208. Williams, Roger R., Stegens, N.L., Goldsmith, J. R. (1977). Associations of cancer site and type with occupation and industry from the Third National Cancer Survey. J. Natl. Cancer Inst. 59, 1147–1185.

209. Milham, S. (1976) Occupational mortality in Washington state, 1950–1971, Vol. I, II, III. Washington, D. C.: U. S. Department of Health, Education, and Welfare, Public Health Service Pub. No. 76–175.

210. Rotkin, I. D. (1977) Studies in the epidemiology of prostatic cancer: Expanded sampling. Cancer Treat. Rep. 61, 173–180.

211. Guralnick, L. (1963) Mortality by occupation and industry among men 20 to 64 years of age, United States, 1950. Washington: U. S. Department of Health, Education and Welfare, Vital Statistics Special Reports, Vol. 53, No. 22.

212. Valle, B. L. (1959) Biochemistry, physiology and pathology of zinc. Physiol. Rev. 39, 443–490.

213. MacKenzie, A. R., Hall, T., Whitmore, W. F. (1972) Zinc content of expressed human prostatic fluid. Nature 193, 72–73.
214. Schroeder, H. A., Nason, A. P., Tipton, T. H., Ballasa, J. J. Essential trace metals in man—zinc. Relation to environmental cadmium. J. Chron. Dis. 20, 179–210.
215. Furst, A., Haro, R. T. (1969) A survey of metal carcinogenesis. Progr. Exp. Tumor Res. 12, 102.
216. Kar, A. B., Chowdbury, A. R. (1968) The distribution of zinc in the subcellular fractions of human prostate. Curr. Sci. 37, 375–380.
217. Mawson, C. A., Fischer, M. I. (1951) Zinc content of the genital organs of the rat. Nature 167, 859.
218. Sternberg, S. S., Cronin A. P., Philips, F. S. (1965) Histochemical demonstration of zinc in the dorsolateral prostate of the rat. Am. J. Pathol. 47, 325–337.
219. Kerr, W. K., Keresteci, A. G., Mayoh, H. (1960) The distribution of zinc within the human prostate. Cancer 13, 550–554.
220. Mawson, C. A., and Fischer, M. I. (1952) The occurrence of zinc in the human prostate gland. Can. J. Biochem. Phys. 30, 336–339.
221. Daniel, O., Haddad, F., Prout, G., Whitmore, W. F. (1956) Some observations on the distribution of radioactive zinc in prostatic and other human tissues. Br. J. Urol. 28, 271–278.
222. Hoare, R., Delory, G. E., Penner, D. W. (1956) Zinc and acid phosphatase in the human prostate. Cancer 9, 721–726.
223. Schrodt, G. R., Hall, T., Whitmore, W. R., Jr. (1964) The concentration of zinc in diseased human prostate glands. Cancer 17, 1555–1566.
224. Rosoff, B., Spencer, R. H. (1965) Tissue distribution of $Zinc^{65}$ in tumor tissue and normal tissue in man. Nature 207, 652–653.
225. Gyorkey, F., Min, K. W., Huff, J. A., Gyorkey, P. (1967) Zinc and magnesium in human prostate—normal, hypertrophic and neoplastic. Cancer Res. 27, 1348–1353.
226. Dhar, N. K. Goel, T. C., Dube P. C., Chowdhury, A. R., Kar, A. B. (1973) Distribution and concentration of zinc in the subcellular fractions of benign hyperplastic and malignant neoplastic human prostate. Exp. Molecular Pathol. 19, 139–142.
227. MacKenzie, A. R., Hall, T., Lo, M. C., Whitmore, W. F., Jr. (1963) Influence of castration and sex hormones on size, histology and zinc content of the canine prostate. J. Urol. 80, 864–874.
228. Gunn, S. A., Gould, T. C. (1956) The relative importance of androgen and estrogen in the selective uptake of ZN^{65} by the dorsolateral prostate of the rat. Endocrinology 58, 443–452.
229. Wilden, E. G., Robinson, M. R. G. (1975) Plasma zinc levels in prostatic disease. Br. J. Urol. 47, 295–299.
230. Gunn, S. A., Gould, T. C., Anderson, W. A. D, (1967) Specific response to mesenchymal tissue to carcinogenesis by cadmium. Arch. Pathol. 83, 493–498.
231. Heath, J. C., Daniel, M. R., Dingle, J. T., Webb, M. (1962) Cadmium as a carcinogen. Nature (London) 193, 592–593.
232. Kazantzis, G. (1963) Induction of sarcoma in the rat by cadmium sulfide pigment. Nature (London) 198, 1312–1314.
233. Gunn, S. A., Gould, T. C., Anderson, W. A. D. (1964) Comparative study of interstitial cell tumors of rat testis induced by cadmium injection and vascular ligation. J. Natl. Cancer Inst. 35, 329–337.
234. Haddow, A., Roe, F. J. C., Dukes, C. E., Mitchley, B. C. V. (1964) Cadmium neoplasia: Sarcomata at the site of injection of cadmium sulfate in rats and mice. Br. J. Cancer 18, 667–673.
235. Roe, F. J. C., Dukes, C. E., Cameron, K. M., Pugh, R. C. B., Mitchley, B. C. B. (1964) Cadmium neoplasia: Testicular atrophy and Leydig cell hyperplasia and neoplasia

in rats and mice following the subcutaneous injection of cadmium salts. Br. J. Cancer 18, 674–681.

236. Kazantzis, G., Hanbury, W. J. (1966) The induction of sarcoma in the rat by cadmium sulfide and by cadmium oxide. Br. J. Cancer 20, 190–199.
237. National Institute for Occupational Health and Safety. (1976) Occupational Exposure to Cadmium. Washington: U. S. Department of Health, Education and Welfare.
238. World Health Organization—International Agency for Research on Cancer (1973) IARC Monographs on the evaluation of Carcinogenic Risk of Chemicals to Man. Vol. 2: Some inorganic and organometallic compounds. Lyon, France: International Agency for Research on Cancer.
239. Gunn, S. A., Gould, T. C., Anderson, W. A. D. (1961) Competition of cadmium for zinc in rat testis and dorsolateral prostate. Acta Endocrinol. 37, 24–30.
240. Gunn, A., Gould, T. C., Anderson, W. A. D. (1963) Cadmium induced interstitial cell tumors in rats and mice and their prevention by zinc. J. Natl. Cancer Inst. 31, 745–753.
241. Schroeder, H. A. (1965) Cadmium as a factor in hypertension. J. Chron, Dis. 18, 647–656.
242. Levy, L. S., Roe, F. J. C., Malcolm, D., Kazantzis, G., Clark, C., Platt, H. S. (1973) Absence of prostatic cancer changes in rats exposed to cadmium. Ann. Occup. Hyg. 16, 111–118.
243. Levy, L. S., Clark, C. (1975) Further studies on the effect of cadmium on the prostate gland. I. Absence of prostatic changes in rats given oral cadmium sulphate for two years. Ann. Occup. Hyg. 17, 205–211.
244. Levy, L. S., Clark, D., Roe, F. J. C. (1975) Further studies on the effect of cadmium on the prostate gland. II. Absence of prostatic changes in mice given oral cadmium sulphate for eighteen months. Ann. Occup. Hyg. 17, 213–220.
245. Boyland, E. (1968) The correlation of experimental carcinogenesis and cancer in man. Prog. Exp. Tumor Res. 11, 222–234.
246. Kolonel, L., Winkelstein, W. (1977) Cadmium and prostatic carcinoma. Lancet, 566–567.
247. Wiederanders, R. E., Evans, G. W. (1969) The copper concentration of benign prostatic hyperplasia and cancer. Invest. Urol. 6, 531–533.
248. Hagstrom, R. M., Sprague, H. A., Landau, E. (1967) The Nashville air pollution study. VII. Mortality from cancer in relation to air pollution. Arch. Environ. Health 15, 237–248.
249. Wilkenstein, W., Kantor, W. (1969) Prostatic cancer. Relationship to suspended air pollution. Am. J. Pub. Health 59, 1134–1138.
250. Stocks, P. (1973) Mortality from cancer and cardiovascular disease in England. J. Hyg. (Cambridge), 71, 237–252.
251. Upton, A. C., Kimball, A. W., Furth, J., Christenberry, K. W., Benedict, W. M. (1960) Some delayed effects of atomic bomb radiation in mice. Cancer Res. 20, No. 8, Part 2, 1–59.
252. Hirose, F., Takizawa, S., Watanabe, H., Takeichi, N. (1976) Development of adenocarcinoma of the prostate in ICR mice locally irradiated with X-rays. Gann 67, 407–411.
253. Brown, C. E. Warren S. (1978) Carcinoma of the prostate in irradiated parabiotic rats. Cancer Res. 38, 159–162.
254. Bean, M. A., Yatami, R., Liu. P. I., Fukazawa, K., Ashley, F. W. (1973) Prostatic carcinoma at autopsy in Hiroshima and Nagasaki Japanese. Cancer 32, 498–506.
255. Angevine, D. M., Jablon, S. (1964) Late radiation effects of neoplasia and other diseases in Japan. Ann. N. Y. Acad. Sci. 114, 2, 823–831.
256. Watanabe, S. (1974) Neoplasms among the atomic bomb survivors in Japan. *In:*

Cancer Epidemiology: Environmental Factors. Florence: Proceedings of the Eleventh International Cancer Congress, Amsterdam: Vol. 3, 1974. Exerpta Medica.

257. Dorn, H. F. (1959) Tobacco consumption and mortality from cancer and other diseases. Publ. Health Rep. 74, 581–593.

258. Doll, R., Peto, R. (1976) Mortality in relation to smoking: 20 years' observations on male British doctors. Br. Med. J. 2, 1525–1536.

259. Sundby, P. (1967) Alcoholism and Mortality. National Institute for Alcohol Research, Pub. No. 6, Oslo: Universitetsforlaget.

260. Schmidt, W., De Lint, J. (1972) Causes of death of alcoholics. Quart. J. Stud. Alcohol, 33, 171–185.

261. Pell, S., D'Alonzo, C. A. (1973) A five-year mortality study of alcoholics. J. Occup. Med. 15, 120–125.

262. Monson, R. J., Lyon, J. L. (1975) Proportional mortality among alcoholics. Cancer 36, 1077–1079.

263. Williams, R. R., Horm, J. W. (1977) Association of cancer sites with tobacco and alcohol consumption and socioeconomic status of patients: Interview study from the Third National Cancer Survey. J. Natl. Cancer Inst. 58, 525–547.

264. Breslow, N. E., Enstrom, J. E. (1974) Geographic correlations between cancer mortality rates and alcohol—tobacco. J. Natl. Cancer Inst. 50, 631–639.

265. Badr. F. M., Barthe, A. (1974) Effect of ethyl alcohol on plasma testosterone level in mice. Steroids 23, 921–928.

266. Van Thiel, D. H. Gavaler, J. S., Lester, R., Goodman, M. D. (1975) Alcohol-induced testicular atrophy: An experimental model for hypogonadism occurring in chronic alcoholic men. Gastroenterology 69, 326–332.

267. Adlercreutz, H. (1974) Hepatic metabolism of estrogens in health and disease. N. Engl. J. Med. 290:3, 1081–1083.

268. Ylikahri, R., Huttunen, M., Harkonen, M., Adlercreutz, H. (1974) Hangover and testosterone. Br. Med. J. 2, 445.

269. Ylikahri, R., Huttunen, M., Harkonen, M., Seuderling, U., Onikki, S., Karonen, S. L., Adlercreutz, H. (1974) Low plasma testosterone values in men during hangover J. Steroid Biochem. 5, 655–658.

270. Gordon, G. G., Olivo, J., Rafii, F. Southern, A. L. (1975) Conversion of androgens to estrogens in cirrhosis of the liver. J. Clin. Endriconol. Metab. 40, 1018–1026.

271. Rubin, E., Lieber, C. S., Altman, K., Gordon, G. G., Southren. A. L. (1976) Prolonged ethanol consumption increases testosterone metabolism in the liver. Science 191, 563–564.

272. Liegel J., Fabre, L. F., Howard, P. Y., Farmer, R. W. (1972) Plasma testosterone and sex hormone binding globulin (SBG) in alcoholic subjects. Physiologist 15, 198.

273. Chopra, I. J., Tulchinsky, D., Greenway, D. I. (1973) Estrogen–androgen imbalance in the hepatic cirrhosis. Studies in 13 male patients. Ann. Intern. Med. 79, 198–203.

274. Southren, A. I., Gordon, G. G., Olivo, J., Rafii, F., Rosenthal, W. S. (1973) Androgen metabolism in cirrhosis of the liver. Metabolism 22, 695–702.

275. Zondek, B. (1934) The fate of follicular hormone in the living body. Lancet, 227, 356.

276. Israel, S. L., Merenze, D. R., Johnston, C. G. (1937) The inactivation of estrogen by the liver. Am. J. Med. Sci. 194, 835.

277. Golden, J. B., Sevringhaus, E. L. (1938) Inactivation of estrogenic hormone of the ovary by the liver. Proc. Soc. Exp. Biol. Med. 39, 361–362.

278. Talbot, N. B. (1939) The inactivation of endogenous estrogen by the liver. Endocrinology 25, 601–604.

279. Edmondson, H. A., Glass, S. J., Soll. S. N. (1939) Gynecomastia associated with cirrhosis of the liver. Proc. Soc. Exp. Biol. Med. 42, 97–99.

280. Pincus, G., Martin, D. W. (1940) Liver damage and endogen inactivation. Endocrinology 27, 838–839.
281. Pincus, I. J., Rahoff, A. E., Cohen, E. M., Tumen, H. J. (1951) Hormonal studies in patients with chronic liver disease. Gastroenterology 19, 735–754.
282. Moore, G. F., Wattenberg, C. A., Rose, D. K. (1945) Breast changes due to diethylstilbestrol during treatment of cancer of the prostate gland. J.A.M.A. 127, 60–62.
283. Lloyd, C. W., Williams, R. H. (1948) Endocrine changes associated with Laennac's cirrhosis of the liver. Am. J. Med. 4, 315–330.
284. Schwartz, M. (1946) The effect of stilbestrol on the testis and breast of patients treated for carcinoma of the prostate gland. Rocky Mt. Med. J. 43, 643.
285. Rupp, J., Cantarow, A., Rakoff, A. E., Paschkis, K. E. (1951) Hormone excretion in liver disease and in gynecomastia. J. Clin. Endocrinol. 11, 688–699.
286. Bennett, H. S., Baggenstors, A. H., Butt, H. R. (1950) The testis, breast and prostate of men who die of cirrhosis of the liver. Am. J. Clin. Pathol. 20, 814–828.
287. Dohan, F. C., Richardson, E. M., Bluemle, L. W., Gyorgy, P. (1952) Hormone excretion in liver disease. J. Clin. Invest. 31, 481–498.
288. Coppage, W. S., Cooner, A. E. (1965) Testosterone in human plasma. N. Engl. J. Med. 273, 902–907.
289. Heard, R. D. H., Saffran, J. C. (1949) The Metabolism of the Estrogen, Part Two. *In:* Recent Progress in Hormone Research. New York: Academic Press, Vol. 4, pp. 43–63.
290. Johns, V. J., Hirst, A. E., Jr. (1950) The incidence of carcinoma of the prostate in cirrhosis of the liver. Cal. Med. J. 73, 503–504.
291. Stumpf, H. H., Wilens, S. L. (1953) Inhibiting effects of portal cirrhosis of the liver on prostatic enlargement. Arch. Intern. Med. 91, 304–309.
292. Glantz, G. M. (1964) Cirrhosis and carcinoma of the prostate gland J. Urol. 91, 291–293.
293. Robson, M. C. (1964) The incidence of benign prostatic hyperplasia and prostate cancer in cirrhosis of the liver. J. Urol. 92, 307–310.
294. Robson M. C. (1966) Cirrhosis and prostatic neoplasms. Geriatrics, 21, 150–154.
295. Wu, S. D. (1942) Anatomic changes in prostate of patients with cirrhosis of the liver. Arch. Pathol. 34, 735–741.
296. Mortanti, G., Gianferrai, L., Cressari, A., Arrigoni, G., Lovati, G. (1956) Recherches clinico-statistiques et genetiques sur les néoplasies de la prostate. Acta Genet. Stat. Med. 6, 304–305.
297. Woolf, G. M. (1960) An investigation of the familial aspects of cancer of the prostate. Cancer 13, 739–743.
298. Lynch, H. T., Larsen, A. L., Magnuson, C. W., Krush, A. J. (1966) Prostate carcinoma and multiple primary malignancies. Cancer 19, 1891–1897.
299. Albert, S., Child, M. (1977) Familial cancer in the general population. Cancer 40. 1674–1679.
300. Steele, R., Lees, R. E. M., Kraus, A. S., Rao, C. (1971) Sexual factors in the epidemiology of cancer of the prostate. J. Chron. Dis. 24, 29–37.
301. Steele, R. (1972) Sexual factors in prostatic cancer. Med. Aspects of Human Sexuality 6, No. 2, 70–81.
302. Bourke, J. B., Griffin, J. P. (1962) Blood groups in benign and malignant prostatic hypertrophy. Lancet ii, 1279–1280.
303. Wajsman, Z., Saroff, J., Murphy, G. (1977) Blood group distribution in prostatic cancer patients. J. Surg. Oncol. 9, 289–291.
304. Swyer, G. J. M. (1944) Postnatal growth changes in human prostate. J. Anat. 78, 130.

305. Wilson, J. D. (1976) Introduction: Benign Prostatic Hyperplasia. Bethesda, Maryland: National Institutes of Health.
306. Brendler, H. (1976) Benign prostatic hyperplasia: Natural history. *In:* Grayhack, J., Wilson, J. Scherbenske, M. (eds) Benign Prostatic Hyperplasia. Bethesda, Maryland: National Institutes of Health.
307. Rotkin, I. D. (1976) Epidemiology of benign prostatic hypertrophy: Review and speculations. *In:* Benign Prostatic Hyperplasia. Bethesda, Maryland: National Institute of Health.
308. Morrison, A. S. (1978) Prostatic hypertrophy in greater Boston. J. Chron. Dis. 31, 357–362.
309. Wynder, E. L., Hyams, I., Shigematsu, T. (1967) Correlations of international cancer death rates. Cancer 20, 113–126.
310. Sommers, S. C. (1957) Endocrine changes with prostatic carcinoma. Cancer 10, 345–358.
311. Schoones, R., Palma, L., D., Gaeta, J. F., Moore, R. H. Murphy, G. P. (1972) Prostatic carcinoma treated at categorical center. N.Y. J. Med. 72, 1021–1027.
312. Armenian, H. K., Lilienfeld, A. M., Diamond, E. L., Bross, I. D. J. (1977) Relation between benign prostatic hyperplasia and cancer of the prostate. Lancet ii, 115–117.
313. Greenwald, P., Kirmss, V., Polan, A. K., Dick, V. S. (1974) Cancer of the prostate among men with benign prostate hyperplasia. J. Natl. Cancer Inst. 53, 335–340.
314. Franks, I., M. (1974) Benign prostatic hyperplasia. Lancet ii, 293.
315. Williams, R. D., Blackard, C. E. (1974) Benign prostatic hyperplasia and cancer of the prostate. Lancet ii, 1265.
316. Byar, D.P. (1975) Benign prostatic hyperplasia and cancer of the prostate. Lancet i, 866.
317. Hutchinson, G. B. (1976) Epidemiology of prostatic cancer. Semin. Oncol. 3. 151–159.
318. Ogawa, M. (1964) Constitutional studies on tumors of the prostate. I. On the measurements of constitution. Acta Urol. Jap. 10. 677–685.
319. Ogawa, M. (1967) Constitutional studies on tumors of the prostate. II. On hair patterns and other features. Acta Urol. Jap. 13, 507–515.
320. Greenwald, P., Damon, A., Kirmss, V., Polan, A. K. (1974) Physical and demographic features of men before developing cancer of prostate. J. Natl. Cancer Inst. 53, 341–346.
321. National Office of Vital Statistics (1956) Mortality from selected causes by marital status, United States, 1949–1951. Vital Statistics—Special Reports. Vol. 39, No. 7.
322. Duffield, T.J., Jacobson, P. H. (1945) Cancer mortality and marital status: An analysis of deaths attributed to cancer among the white population of New York City during 1939–1941. J. Natl. Cancer Inst. 6, 103–112.
323. Lancaster, H. O. (1952) The mortality in Australia from cancer peculiar to the male. Med. J. Aust. 2, 41–44.
324. Martin, C. E. (1966) Marital and Coital Factors in Cervical Cancer. Baltimore: Johns Hopkins University, Ph.D. Thesis.
325. Martin, C. E. (1975) Marital and sexual factors in relation to age, disease and longevity. *In:* Life History Research in Psychopathology. Wirt. R. D., Winokur G. Roff, M. (eds). Minneapolis, Minn.: University of Minnesota Press.
326. Gittes, R. F., Chu, T. M. (1976) Detection and diagnosis of prostate cancer. Semin. Oncol. 3, 123–130.
327. Murphy, G., Karr, J. Chu, T. M. (1978) Prostatic acid phosphatase: Where are we? CA, 28, 258–264.
328. Klein, L. A. (1979) Prostatic carcinoma N. Engl. J. Med. 300, 824–833.
329. Jackson, M. A., Aluwalia, B. S., Attah, E. B., Connolly, C.A., Herson, J., Heshmat,

M. Y., Jackson, A. G., Jones, G. W., Kapoor, S. K., Kennedy, J., Kovi. J., Lucas, A. O., Nkposong, E. O., Olisa, E., Williams, A. O. (1975) Characterization of prostatic carcinoma among blacks: A preliminary report. Cancer Chemother. Rep. 59, 3–15.

330. Schuman, L. M., Mandel, J., Blackard, C., Bauer, H., Scarlett, J., McHugh, R. (1977) Epidemiologic study of prostatic cancer: Preliminary report. Cancer Treat. Rep. 61, 181–186.
331. Slavins, H. B., Gavett, E. (1946) Primary herpetic vulvovaginitis. Proc. Exp. Med. Biol. 63, 343–345.
332. Varga, A., Browell, B. (1960) Viral inclusion bodies in vaginal smears. Obstet. Gynecol. 16, 441–444.
333. Yen, S. S., Reagan, J. W., Rosenthal, M. S. (1965) Herpes simplex infection in female genital tract. Obstet. Gynecol. 25, 475–492.
334. Hutfield, D. C. (1966) History of herpes genitalis Br. J. Bener. Dis. 42, 263–268.
335. Naib, Z. M., Nahmias, A. J., Josey, W. E. (1966) Cytology and histopathology of cervical herpes simplex infection. Cancer 19, 1026–1031.
336. Tannenbaum, M. Spiro, D., Lattimer, J. K. (1967) Biology of the prostate gland: the electron microscopy of cytoplasmic filamentous bodies in human benign prostatic cells adjacent to cancerous cells. Cancer Res. 27, 1415–1421.
337. Tannenbaum, M., Lattimer, J. K. (1970) Similar virus–like particles found in cancers of the prostate and breast. J. Urol. 103, 471–475.
338. Morrisseau, P. M., Phillips, C. A., Leadbetter, G. W. (1970) Viral prostatitis. J. Urol. 103, 767–769.
339. Centifanto, Y. M., Drylie, D. M., Deardourff, S. L., Kaufman, E. (1972) Herpesvirus type 2 in the male genitourinary tract. Science 178, 318–320.
340. Centifanto, Y. M. Kaufman, H. E., Zam, F. S., Drylie, D. M, Deardourff, S. L. (1973) Herpesvirus particles in prostatic carcinoma cells, J. Virol. 12, 1608–1611.
341. Centifanto, Y. M., Zam, Z. S., Kaufman, H. E., Drylie, D. M. (1975) In vitro transformation of hamster cells by herpes simplex virus type 2 from human prostatic cancer cells. Cancer Res. 35, 1880–1886.
342. Jeannson, S., Molin, L. (1974) On the occurrence of genital herpes simplex virus infection. Clinical and virological findings and relation to gonorrhea. Acta Dermatol. Venereal. 54, 479–485.
343. Deardourff, S. L., Deture, F. A., Drylie, D. M., Centifanto, Y. M., Kaufman, H. (1974) Association between herpes hominis type 2 and the male genitourinary tract. J. Urol. 112, 126–129.
344. Deture, F. A., Drylie, D. M., Kaufman, H. E., Centifanto, Y. M. (1976) Herpesvirus type 2: Isolation from seminal vesicle and testes. Urology 7, 541–544.
345. Sabin, A. B., Tarro, G. (1973) Herpes simplex and herpes genitalis viruses in etiology of some human cancers. Proc. Natl. Acad. Sci. 70, 3225–3229.
346. Deture, F. A., Drylie, D. M., Kaufman, H. E., Centifanto, Y. M. (1978) Herpesvirus type 2: Study of semen in male subjects with recurrent infections. J. Urol. 120, 449–451.
347. Herbert, J. T., Birkhoff, J. D., Feorino, P. M., Caldwell, G. (1976) Herpes simplex virus type 2 and cancer of the prostate. J. Urol. 116, 611–612.
348. Paulson, D. F., Fraley, E. E., Rabson, A. S., Ketcham, A. S. (1968) SV–40 transformed hamster prostatic tissue. Surgery 64, 241–247.
349. Paulson, D. F., Rabson, A. S. Fraley, E. E. (1968) Viral neoplastic transformation of hamster prostate tissue in vitro. Science 159, 200–201.
350. Fraley, E. E., Paulson, D. F. (1969) Morphological and biochemical studies of virus (SV40) transformed prostatic tissue. J. Urol. 101, 735–740.
351. Abdalla, A. M., Oliver, J. A. (1971) SV40 transformed prostatic carcinoma in the hamster: effect of hormonal manipulation on the growth rate. Cancer 27, 468–470.
352. Paulson, D. F., Bonar, R. A., Sharief, Y., Vergara, J. R., Reich C., Shah, K. V. (1975)

Properties of prostatic cultures transformed by SV40. Cancer Chemother. Rep. 59, 51–55.

353. Shah, K. V., Palma, L. D., Murphy, G. P. (1971) The occurrence of SV40–neutralizing antibodies in sera of patients with genitourinary carcinoma. J. Surg. Oncol. 3, 443–450.

354. Shah, K. V., Weismann, M., Murphy, G. P. (1972) Occurrence of simian virus 40-reacting antibodies in sera of some patients with prostatic cancer. J. Surg. Oncol. 4, 90–93.

355. Shah, K. V., Daniel, R. W., Stone, K. R., Elliott, A. Y. (1978) Investigation of human urogenital tract tumors for papova virus etiology: Brief communication. J. Natl. Cancer Inst. 60, 579–591.

356. Lang, D. J., Kummer, J. F. (1972) Demonstration of cytomegalovirus in semen. Persistence and demonstration in extracellular fluids. N. Engl. J. Med. 287, 756–758.

357. Lang D. J., Kummer, J. F., Hartley, D. P. (1975) Cytomegalovirus in semen. N. Engl. J. Med. 291, 121–124.

358. Albrecht, T., Rapp, F. (1973) Malignant transformation of hamster embryo fibroblasts following exposure to ultraviolet irradiated human cytomegalovirus. Virology 55, 53–61.

359. Sanford, E. J., Geder, L., Laychock, A., Rohner, T. J., Rapp, F. (1977) Evidence for the association of cytomegalovirus with carcinoma of the prostate. J. Urol. 118, 789–792.

360. Geder, L., Sanford, E. J., Rohner, T. J., Rapp F. (1977) Cytomegalovirus and cancer of the prostate: In vitro transformation of human cells. Cancer Treat. Rep. 61, 139–146.

361. Ablin, R. J. (1972) Immunologic studies of normal, benign and malignant human prostatic tissue. Cancer 29, 1570–1574.

362. Webber, M. M., Stonington, O. G., Lehman, J. (1973) Virus in prostatic epithelium of man. Urology. 1, 561–567.

363. Dmochowski, L., Maruyama, K., Ohtsuki, Y., Seman, G., Bowen, J. M., Newton, W. A., Johnson, D. E. (1975) Virologic and immunologic studies of human prostatic carcinoma. Cancer Chemother. Rep. 59, 17–31.

364. Ablin, R. J. (1976) Serum antibody in patients with prostatic cancer. Br. J. Urol. 48, 355–361.

365. Dmochowski, L., Ohtsuki, Y., Seman, G., Maruyama, K., Knesek, J. E., East, J. L., Bowen, J. M., Yoshida, H., Johnson, D. E. (1977) Search for oncogenic viruses in human prostatic cancer. Cancer Treat. Rep. 61, 119–127.

366. McCombs, R. M. (1977) Role of oncornaviruses in carcinoma of the prostate. Cancer Treat. Rep. 61, 131–132.

367. Mickey, D. D., Stone, K. R., Stone, M. P., Paulson D. F. (1977) Morphologic and immunologic studies of human prostatic carcinoma. Cancer Treat. Rep. 61, 133–138.

368. Ohtsuki, Y., Seman, G., Dmochoski, L., Bowen, J. M., Johnson, D. E. (1977) Virus–like particles in a case of human prostate carcinoma. J. Natl. Cancer Inst. 58, 1493–1496.

369. Sanford, E. J., Rohner, T. J., Rapp, F. (1975) Virology of prostatic cancer. Cancer Chemother. Rep. 59, 33–38.

370. Zeigel, R. F., Arya, S. K., Horoszewicz, J. S., Carter, W. A. (1977) A status report. Human prostatic carcinoma with emphasis on potential for viral etiology. Oncology, 34, 29–44.

371. Ravich, A. (1942) Relationships of circumcision to cancer of the prostate. J. Urol. 48, 298–299.

372. Ravich, A., Ravich, R. A. (1951) Prophylaxis of cancer of the prostate, penis and cervix by circumcision. N. Y. State J. Med. 51, 1519–1520.

373. Gibson, E. C. (1954) Carcinoma of the prostate in Jews and circumcised Gentiles. Br. J. Urol. 26, 227–229.

374. Kaplan, G. W., O'Connor, V. J., Jr. (1966) The incidence of carcinoma of the prostate in Jews and Gentiles. J.A.M.A. 196, 803–804.

375. Apt., A. (1965) Circumcision and prostatic cancer. Acta Med. Scand. 178, 493–504.

376. Ravich, A. (1971) Viral carcinogenesis in venereally susceptible organs. Cancer 27, 1493–1496.

377. Diamond, E. L., Lilienfeld, A. M. (1962) Effects of errors in classification and diagnosis in various types of epidemiological studies. Am. J. Pub. Health, 52, 1137–1144.

378. Feminella, J. G., Lattimer, J. K. (1973) An apparent increase in genital carcinomas among wives of men with prostatic cancer. Pirquet Bull. Clin. Med. 20, 3–10.

379. Greenwald, P. Kirmss, V., Burnett, W. S. (1979) Prostate cancer epidemiology: Widowhood and cancer in spouses. J. Natl. Cancer Inst. 62, 1131–1136.

380. Armstrong, B., Doll, R. (1975) Environmental factors and cancer incidence and mortality in different countries, with special reference to dietary practices. Int. J. Cancer, 15, 617–631.

381. Wynder, E. L. (1975) Overview: Nutrition and cancer. Prev. Med. 4, 322–327.

382. Wynder, E. L. (1976) Nutrition and cancer. Fed. Proc. 35, 1309–1315.

383. Weisburger, J. H., Cohen, L. A., Wynder, E. L. (1977) On the etiology and metabolic epidemiology of the main human cancers. *In*: Origins of Human Cancer, Hiatt, H. H., Watson, J. D., Winsten, J. A. (ed). Cold Harbor Spring Laboratory.

384. Lipsett, M. B. (1979) Interaction of drugs, hormones, and nutrition in the causes of cancer. Cancer 43, 1967–1981.

385. Weisburger, J. H. (1979) Mechanism of action of diet as a carcinogen. Cancer 43, 1987–1995.

386. Wynder, E. L. (1975) Introductory remarks. Cancer Res. 35, 3238–3239.

387. Wynder, E. L., Bross, I. J., Hirayama, T. (1960) A study of the epidemiology of cancer of the breast. Cancer 13, 559–601.

388. Caroll, K. K. (1975) Experimental evidence of dietary factors and hormone dependent cancers. Cancer Res. 35, 3374–3383.

389. Caroll, K. K., Khor, H. T. (1975) Dietary fat in relation to tumorigenesis. Prog. Biochem. Pharmacol. 10, 308–353.

390. Alcantara, E. N., Speckmann, E. W. (1976) Diet, nutrition and cancer. Am. J. Clin. Nutr. 29, 1035–1047.

391. Hill, P., Chan, P., Cohen, L. A., Wynder, E., Kuno, K. (1977) Diet and endocrine related cancer. Cancer 39, 1820–1826.

392. Price, D. (1963) Comparative aspects of development and structure in the prostate. *In*: Vollmer, E., Kauffmann, G. (eds.). Biology of the Prostate and Related Tissue. National Cancer Institute Monograph 12.

393. Brandes, D., Bourne, G. H. (1963) Histochemistry of some aspects of prostate pathology. *In*: Vollmer, E., Kauffmann, G. (eds.). Biology of the Prostate and Related Tissue. National Cancer Institute Monograph 12.

394. Clayson, D. B. (9162) Chemical Carcinogenesis. London: Churchill Livingston.

395. Arffmann, E. (1960) Heated fats and allied compounds as carcinogens. A critical review of experimental results. J. Natl. Cancer Inst. 25, 893–926.

396. O'Gara, R. W., Stewart, L., Brown, J., Hueper, W. C. (1969) Carcinogenicity of heated fats and fat fractions. J. Natl. Cancer Inst. 42, 275–287.

397. Watson, A. F., Mellanby, E. (1930) Tar cancer in mice, II. The condition of the skin when modified by external treatment or diet, as a factor in influencing the cancerous reaction. Br. J. Exp. Pathol. 11, 311–322.

398. Bauman, C. A., Rusch, H. P. (1939) Effect of diet on tumors induced by ultraviolet light. Am. J. Cancer 35, 213–221.
399. Lavik, P. S., Baumann, C. A. (1941) Dietary fat and tumor formation. Cancer Res. 1, 181–187.
400. Tannenbaum, A. (1942) The genesis and growth of tumors. III. Effects of a high fat diet. Cancer Res. 2, 468–475.
401. Silverstone, H., Tannenbaum, A. (1950) The effect of the proportion of dietary fat on the rate of formation of mammary carcinoma in mice. Cancer Res. 10, 448–453.
402. Silverstone, H., Tannenbaum, A. (1951) The influence of dietary fat and riboflavin on the formation of spontaneous hepatomas in the mouse. Cancer Res. 11. 200–203.
403. Szepsenwol, J. (1964) Carcinogenic effect of ether extract of whole egg, alcohol extract of egg yolk and powdered egg free of the ether extractable part in mice. Proc. Soc. Exp. Biol. Med. 116, 1136–1139.
404. Cutts, H. J., Nobel, R. L. (1964) Estrone induced mammary tumors in the rat. Cancer Res. 24, 1116–1123.
405. Furth, J. (1972) Prolactin and carcinogenesis. *In*: Prolactin and Carcinogenesis. Boyns, A. R., Griffiths, K. (eds.). Proceedings of the Fourth Tenovus Workshop. Alpha Omega Alpha Pub. Co., Cardiff, Wales.
406. Meites, J. (1972) Relation of prolactin and estrogen to mammary tumorigenesis in the rat. J. Natl. Cancer Inst. 48, 1217–1224.
407. Muhlbock, O. (1973) Role of hormones in the etiology of breast cancer. J. Natl. Cancer Inst. 48, 1213–1216.
408. Sinha, D., Cooper, D., Dao, T. L. (1973) The nature of estrogen and prolactin effect on mammary tumorigenesis. Cancer Res. 33, 411–414.
409. Chan, P. C., Cohen, L. A. (1974) Effect of dietary fat antiestrogen and antiprolactin on the development of mammary tumors in rats. J. Natl. Cancer Inst. 52, 25–30.
410. Chan, P. C., Cohen, L. A. (1975) Dietary fat and growth promotion of rat mammary tunors. Cancer Res. 35, 3384–3386.
411. Chan, P. C., Didato, F., Cohen, L. A. (1975) High dietary fat, elevation of fat, serum prolactin and mammary cancer. Proc. Soc. Exp. Biol. Med. 149, 133–135.
412. Howell, M. A. (1974) Factor analysis of international cancer mortality data and per capita food consumption. Br. J. Cancer 29, 328–336.
413. Howell, M. A. (1975) Diet as an etiological factor in the development of cancers of the colon and rectum. J. Chron. Dis. 28, 67–80.
414. Lea, A. J. (1967) Neoplasms and environmental factors. Ann. Roy. Coll. Surg. 41, 432–438.
415. Takashashi, E. (1964) Coffee consumption and mortality for prostate cancer. Tohoku J. Exp. Med. 82, 218–223.
416. Oiso, T. (1975) Incidence of stomach cancer and its relation to dietary habits and nutrition in Japan between 1900 and 1975. Cancer Res. 35, 3254–3258.
417. Hirayama, T. (1977) Changing patterns of cancer in Japan with special reference to the decrease in stomach cancer mortality. *In*: Hiatt, H. H., Watson, J. D., Winsten, J. A. (eds.). Origins of Human Cancer. Book A. Cold Spring Harbor Laboratory.
418. Hirayama, T. (1974) Prospective studies on cancer epidemiology based on census population in Japan. *In*: Cancer Epidemiology: Environmental Factors. Proceedings of the Eleventh International Cancer Congress, Florence, Vol. 3. Amsterdam: Excerpta Medica.
419. Hankin, J. H., Nomura, A., Rhoads, G. G. (1975) Dietary patterns among men of Japanese ancestry in Hawaii. Cancer Res. 35, 3259–3264.
420. Shanmugaratnam, K., Wee, A. (1973) "Dialect group" variations in cancer incidence among Chinese in Singapore. *In*: Host Environment Interactions in the Etiology of Cancer in Man. International Agency for Research on Cancer. Lyon, France.

421. Martinez, I., Torres, R., Frias, Z. (1975) Cancer incidence in the United States and Puerto Rico. Cancer Res. 35, 3265–3271.
422. Fernandez, N. A. (1975) Nutrition in Puerto Rico. Cancer Res. 35, 3272–3291.
423. Lea, A. J. (1966) Dietary factors associated with death rates from certain neoplasms in man. Lancet ii, 332–333.
424. Wynder, E. L., Shigematsu, T. (1967) Environmental factors of cancer of the colon and rectum. Cancer 20, 1520–1561.
425. Wynder, E. L., Kajitani, T., Ishikawa, S., Dodo, H., Takano, A. (1969) Environmental factors of cancer of the colon and rectum. II. Japanese epidemiological data. Cancer 23, 1210–1220.
426. Drasar, B. S., Irving, D. (1973) Environmental factors and cancer of the colon and breast. Br. J. Cancer 27, 167–172.
427. Haenszel, W., Berg, J. W., Segi, M., Kurihara, M., Locke, F. B. (1973) Large bowel cancer in Hawaiian Japanese. J. Natl. Cancer Inst. 51, 1765–1779.
428. Wynder, E. L., Hirayama, T. (1977) Comparative epidemiology of cancer of the United States and Japan. Prev. Med. 6, 567–594.
429. Bjelke, E. (1973) Epidemiologic Studies of Cancer of the Stomach, Colon and Rectum: With Special Emphasis on the Role of Diet. Vols. 1–5. Minneapolis: University of Minnesota, Ph.D. thesis.
430. Berg, J. W. (1975) Can nutrition explain the pattern of international epidemiology of hormone-dependent cancers? Cancer Res. 35, 3345–3350.
431. Thiessen, E. U. (1974) Concerning a familial association between breast cancer and both prostatic and uterine malignancies. Cancer 34, 1102–1107.
432. Halberg, F., Cornelissen, G., Sothern, R. B., Wallach, L. A., Halberg, E., Ahlgren, A., Kuzel, M., Radke, A., Barbosa, J., Goetz, F., Buckley, J., Mandel, J. S., Schuman, L. M., et al. (1979) International geographic studies of oncological interest on chronobiological variables. *In*: Kaiser, H. (ed.). Comparative Pathology of Growth in Animals, Plants, and Man. Baltimore: Williams and Wilkins.
433. Lilienfeld, D., Garagliano, C. F., Lilienfeld, A. M. (1976) Gastric cancer. J. Natl. Cancer Inst. 57, 9.
434. Morgan, R. W., Jain, M., Miller, A. B., Choi, N. W., Matthews, V., Munan, L. M., Burch, J. O., Feather, J., Howe, G. R., Kelley, A. (1978) A comparison of dietary methods in epidemiologic studies. Am. J. Epidemiol. 107, 488–498.
435. Graham, S., Mettlin, C. (1979) Diet and colon cancer. Am. J. Epidemiol. 109, 1–20.
436. Wynder, E. L. (1979) Dietary habits and cancer epidemiology. Cancer 43, 1955–1961.

EPIDEMIOLOGY OF PANCREATIC CANCER

LEON GORDIS, M.D., Dr. P.H.

CONTENTS

INTRODUCTION

Pancreatic cancer is the fourth leading cause of death from cancer in the United States (1) and is exceeded only by cancer of the lung, colon and rectum, and breast. About 20,000 people in this country die each year from pancreatic cancer (2). In considering only carcinomas of the digestive tract, carcinoma of the pancreas is second only to carcinoma of the colon and rectum in frequency. In males, it is exceeded by lung, colon and rectum, and prostate. Age-adjusted mortality rates have increased from 2.9 per 100,000 in 1920 to 9 per 100,000 in 1970. In terms of incidence, pancreatic cancer now ranks tenth among cancers in the United States. Thus, both by its rank and by its pattern of increasing mortality and incidence, it represents a major community health problem in the United States today.

Its importance is further emphasized by its extremely bleak prognosis. Median survival time, regardless of therapy is 2–3 months after diagnosis. The 1-year relative survival rate is about 8% and the 5-year rate is about 2% (3). When first seen, 90% of patients have regional lymph node metastases and 80% have liver metastases (4). There is no evidence thus far that the prognosis is significantly better in patients whose disease is diagnosed earlier. Consequently, it seems clear that the main hope for improving the picture regarding pancreatic cancer will be through the development of effective measures for prevention.

Prevention of pancreatic cancer will require identification of specific etiologic factors and of those associated with a high risk. If exposure to specific factors can be ascertained, and such exposure can be reduced or eliminated, there will be real hope for prevention. This requires intensive epidemiologic study as a crucial first step in elucidating the etiology of this disease.

METHODOLOGIC ISSUES

Gudjonson et al. (5) reviewed the reliability of diagnosis of pancreatic cancer in 100 patients. At the first operation, a positive biopsy was obtained in only 72.6% of patients who later proved to have pancreatic cancer. Furthermore, a tissue diagnosis was often not made because of the surgeons' reluctance to biopsy the pancreas or because of inadequate biopsy techniques. Of the 41 patients proved at autopsy to have pancreatic cancer, 16 (39%) had been surgically explored once or twice without a positive biopsy.

The fact that fewer and fewer diagnosed cases are histologically confirmed is an increasingly important problem in the epidemiologic study of pancreatic cancer. This is a result of the fact that more diagnoses are being made without surgery or biopsy and that autopsies are often not obtained. In addition, even when a surgical operation is carried out, a biopsy is often not obtained because of the clinical complications that may ensue following this procedure.

From the Department of Epidemiology, Johns Hopkins School of Hygiene and Public Health, Baltimore, Maryland 21205.

Preparation of this chapter was supported in part by Grant No. 5 R26 CA21642 from the National Institutes of Health.

A number of diagnostic tests are utilized for establishing the presence or absence of pancreatic cancer and these include radionuclide scanning, ultrasonography, computerized axial tomography, retrograde cholangiopancreatography (ERCP), and arteriography. Laboratory assays of carcinoembryonic antigen, alpha-fetoprotein, pancreatic oncofetal antigen, and serum ribonuclease have been explored as possible biological markers for detecting pancreatic cancer (6–9), but none is sufficient for making the diagnosis in and of itself.

TUMOR HISTOLOGY AND LOCATION

Most malignant tumors of the pancreas are adenocarcinomas (90%) of which most arise from ductal epithelium and the remainder from acinar tissue. Islet cell tumors occur infrequently, and cystadenomas and cystadenocarcinomas are extremely rare. Most islet cell tumors are functional, and about 10% of these are malignant. Nonfunctioning islet tumors are very rare. The present review will focus primarily on tumors of the exocrine pancreas.

The most frequent location of pancreatic carcinomas varies in different reports of series of patients. The head (including the periampullary region) is the most frequent site in clinical series (10), but in autopsy material the body and tail predominate (11).

In a survey (from 1943 to 1964) of the records of 289 patients with malignant tumors of the pancreas at Charity Hospital and at the Veterans Administration Hospital in New Orleans, Richard and Cohn (12) found that 66% were located in the head of the pancreas, 17% in the body, 10% in the tail, and 7% were diffuse. Abdominal pain was most frequently the initial symptom and jaundice the second most common followed by weight loss. These investigators found no difference between males and females or between blacks and whites in the initial clinical characteristics of the disease.

In an autopsy study, ductal hyperplasia was found in 41% of 141 patients with pancreatic carcinoma (13). The findings suggested that there may be a sequential relationship between ductal hyperplasia and pancreatic cancer. A study by Cubilla and Fitzgerald (14) of 227 patients with pancreatic cancer found that ductal papillary hyperplasia was three times more prevalent in the pancreatic cancer cases than in a group of 100 autopsies of patients with non-pancreatic cancer. The finding that a marked degree of atypia was observed in 20% of the cancer patients and carcinoma in situ in 18%, suggests by analogy with other cancers that these may be precursor lesions and consequently that there may be a potential for diagnosing the disease at some early preinvasive state. Animal data support such a possibility in that, when pancreatic cancer had been induced in hamsters by carcinogens, a specific secretory abnormality developed before any ductal obstruction developed (15).

Islet cell carcinomas accounted for 2% of cases in the End Results Group Report (3). Patients with islet cell carcinomas differed from those with other types of pancreatic cancer in that the median age was younger at the time of diagnosis, with two-thirds being under 60 years. In contrast, two-thirds of other types of pancreatic cancer occurred in patients over age 60. Islet cell carcinomas also accounted for 11% of the pancreatic cancers seen in patients between 20 and 40 years of age.

DEMOGRAPHIC AND GEOGRAPHICAL PATTERNS

International Differences

The age-adjusted mortality rates from pancreatic cancer are low in Italy and Japan in both males and females, and in general the ratio of the highest rate to the lowest rate is approximately 2 (16). (Figure 1) Although the incidence rates of pancreatic carcinoma are greatest in western and industrialized countries, noteworthy exceptions are the high rates among the Maioris in New Zealand and in female native Hawaiians and black Americans (17) (Figure 2).

Migrant Studies

Migrant studies, especially those focusing on migrants from Japan to the United States and their descendants, have been extremely valuable in assessing the relative contributions of genetic and environmental factors to the etiology of a variety of cancers. However, the picture for cancer of the pancreas is not clear. As seen in Table 1, (19) mortality rates of pancreatic cancer are about twice as high in the United States as in Japan. When data for migrants from Japan to the United States are examined (Table 2) (20), Issei (migrants from Japan) have higher risks than either Nisei (U.S.-born children of migrants from Japan) or U.S. whites. Although there is no progressive sequence from country of origin to country of adoption, the rates among the Issei (and among the Nisei where the data are available) suggest some increase over the mortality rates for native Japanese living in Japan (21). At least part of the problem might be due to misclassification of some cases of pancreatic

FIGURE 1. Mortality rates from pancreatic cancer in selected countries 1972 (rates per 100,000).

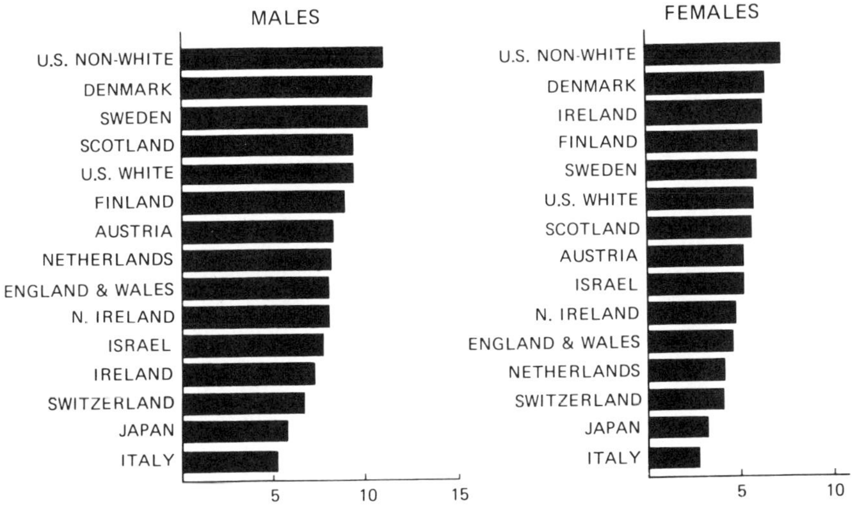

* U.S. WHITE AND NON-WHITE RATES ARE FOR 1973-74

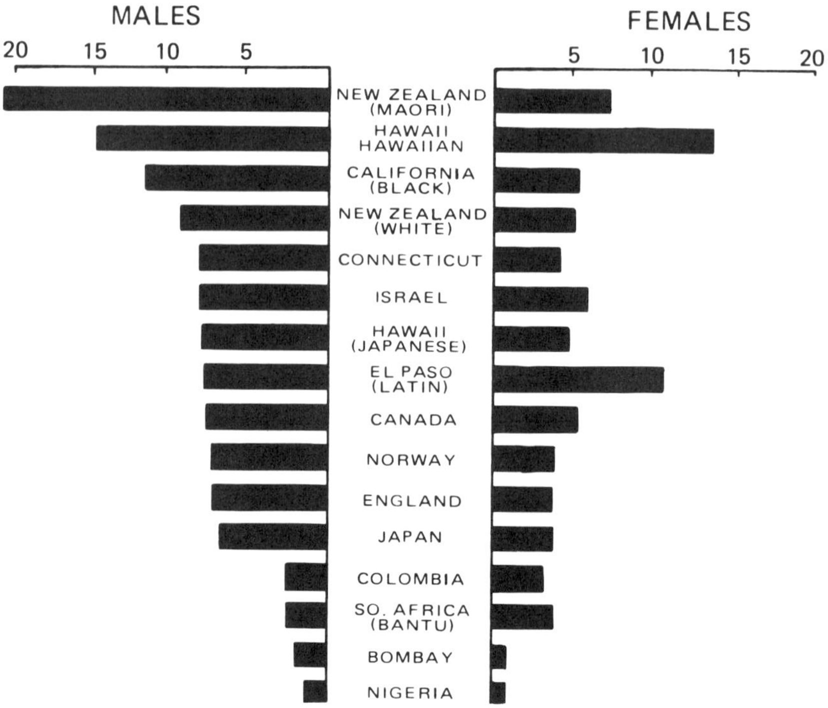

FIGURE 2. International variation in incidence rates for pancreas cancer (per 100,000 per annum age-standardized to world population).

Source: Fraumeni (18).

cancer in Japan as stomach cancer. This possibility has, in fact, been suggested by a study of the causes of death reported on death certificates in Hiroshima and Nagasaki (22).

In a study of cancer mortality in Japanese residents in Hawaii and in the continental United States, both groups of Japanese were found to have an excess of deaths from cancers of the pancreas and of the lung and from lyphosarcoma as compared to U.S. whites and nonwhites, although the difference was not statistically significant (23).

In a study focusing on migration within the United States, Mancuso and Sterling (24) assessed cancer mortality in Ohio residents from 1959 to 1967 comparing those born in Ohio with those who had been born elsewhere. The age-adjusted rates for cancer of the pancreas among southern-born nonwhite males were high, even though on a regional basis the lowest rate for nonwhites was in the South. The age-specific rates of those born in the South were consistently higher than for those born in Ohio and markedly so above age 45. Similarly, the pancreatic cancer mortality rate for southern-born nonwhite females was 2.5 times the rate for Ohio-born non-whites. The authors proposed that some exogenous factor may be affecting southern-born nonwhite males and females in regard to pancreatic cancer.

TABLE 1. Crude Death Rate from Pancreatic Cancer per 100,000 in the United States and Japan, by Sex

	U.S. whites, 1970	Japanese, 1972
Males	10.4	5.5
Females	7.7	3.8
Ratio (M:F)	1.4	1.4

Source: Wynder, E. L., Hirayama, T., Comparative epidemiology of cancers of the United States and Japan, Prev. Med. 6, 567–594, 1977. Copyright 1980, Appleton-Century-Crofts, a Publishing Division of Prentice-Hall, Inc.

TABLE 2. Standardized Mortality Ratios for Pancreatic Cancer for Issei (1959–1962), Nisei (1958–1962), U.S. Whites (1959–1961), and Japanese (1960–1961)

	Japanese	Issei	Nisei (>65 years)	U.S. whites
Males	100	475	167	274
Females	100	349	104	270

Source: Haenzel, W., Kurihara, M., Studies of Japanese migrants. Mortality from cancer and other diseases among Japanese in the United States, J. Nat. Cancer Inst. 40, 43–68, 1968.

Time Trends

Rates of pancreatic cancer in the United States have been increasing at least since 1950, although there appears to have been a leveling off of this trend in recent years. The time trends in mortality from pancreatic cancer in the United States from 1950 to 1967 are presented in Figure 3 (25). The highest rates are seen in nonwhite males in whom rates of pancreatic cancer doubled from 1950 to 1967, with the next highest rates in white males followed by nonwhite females and white females. Examination of time trends in mortality rates from pancreatic cancer reported by the New York State Cancer Registry shows a minimal if any change in mortality from 1961 to 1973 (Table 3) (26).

In examining mortality trends over time, the possibility must be considered that an apparent trend could result from artifacts. For example, changes in the quality of diagnosis and specifically a reduction in the number of underdiagnosed deaths may produce an *apparent* increase in carcinoma of the pancreas, even if the true rate has not changed. This is, in fact, suggested by the observation that the increase in mortality from pancreatic cancer in recent years has been more pronounced in blacks than in whites. Although this may reflect a selective exposure of blacks to a carcinogenic agent or agents, it could also result from better diagnosis of the disease associated with improved quality and availability of medical care to the black population.

Another possibility that must be considered in interpreting the increase in pancreatic cancer mortality over time is that it could be an artifact resulting from the periodic revisions of the International Classification of Diseases. However, classification revisions do not appear to be major factors in this increase. For example, Klebba (27) compared mortality statistics based on the

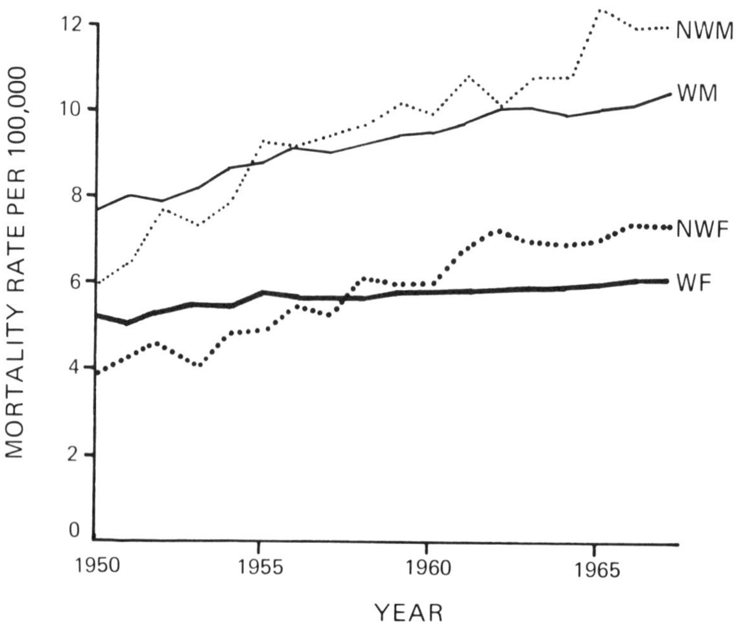

FIGURE 3. Age-adjusted mortality rates for pancreatic cancer, by race, sex, and calendar time.

seventh and eighth revisions of the International Classification of Diseases. In this study, a random sample of all deaths in 1966, stratified by cause, were coded by both the seventh and eighth revisions. Of 16,360 deaths in 1966 coded as cancer of the pancreas by the seventh revision, 112 (0.7%) went to other causes when coded by the eighth revision. The difference was due to changes in coding procedures between the seventh and eighth revisions rather than to changes in the ICD classification of pancreatic cancer. However, the difference is minimal and cannot be a significant factor in accounting for the increases observed in deaths from pancreatic cancer in the United States in recent years.

The increase in mortality from pancreatic cancer is observed in all age

TABLE 3. Time Trends in Age-Adjusted Pancreatic Cancer Mortality Rates (per 100,000 population), New York State (Exclusive of New York City), 1967–1973[a]

	1961	1964	1967	1969	1973
Males	11.51	10.73	11.06	12.66	11.77
Females	6.59	7.02	6.94	6.70	7.47

Source: Greenwald P. et al., Cancer Incidence and Mortality in New York State (Exclusive of New York City), Bureau of Cancer Control, New York State Department of Health, 1976.

[a]Adjusted to 1970 population.

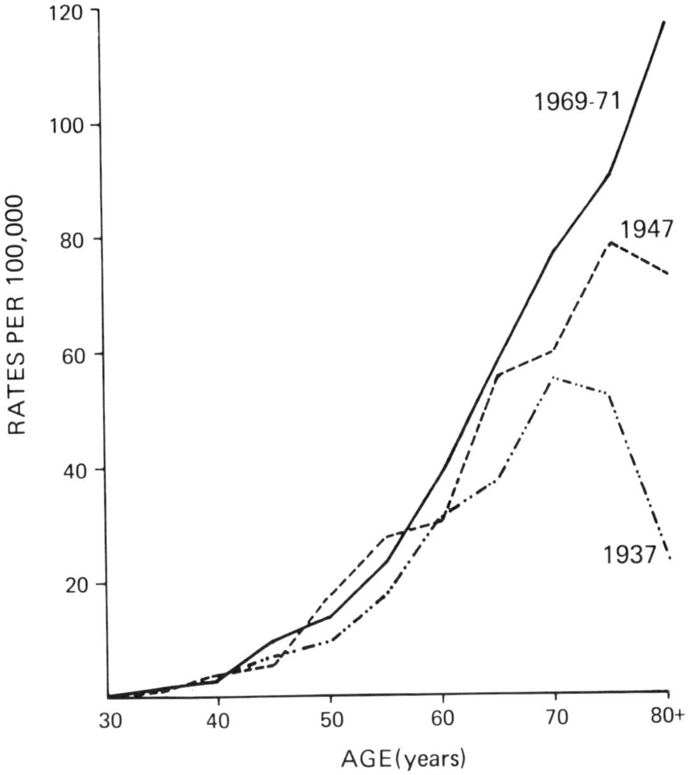

FIGURE 4. Time trends in age-specific incidence rates of pancreatic cancer, United States, 1937–1969.

Source: Dorn and Cutler (1959).

groups over 44 and in both sexes among whites. Another observation is that the age-adjusted death rate from pancreatic cancer first exceeded that of stomach cancer in 1968 (28, 29). Although part of the apparent increase in pancreatic cancer might be attributable to misclassification of pancreatic cancer as stomach cancer in earlier years, various analyses of the data indicate that the rise in pancreatic cancer is nevertheless real (30).

As seen in Figure 4 (31, 32), the incidence of pancreatic cancer appears to have increased in older ages in white males from the First (1937) to the Second National Cancer Survey (1947) in the United States, with an increase in the Third National Cancer Survey (1969–1971) for those over the age of 70. At young ages there is no consistent trend, probably because of the small number of cases at these ages. The increase in incidence from 1937 to 1969 is observed in each race and sex group in the United States (Table 4) (33), with rates in black males and black females now exceeding those in white males and white females, respectively. Tables 5, 6, and 7 show time trends in incidence rates based on data from cancer registries in New York State, Connecticut, and Alameda County, California (26, 34).

TABLE 4. Incidence Rates, by Race and Sex, for Cancer of the Pancreas

Race and Sex	1937	1947	1969
White male	7.0	9.3	11.3
White female	4.9	5.5	6.7
Black male	5.0	11.6	15.0
Black female	3.4	6.4	14.5

Source: Pledger, R. A., et al., Introduction: National Cancer Institute Pancreatic Carcinogenesis Program, Cancer Res. 35, 2226–2227, 1975.

TABLE 5. Time Trends in Age-Adjusted Pancreatic Cancer Incidence Rates, New York State (exclusive of New York City), 1967–1972[a]

	1961	1964	1967	1969	1972
Males	11.36	10.15	11.11	12.49	10.55
Females	6.13	6.66	6.41	6.69	6.62

Source: Greenwald, P., et al., Cancer incidence and mortality in New York State (exclusive of New York City), Bureau of Cancer Control, New York State Department of Health, 1976.

[a]Adjusted to 1970 population; rates per 100,000 population.

TABLE 6. Time Trends in Age-Adjusted Pancreatic Cancer Incidence Rates, Connecticut, 1961–1969[a]

	1961	1964	1967	1969
Males	9.6	8.9	10.1	10.2
Females	5.9	5.5	6.8	6.4

Source: Arellano, M.G., et al., Cancer patterns in Alameda County, California, Br. J. Cancer 26, 473–482, 1972.

[a]Rates per 100,000 population.

TABLE 7. Time Trends in Age-Adjusted Pancreatic Cancer Incidence Rates, Alameda County, California, 1960–1969[a]

	1960–162	1963–1965	1966–1967	1968–1969
Males	9.1	10.6	10.6	11.9
Females	6.0	6.4	6.6	7.4

Source: Arellano, M. G., et al., Cancer pattern in Alameda County, California, Br. J. Cancer 26, 473–482, 1972.

[a]Rates per 100,000 population.

Race

In the United States, mortality rates from pancreatic cancer in blacks have been reported to be higher than in whites and all other ethnic groups except Japanese (Table 8) (18). Mortality rates in U.S. blacks are also higher than those in African blacks. Both U.S. whites and blacks show higher age standardized incidence rates of pancreatic cancer than do Africans (35). Rates for

TABLE 8. Average Annual Age-Adjusted Mortality Rates for Pancreas Cancer in the United States by Sex and Race, 1950 to 1969

	Males	Females
White	9.63	5.83
Black	10.40	6.23
Amerind	6.66	6.03
Chinese	8.87	3.59
Japanese	10.64	5.68

Source; Fraumeni, J. F., Cancers of the pancreas and biliary tract; epidemiological considerations, Cancer Res. 35, 3437–3446, 1975.

[a]Rates per 100,000 population.

TABLE 9. Age-Adjusged Pancreatic Cancer Incidence Rates By Race and Sex Alameda County, California, 1960–1969[a]

	White	Black	Chinese	Japanese
Males	10.0	13.9	9.8	14.8
Females	6.3	8.5	0.0	4.2

Source: Arellano et al., Cancer patterns in Alameda County, California, Br. J. Cancer 276, 473–482, 1972.

[a]Rates per 100,000 population.

U.S. nonwhites have exceeded those for whites in both males and females since the 1950s. Data from the Alameda County, California, Cancer Registry show incidence rates in black males to be exceeded only by those in Japanese males. In females, the highest incidence rates were seen in blacks (Table 9) (34).

The increase in pancreatic cancer seen in the United States population over the last several decades appears to have been greater in blacks than in whites. This may be a true increase in incidence or could primarily reflect improved availability and quality of medical care for blacks (35).

Mortality rates of pancreatic cancer increase with age in both white males and females, but in blacks they appear to decline after age 70 (Figure 5) (18). The incidence rates of pancreatic cancer also increase with advancing age, but in blacks they decline in older males and females (Figure 6) (31). Parkash (37), however, found that the increase with age occurred in both sexes with the male preponderance persisting in each age group. The higher rates at younger ages in nonwhites and the lower rates in nonwhites at older ages, may be a true racial difference or an artifact resulting from inaccuracies in the ascertainment of either pancreatic cancer cases of deaths or in the estimates of the black population which serve as denominators for the incidence and mortality rates.

Age

Approximately 80% of cases of pancreatic cancer occur between ages 60 and 80, and cases below age 40 are extremely rare, although they have been seen in children as young as 3 months of age (38). A case of adenocarcinoma of the

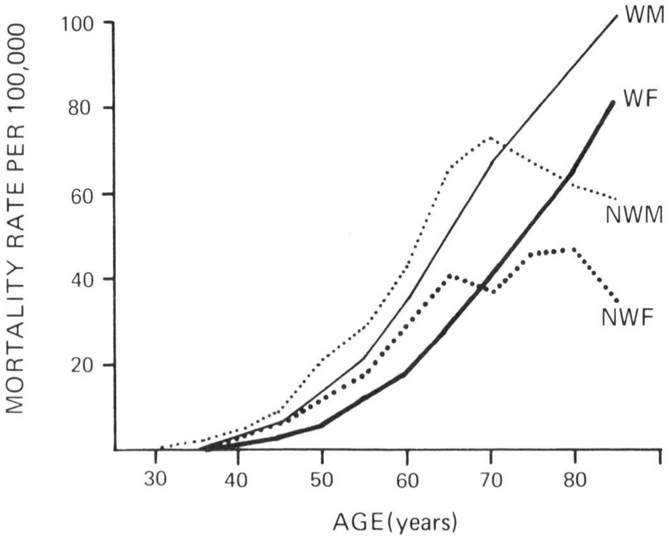

FIGURE 5. Age-specific mortality rates per 100,000 pancreatic cancer, by race and sex, United States, 1950–1969.
Source: Fraumeni (18).

head of the pancreas was reported by Tsukimoto (39) in a 4-year-old Japanese girl and one of adenocarcinoma at the head of the pancreas was reported in a 13-year-old girl by Taxy (40) who also reviewed the English language literature of case reports of pancreatic cancer in children. From 1918 to 1962, less than 2% of the 600 patients with pancreatic cancer seen at the Charity Hospital in New Orleans were under 40 years of age (41).

The epidemiology of pancreatic cancer as reported in the Connecticut Tumor Registry was reviewed by Moldow and Connelly (42). From 1957 to 1963, 865 cases of pancreatic cancer were identified; they comprised 10% of all digestive system tumors and had an average age of 64.4 years, at time of diagnosis. There were more men than women and the women were significantly older at time of diagnosis. They also identified a season variation with peaks in May and August for onset of symptoms.

Sex

Pancreatic cancer occurs more frequently in males in both whites and nonwhites. The male : female ratios of incidence rates from various cancer registries are 1.5 for California whites, 2.2 for California blacks, and 1.2 in Connecticut. The sex ratio exceeds one at every age in both whites and nonwhites, and the sex ratio of age-adjusted rates is similar in whites and nonwhites (1.68 and 1.67). Whether the male excess in this disease is due to some host characteristic of males or to a selective environmental exposure, perhaps occupational, is an important issue for further investigation.

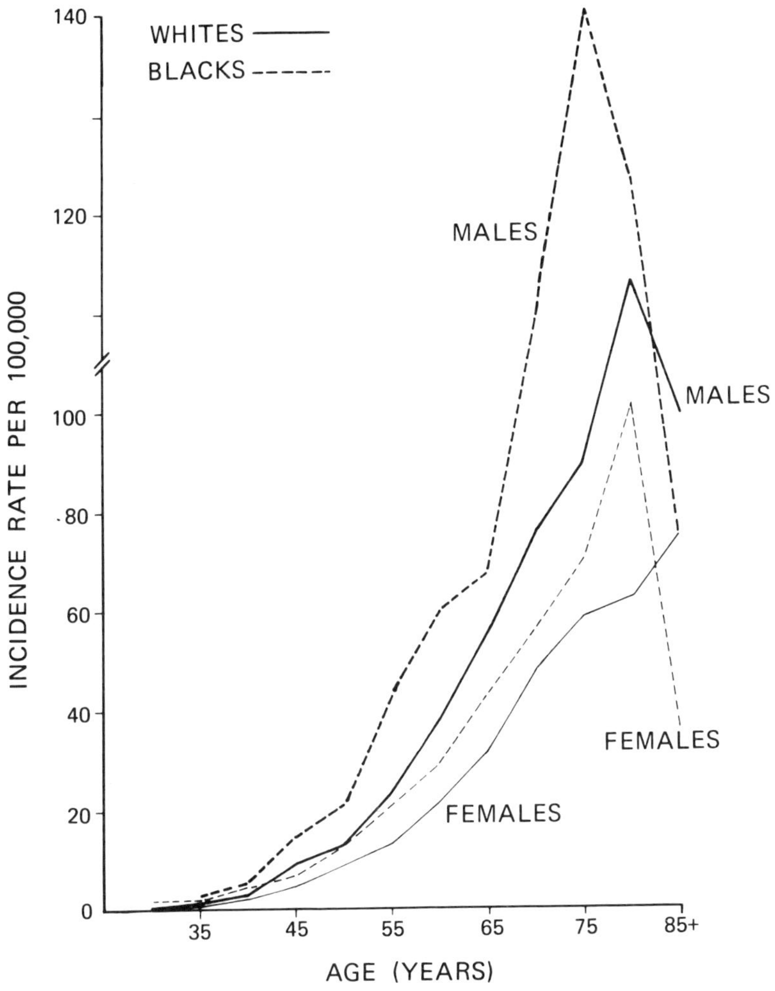

FIGURE 6. Average annual age-specific incidence rates (per 100,000) for pancreas cancer by sex and race.

Grieve (10) studied all cases of pancreatic cancer admitted to Western General Hospital in Edinburgh from 1956–1970, and observed that the ratio of the number of male cases to female cases was 1.1. However, when the ratios were examined for different tumor locations, they were found to be 1.5 for carcinoma of the head of the pancreas and 0.6 for carcinoma of the body and tail. This interesting observation requires confirmation by use of the ratio of sex-specific incidence rates by region and could provide a valuable clue to etiologic differences.

Lilienfeld et al. (43) examined cancer rates by state in the United States and focused on the sex ratio (male to female). On the basis of their analysis, they grouped cancer sites into three categories: those in which the states showed a positive relationship between male and female rates, those which showed rates varying widely in males but only slightly in females and those showing no particular pattern. Cancer of the pancreas was shown to be in the second category. It is of interest that those cancers in which environmental agents such as cigarette smoking have been etiologically implicated also generally tended to fall into this category.

Urban-Rural Differences

Mortality rates from pancreatic cancer are generally higher in urban than in nonurban areas among whites, and the difference is even more pronounced among nonwhites. Whether this is due to environmental factors associated with urbanization or to better availability of medical care remains to be determined. In Sweden, Cederlof (44) found that mortality from pancreatic cancer was higher in urban than in rural residents and not related to alcohol use or to income. Urban residents had a relative risk of 2.5 compared to rural residents.

The geographic distribution of mortality from pancreatic cancer in the United States shows no consistent pattern. A detailed analysis of the geographic distribution of pancreatic cancer within the United States identified only one cluster in an area including parts of Louisiana and Mississippi (45). A correlation of mortality patterns for both pancreatic and lung cancers in males is consistent with an implication of tobacco consumption in the etiology of both cancers. In females, mortality from pancreatic cancer was found to be correlated geographically with that of diabetes.

Religion

Using mortality data from New York City, MacMahon (46) and Newill (47) found that pancreatic cancer was from 25 to 50% more frequent among Jews than among Catholics or Protestants. Similar findings were reported by Seidman (48) for women. The incidence of pancreatic cancer is also higher among Jews than among non-Jews in Israel (17). However, these findings indicating higher risks in Jews were not confirmed in a study utilizing the Connecticut Cancer Registry (42).

Lyon et al. (49) recently analyzed cancer incidence for Mormons and non-Mormons in Utah utilizing the Utah State Cancer Registry, which contains information on more than 40,000 cancer patients. Although Mormons had a lower incidence of a number of smoking-related cancers, as well as of cancer of the breast, cervix, and ovary in females and cancer of the stomach in males and of the colon in both sexes, pancreatic cancer rates were also low both in Mormons and in non-Mormons, compared with the 1969–1971 incidence rates reported by the U.S. Third National Cancer Survey (31).

In a separate study, Enstrom (50) used church records to study cancer and total mortality among California Mormons from 1968 to 1975, Utah Mormons from 1970 to 1975, and a National Center for Health Statistics sample of nonsmoking white males. Standardized mortality ratios (SMRs) were calculated using 1970 U.S. white male rates. The SMRs for pancreatic cancer were 47% for California Mormon males over 35 years of age, 72% for Utah Mormon males over 35 years of age, and 54% for the sample of U.S. white males, aged 35 to 84 who had never smoked cigarettes. When the SMR was calculated for combined smoking-related cancer sites (buccal cavity, pharynx, esophagus, lung, and bladder), it was 26% in California and 20% in Utah. In this study, comparisons of cancer mortality between Mormons and non-Mormons living in the same state were not reported.

Rates of pancreatic cancer have also been reported to be lower than expected in Seventh Day Adventists. The SMR for males was 50% and for females 76% in Adventists 35 years of age or over (51). Because Seventh Day Adventists abstain from smoking and drinking and many avoid meat and coffee, these factors have been regarded as etiologic clues with regard to cancer of the pancreas. Rates of cancer of the colon and cancer of the stomach are also lower than expected among the Adventists.

Socioeconomic Status

Although increased pancreatic cancer risks have been reported among low socioeconomic populations (52), other studies have not consistently demonstrated any relationship of pancreatic cancer with socioeconomic status (43, 53, 54). In a study of occupational mortality in England and Wales by the Registrar General, (55) no relationship with social class gradient was observed even when the cancers were separated by location into head of the pancreas, other specified parts of the pancreas, and unspecified location.

POSSIBLE ETIOLOGIC FACTORS

Familial and Genetic Factors

Familial occurrence of pancreatic cancer is rare. However, Friedman and Fialkow (56) reported four brothers who developed pancreatic cancer between the ages of 66 and 77 years. All four were cigarette smokers, and none was alcoholic or had a history of pancreatitis. Another family cluster was reported by MacDermott and Kramer (57). Three brothers and a sister developed adenocarcinoma of the pancreas between ages 69 and 72. Again there was no evidence of pancreatitis in this family. These reports suggest that there may be a hereditary predisposition to pancreatic cancer in later life but there is no evidence to date to suggest such a predisposition for pancreatic cancer occurring at earlier ages.

Pancreatic cancer has been reported in association with Gardner's syndrome, which is inherited as an autosomal dominant (58). The syndrome as outlined by Gardner (59) consists of polyposis, osteomatosis, epidermal and sebaceous cysts, and fibromatosis. Carcinoma of the pancreas has also been reported in association with hereditary pancreatitis, also inherited as an autosomal dominant condition. Lynch et al. (60) reported five melanoma-prone families in which an excess of several types of cancer was found. Pancreatic cancer occurred in two. An occult adenocarcinoma of the pancreas has been reported in association with Lindau's disease—defined as an association of cerebellar hemangioblastomas with one or more of the following: retinal angiomata; spinal cord hemangioblastoma; syringomyelia; pancreatic cysts; pulmonary cysts; and hepatic, renal, adrenal, and epididymal abnormalities (61). Adenocarcinoma of the pancreas has also been reported in association with neurofibromatosis (62).

The autosomal dominant disorder, multiple endocrine neoplasia, type 1 (MEN 1) of Wermer, consists of adenomas or adenocarcinomas of the pituitary, parathyroid, pancreas, and adrenal cortex. The pancreatic tumors are of the islet cell variety and may be functional insulinomas, glucagonomas or gastrinomas. Rashad (63) reported a family in Hawaii in which there appeared to be an unusual aggregation of several cancer cases due to the von Hippel–Lindau syndrome, one of which was pancreatic carcinoma.

Newell et al. (64) studied diagnostically confirmed cases of cancer of the pancreas (and other malignancies) obtained from the Charity Hosptial of Louisiana Tumor Registry and compared their ABO blood group distribution to a sample of 5000 individuals who voluntarily donated blood to the same hospital. Their findings supported previous reports that blood group A was associated with cancer of the pancreas among black males and white females. However, blood donor groups often are not representative of the general population, and biases may therefore result in using them for deriving expected percentages. The conclusions of the study must therefore be viewed with caution.

The relationship of Rh type to pancreatic cancer was explored by Vogel (65). The relative risk for pancreatic cancer [D(+): D(−)] was 0.72. The relative risk for pancreatic cancer for blood group A compared to group O subjects was 1.23.

Studies of blood groups are subject to a number of methodological problems so that associations may be spuriously found or, conversely, a lack of association may be artifactually observed. Such findings may result from biases in selection of control groups and from the fact that, in general, positive findings tend to be published while negative findings may remain unpublished. In addition, there is often a failure to subdivide the disease category by histologic type and other characteristics, so that in actuality different conditions may be inappropriately grouped together in a given study.

Terasaki et al. (66) studied the frequencies of HLA antigens in 2005 cancer patients and 1536 healthy controls who were HLA typed from 1973 to 1975 and in a group of 4017 cancer patients and 3896 healthy controls who had been typed from 1970 to 1975. There was no evidence to suggest any association of a specific HLA type with pancreatic cancer.

An interesting area of study has been the risk of cancer in persons with immunodeficiency syndromes. One such disease is ataxia-telangiectasia, an autosomal recessive condition in which there are defects of the lymphoid system, central nervous system, skin, and blood vessels. One preliminary study has suggested that pancreatic carcinoma is 15 times more frequent in persons presumed to be heterozygotes for ataxia-telangiectasia than in control relatives. However, immunologic data were not available, and the association between immunodeficiency and cancer in family members is not conclusive (67).

Rashad (68) has reported a study in which the Hawaii Household Registration File and death record file were linked. Included in the information extracted were the dermatoglyphic traits of the subject. Each cancer death was matched with another individual for sex, age, and race and both dermatoglyphic characteristics, and ABO blood groups in cases and controls were investigated. Rashad (63) reported an excess of true-whorls in patients with cancer of the pancreas although the actual data were not presented.

Diabetes

An apparent association of diabetes and pancreatic cancer has been reported by many investigators (69–72). Populations which are at high risk for pancreatic cancer are generally at high risk for diabetes. Both diabetes and pancreatic cancer have a declining sex ratio with increasing age, a phenomenon that is not observed in other digestive tract cancers or other tobacco-related malignancies.

Kessler (73) studied cancer mortality among 21,447 diabetic patients registered at the Joslin Clinic in Boston during a 26-year period ending in 1956. No control population was used. Instead, standardized mortality ratios were calculated using the general Massachusetts population. Male diabetics were found to have lower than expected mortality from cancer of all types combined and female diabetics showed no statistically significant difference from the exptected rate. Among the 15 specific types of cancer examined in this study, a statistically significant excess of deaths in diabetics was observed only for pancreatic cancer, in both males and females. However, on further analysis, when deaths were excluded in patients for whom it could not be established that the diabetes had, in fact, preceeded the pancreatic cancer, the standardized mortality ratio in males fell from 1.47 to 1.27 and was no longer statistically significant, whereas in females the ratio fell from 2.13 to 1.82 but remained statistically significant. Although these findings suggest an association between diabetes and pancreatic cancer, a question must be raised whether the general Massachusetts population was indeed an appropriate comparison group for the patient population seen at the Joslin Clinic.

Karmody and Kyle (74) studied patients admitted to the Aberdeen Royal Infirmary from 1955 through 1967. They found 265 proved carcinomas of the pancreas during this period, of whom 51 also had diabetes. When they examined the interval between diagnosis of diabetes and carcinoma, it was found to be less than 3 months in 25 of the 51 patients. In only six patients was the interval over 2 years.

Wynder et al. (75) found a significant association with prior diabetes in females with pancreatic cancer but not in males. The relationship in females persisted even after the cases with recent onset diabetes were eliminated from the analysis.

Tobacco

There appears to be an increased risk of cancer of the pancreas in cigarette smokers. Histologic evidence shows that hyperplastic changes in pancreatic duct cells with atypical changes in their nuclei have been observed among smokers coming to autopsy and the extent of such changes appears to increase with the amount smoked (18). In addition, data from animal studies suggest that nitrosamines present in tobacco smoke are carcinogenic for the pancreas (76).

Six prospective studies of cigarette smokers specifically investigated mortality of pancreatic cancer. As shown by Table 10 (77), the ratios for pancreatic cancer deaths in current cigarette-only smokers compared to nonsmokers ranged from 1.6 in British physicians to a high of 3.1 in Swedish male subjects. In three of the six studies, the ratio was less than 2. The relative risk of pancreatic cancer in smokers compared with nonsmokers in the American Cancer Society Survey is estimated at 2.69 in males aged 45–64 and 2.17 in males aged 65–79 (78). Best (79) followed up 78,000 Canadian veterans and found an increased relative risk of pancreatic cancer with cigarette smoking. There was a dose-response relationship, with the relative risk for less than 10 cigarettes a day being 1.4 and for over 20 cigarettes per day being 2.37. Other studies showing increased risk of pancreatic cancer in cigarette smokers are those of Dorn reported by Kahn (80), Hirayama (81), and Weir and Dunn (82).

The Dorn study also suggested a dose-response relationship with the mortality ratio for smokers of 10–20 cigarettes a day compared to nonsmokers being 1.79 and for those smoking 21–39 cigarettes a day 2.15. Ex-smokers (excluding those who stopped because of doctors' orders) had a mortality ratio of 1.32.

Wynder et al. (75) carried out a case-control study of pancreatic cancer. The cases comprised 100 males and 42 females who had adenocarcinoma of the pancreas and who were interviewed at seven hospitals in New York, Houston,

TABLE 10. Mortality Ratios from Pancreatic Cancer in Current Cigarette-Only Smokers in Six Prospective Studies[a]

Reference	Study population	Mortality ratio
Doll and Peto (1976)	British male physicians	1.6
Hammond (1966)	U.S. males (age 45–64)	2.69
	U.S. males (age 65–79)	2.17
Kahn (1866)	U.S. veterans	1.84
Hirayama (1972)	Japanese males and females	1.83
Best (1966)	Canadian veterans	2.1
Cederlof et al. (1975)	Swedish males	3.1
	Swedish females	2.5

[a]Morbidity and Mortality Weekly Report, 1979.

and Los Angeles. All the patients had histologically proved cancer of the pancreas. Data on these patients were compared with those on controls "which were selected from patients interviewed for other epidemiologic studies conducted by our group during the same period and for which the same questionnaire was used." No further description of the pool from which the controls were chosen was given in their paper. Two controls were selected for each male pancreatic adenocarcinoma patient and three controls for each female patient matched for age, sex, race, and hospital. To be eligible as a control, the patient had to have no tobacco-related cancers (lung, larynx, mouth, esophagus, bladder, or kidney) or tobacco-related disease (chronic bronchitis, emphysema, or coronary heart disease). This exclusion of people with known or putative tobacco-related conditions from the control group may have increased the likelihood that an association with tobacco would be found for the cases.

Compared to the controls, the percentage of cigarette smokers was significantly greater in the male cancer patients, but in the female patients the difference was only of borderline statistical significance. Data were not presented regarding the length of time the patients had been smoking or how recently they might have taken up the smoking habit. The interviewers were apparently not masked as to the diagnostic classification of the subjects, and the question of whether there were any refusals to cooperate among the cases identified was not addressed in the paper.

Autopsy studies of smokers show hyperplastic changes in the pancreatic duct. Hammond (78) suggested that the male preponderance in pancreatic cancer may be entirely due to cigarette smoking because no sex difference for pancreatic cancer was observed among nonsmokers. On the other hand, in contrast to other malignancies that have been related to tobacco use, the sex ratio for pancreatic cancer declines with advancing age. Levin and Connelly (36) have therefore suggested that either smoking plays a small role in the etiology of pancreatic cancer or the population of males susceptible to pancreatic cancer may be dying of other smoking-related diseases first.

Stocks (83) compared age-adjusted death rates in 1964–1965 from cancers of different sites with the annual consumption of cigarettes, tea, and coffee in 20 countries. Coffee consumption appeared to correlate positively with cancer of the pancreas as well as with prostatic cancer and leukemia in males. No such relationship for pancreatic cancer was found in females nor was this malignancy related to cigarette consumption in this analysis.

The rise in pancreatic cancer deaths has been much less than the rise in deaths from lung cancer during the same period. If cigarette smoking plays as strong an etiologic role in the development of pancreatic cancer as it does in lung cancer, one might have expected to see a greater increase during this period. However, the lung probably has a more intense exposure to cigarette smoke than the pancreas, as the pancreas is exposed to the by-products of cigarette smoke which reach it through the circulation and through the secretion of bile. Thus, in a given smoker the pancreas may be exposed to a much lower concentration of any carcinogenic agent present in tobacco. Furthermore, lung and pancreatic tissue may differ in their relative susceptibilities to carcinogenesis by specific components of tobacco smoke.

Wynder et al. (75) have suggested as one hypothesis that cigarette smoking may lead to the development of pancreatic cancer through metabolites of tobacco being excreted from the liver into the bile and refluxed into the pancreatic duct. Two other possibilities they suggest are that components of tobacco smoke may increase blood lipids and that tobacco smoking may contain certain nitrosamines that may be metabolically activated in the pancreas.

Alcohol Intake

Alcoholism appears to predispose to cancers of the mouth, pharynx, esophagus, larynx, liver, and possibly pancreas (84–86). However, the evidence relating alcoholism to pancreatic cancer is fairly weak and inconsistent, and the data currently available suggest that any increased risk from alcoholism is fairly small.

Burch and Ansari (85) studied 83 patients with pancreatic cancer in the Veterans Administration Hospitals in New Orleans and found that 65% had histories of moderate to heavy alcohol intake as compared to 14% in a hospital control group dying from other causes. Details of selection of the control group were not presented.

Hakulinen et al. (84) investigated the relationship between alcohol consumption and cancer morbidity in two male Finnish populations. The files on a group of chronic skid-row alcoholics which numbered about 4,370 annually in 1967–1970 were checked against the Finnish Cancer Registry for the same period. Excess morbidity was observed from cancer of the pharynx, esophagus and lung. An excess of pancreatic cancer was also observed (4 observed versus 2.21 expected), but because of the small numbers the finding was not statistically significant. Monson and Lyon (87) tested the same hypothesis by studying the mortality experience of 1,382 chronic alcoholics. The patients studied were chronic alcoholics admitted to mental institutions in Massachusetts in 1930, 1935, or 1940. These individuals were traced until death or January 1, 1971. They compared observed and expected proportional mortality percentages of different causes of death in 894 whites who were known to have died. Three deaths from carcinoma of the pancreas were observed compared to 5.2 expected, but the results were difficult to interpret because of the large number of individuals lost to follow-up.

One of the problems in studying the relationship of alcoholism to pancreatic cancer is the difficulty in discriminating between the possible effects of alcohol and of tobacco, because of the positive correlation between tobacco use and alcohol consumption. The few studies that have tried to control for the effect of tobacco have contradictory findings in relation to alcohol. Wynder et al. (75) attempted to standardize for tobacco usage in a case-control study from Memorial Hospital, New York City, and found no association between alcohol consumption and pancreatic cancer.

Pancreatitis

The relationship of chronic pancreatitis to pancreatic cancer is of considerable interest. A family with a hereditary form of pancreatitis was described by Comfort and Steinberg (88) in 1952, and other kindreds have since been reported (89–93). It appears to be a non-sex-linked dominant trait perhaps with incomplete penetrance. In these families, there is an increased risk of pancreatic carcinoma with about 30% of deceased patients in these families who had definite or suspected hereditary pancreatitis having developed pancreatic cancer (94). However, in these families, development of carcinoma of the pancreas is not limited to the patients with pancreatitis.

The picture is less clear, however, with nonhereditary pancreatitis. Although there is a correlation of acute and chronic pancreatitis with alcoholism, the question of the relationship of either alcoholism or chronic pancreatitis (of a nonfamilial form) to pancreatic cancer remains unresolved.

Chronic pancreatitis is most frequently associated with alcoholism or biliary tract disease and sometimes with both. The mechanism by which excess alcohol intake leads to pancreatitis is not understood. There is no evidence for a direct effect of alcohol on the pancreas or on pancreatic function, although it does stimulate gastrin release and the gastric secretion thus indirectly stimulates pancreatic secretion. In the presence of duodenitis perhaps with some edema, there might be increased pancreatic secretion against partially obstructed outflow. However, whether this is the mechanism by which alcohol produces pancreatitis, is not understood.

Pancreatitis is also known to occur as a complication of hyperparathyroidism; about 10–15% of patients with hyperparathyroidism have pancreatitis (95). Pancreatitis is also associated with hypercalcemia of multiple myeloma and has been reported in a patient without parathyroid glands who was poisoned by excessive does of Vitamin D (96). Pancreatitis may also be associated with hyperlipemia (97) and in some cases the lipid disorder is primary familial, particularly type I hyperlipidemia. In other cases the lipid abnormality appears to be secondary to the pancreatitis.

Are patients with pancreatitis at increased risk for carcinoma of the pancreas and, if so, is it because pancreatitis predisposes them to pancreatic cancer or do both conditions share common etiologies? A number of problems are involved in exploring this relationship. In patients with long-standing chronic pancreatitis, the diagnosis of pancreatic cancer may be difficult because of the similarity of symptoms. In addition, although carcinoembryonic antigen has been reported to be elevated in patients with pancreatic cancer, it has also been reported to be elevated in over half the patients with chronic pancreatitis (98). Many patients who die from pancreatic cancer have evidence of pancreatitis, but this may be a result of obstructive changes resulting from the cancer itself.

In a report of 100 cases of carcinoma of the pancreas, Mikal and Campbell (99) found pancreatitis in 49. However, the association of inflammatory changes with carcinoma are well known. The delayed occurrence of pancreatic cancer in patients with chronic pancreatitis has been reported relatively frequently. In many of the reported cases, the time interval between the pancreatitis and the diagnosis of pancreatic carcinoma is not stated. Bartholomew et al. (100) considered the occurrence of carcinoma in cases of chronic pancreatitis to be coincidental.

In one study of 255 patients with pancreatic carcinoma, 26 had associated pancreatitis (101), and in another 100 patients with chronic relapsing pancreatitis, 6 were found to have carcinoma of the pancreas (102). In another report, 7.8% of 385 cases of cancer of the pancreas were preceded by chronic pancreatitis; in addition, 7.5% had histories of peptic ulcer, 6.5% of chronic hepatitis, 5.2% of cholelithiasis, 10.1% chronic cholecystitis and 11.9% chronic gastritis (103). Morphologic changes in the pancreatic tissue outside the tumor area suggested that chronic pancreatitis often precedes cancer of the pancreas. Paulino-Netto et al. (102) reported an increased risk of pancreatic cancer in patients with pancreatic calcification and suggested that chronic irritation might therefore be etiologically involved.

Ishii and co-workers (104) compared 150 patients with chronic calcifying pancreatitis with 1,070 patients with carcinoma of the pancreas. The male-to-female ratio was 3.5 in the pancreatitis patients compared to 1.9 in the pancreatic carcinoma patients. Cigarette smoking and alcohol intake were significantly higher in both groups of patients than among a group of controls, but the daily intake of alcohol was greater in the pancreatitis than in the pancreatic carcinoma patients.

Thus, data suggest that a relationship may exist between pancreatitis and pancreatic carcinoma, but the overall picture is unclear. Although pancreatitis is often found at autopsy in patients with pancreatic cancer, some investigators believe that if pancreatitis does predispose to cancer, the association is probably quite weak (75). However, many methodologic difficulties are involved, among which are the need to consider the possible contributions of multiple variables to the etiology and the problem of selecting appropriate comparison groups.

Chemical Exposures

Animal Studies. Over 40 years ago, the observation was made that spontaneous tumors of the pancreas are rare in all species of animals and birds in comparison with their incidence in man (105). This raises the question of whether this is a true species difference or whether human beings are selectively exposed to pancreatic carcinogens. However, Rowlatt (106) pointed out that while there are considerable species differences in mammals in the frequency of spontaneous adenocarcinoma of the pancreas, it has been described quite often in a number of unrelated mammalian species and affects a wide range of animal species.

A number of chemical agents have been shown to produce pancreatic cancer in laboratory animals. *N*-methyl-*n*-nitrosourea administered intragastrically produced pancreatic cancer in inbred NIH guinea pigs (107). Diisopropanol-nitrosamine in a variety of dosages administered subcutaneously to 8-week-old random-bred Syrian golden hamsters, uniformly produced pancreatic adenomas (108). Ductal-type pancreatic adenocarcinomas were found in over 80% of animals at all doses, and a small percentage developed acinar-type pancreatic adenocarcinomas (109). Aflatoxin B_1 has been shown by electron microscopy to be toxic for the pancreas, but did not appear to produce pancreatic cancer (110). Azaserine has been shown to produce hyperplastic nodules and adenomas of the exocrine pancreas but not malignant tumors (111). Pancreatic tumors have been produced in laboratory animals by a number of other agents including acetaminofluorene (112), p-dimethylamino-azobenzene (113), methylcholanthrene (114), and ionizing radiation (115), although the last produced only islet cell tumors. Following administration of 2,2′-dihydroxy-di-N-propylnitrosamine (DHPN), 100% of Syrian golden hamsters developed pancreatic cancer (116) and N-nitroso-bis (2-hydroxypropyl) amine produced neoplasms originating from the ductal epithelium in the same species (117).

In a serial sacrifice experiment, Levitt et al. (118) treated outbred male Syrian golden hamsters weekly for life with subcutaneous injections of N-nitroso-bis (2-hydroxypropyl) amine (DIPN). Nonspecific changes were followed by progressive proliferation of inter- and intralobular ductal cells with subsequent development of multicentric foci of cystic and papillary cystic adenomas, intraductal carcinomas, and invasive ductal neoplasms. These observations were interpreted as being consistent with a multistage process in the development of pancreatic adenocarcinoma of ductal origin.

Druckrey et al. (119) demonstrated that guinea pigs could develop pancreatic adenocarcinoma when given methylnitrosourethane in the drinking water. The incidence rate was low and latent period was long, but the potential value of this animal model is immense, and its implications for the possibility of chemical pancreatic carcinogenesis in man is extremely important.

From 1964 to 1972 pancreatic islet cell tumors were reported in 27 dogs and 2 cats by 11 colleges of veterinary medicine in the United States and Canada. Some of the features were remarkably similar to those of cases reported in humans (120). Pancreatic cancer has also been reported in cattle and horses as well as in dogs and cats. Two dogs had pancreatic carcinoma associated with thyroid adenoma, a combination that has also been reported in man (121).

Human Studies. Evidence suggests that chemical agents may also induce cancers of the pancreas in man. Cancer of the pancreas has been reported to occur excessively among workers exposed to coal gas (122). Redmond et al. (123) found a significant excess in the cancer of the colon and pancreas among workers in a coke plant, but the excess was confined to nonoven workers. Other occupational exposures which have been linked to pancreatic cancer include working in metal industries and aluminum milling, in particular that phase of the operation involving use of coal tar pitch derivatives (124, 125). An increase in cancer deaths in workers in wood-related occupations has been reported with pile-drivers who have an excess frequency of colonic, gastric, and pancreatic cancer (126). In a study of 639 males employed in 1938 or 1939 in a company manufacturing beta-naphthylamine and benzidine and followed to 1965, the mortality rate due to cancer of the pancreas for white men ages 25 to 64 was over five times the expected rate (127).

Of particular interest is a study of the cancer experience of chemists. In a study carried out by Li et al. (128) of the causes of death among 3,637 members of the American Chemical Society who died between 1948 and 1967, a significantly higher proportion of deaths from cancer was found among male chemists in the two age categories, 20–64 years and over 64 years, as compared with professional men in general ($P < 0.001$) and the elderly white male population in the United States ($P < 0.05$). Nearly half the excess cancer deaths were malignant lymphomas and carcinomas of the pancreas. In this study, mortality rates were not calculated because the population at risk could not be accurately determined over the period of study. Instead, the relative frequencies of specific causes of death were derived and compared with "expected" numbers based on the case-specific proportion of the mortality of 9,957 professional men who died between 20 and 64 years of age in 1950. Among chemists aged 20–64 years of age, 36 deaths from cancer of the pancreas were observed, compared to the 22 expected ($P < 0.01$). Among male chemists over 64 years of age, 20 deaths were observed, compared to an expected number of 13, a difference that did not attain statistical significance. The authors themselves point out a number of potential biases in this study. First, 22% of the death certificates were not found. It is also possible that they may have had a preferential reporting of cancer deaths to the Society. Furthermore, the relative frequency method used in this paper is more likely to lead to erroneous inferences than would population-based data. Nevertheless, the data are certainly strongly suggestive of occupationally induced pancreatic cancer among chemists. No data were available, however, regarding the specific chemical exposures involved.

Capurro (129) followed a population of people who lived near or worked in chemical plants where mixtures of solvent vapors were often in the atmosphere. He reported two cases of pancreatic cancer among 120 people whom he was able to follow over a 15-year period. However, specific details were not presented regarding these two cases.

Monson and Fine (130) studied cancer mortality and morbidity among rubber workers at an Akron, Ohio, plant. In two departments, elevators and tire curing, the ratios of observed to expected numbers of deaths were 3.0 and 2.5, respectively. However, the authors question the importance of this finding, as it was based on relatively small numbers and the two departments did not share any common chemical exposure.

Diet

A role for diet in the etiology of pancreatic cancer, possibly in conjunction with other agents has been suggested by Hirayama (131), who reported a prospective study of cigarette smoking in Japan, showing a relative risk of 1.41 for pancreatic cancer in daily cigarette smokers. He estimated the attributable risk at 23%. When the risk was analyzed in relation to meat consumption, a relative risk of 2.54 was found for those consuming meat daily and the attributable risk was estimated at 11%. When both factors, cigarette smoking and meat consumption, were combined, the relative risk was highest. Wynder has also suggested (132, 133) that overnutrition may be related to a number of cancers including that of the pancreas. There is suggestive evidence that a high fat diet may be associated with pancreatic cancer, as seen in Figure 7, which correlates pancreatic cancer mortality by country, based on the mortality data of Segi et al. (134), to total fat intake in selected countries (135).

Such ecologic data have limitations for demonstrating a causal relationship

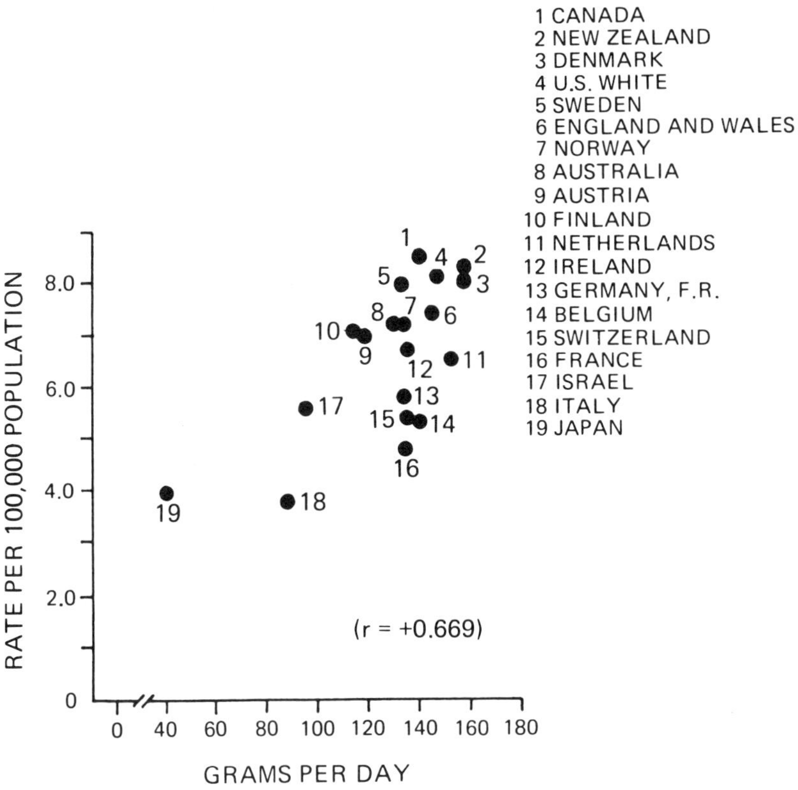

FIGURE 7. Correlation of mortality rates from pancreatic cancer and total fat intake.
Source: Segi et al. (1969); FAO (1969).

between diet and pancreatic cancer. It would be preferable to obtain dietary histories both in patients with pancreatic cancer and in appropriate controls. However, extremely difficult problems are associated with obtaining a valid history of dietary intake, particularly in relationship to the etiology of cancers which may have long latent periods. A significant quantitative error can be expected even in regard to recent food intake. When the focus is on illnesses that may have a latent period of 20–30 years, the problem is further exacerbated, so that history of dietary intake as part of a case-control study will be grossly unreliable (136). In addition, with an insidious disease, a patient's dietary habits may have changed as a result of his illness even before he became aware of the diagnosis. Thus, the temporal relationship between reported dietary characteristics and the development of the disease itself may be unclear. Consequently there is an urgent need to develop more valid measures of both recent and more remote dietary intake. It may well be that biochemical markers will have to be developed to validate dietary recall.

OTHER FACTORS

Soloway and Sommers (121) have reported an endocrinopathy in which pancreatic carcinoma was associated with thyroid adenoma, in an autopsy series. A similar association has been reported in animals (137). A case of ductal adenocarcinoma of the pancreas has been reported in association with Zolinger-Ellison syndrome (138), although this syndrome is classically associated only with islet-cell tumors. One autopsy study of patients with pancreatic cancer revealed a high frequency of endometrial hyperplasia as well as neoplasms of the breast, uterus and ovary. This was interpreted as reflecting excessive pituitary activity. On the basis of their case-control study, Wynder et al. (75) suggested a relationship of pancreatic cancer to cholecystectomy in women, a finding that requires confirmation.

Other Illnesses

In a case-control investigation of pancreatic carcinoma in six major Oklahoma City hospitals, which studied 201 histologically proved cases, the sex ratio declined with age in a pattern similar to diabetes (139). Family history of diabetes, cancer of the digestive tract, pancreatitis, duodenal or gastric ulcer, and chronic constipation were associated with an increased risk of pancreatic cancer. There was also a positive association with a history of appendectomy.

A study of the relationship of asthma to a variety of cancers was carried out by Robinette and Fraumeni (140); 9,550 U.S. Army veterans diagnosed as having bronchial asthma were followed for 29 years. The group was compared with age-matched controls hospitalized for acute nasopharyngitis. A significantly increased mortality from cancer was found which was primarily attributable to cancers of the lung and pancreas. Their findings contrast with those of most other investigators who have found a generally lower than expected risk of cancer in allergic and asthmatic patients (141–146). Three other studies have reported no relationship between cancer and allergies (147–149); one study carried out over 25 years ago suggested a positive association (150). However, none of these previous studies presented data on pancreatic cancer. The excess frequency of pancreatic cancer found in Robinette and Fraumeni's study does not appear to be completely attributable to smoking. The interesting possibility suggested by the authors that certain forms of asthma therapy may contribute to pancreatic carcinogenesis requires further investigation.

Radiation

In a study of survivors of the atomic bombings of Hiroshima and Nagasaki from 1950 to 1966, no radiation effect was suggested for pancreatic cancer (151, 152). However, therapeutically irradiated adults have been reported to have an increased risk of pancreatic cancer (153). No such risk has been reported in children receiving therapeutic radiation.

Rosen et al. (115) observed the long-term effects of ionizing radiation in rats and found that 16% developed islet cell tumors of the pancreas compared to 9.8% of the controls. There was no apparent association with exocrine tumors.

Infection

There is also no evidence so far to support an infectious etiology. In laboratory animals, Rous sarcoma virus has produced pancreatic sarcomas but not carcinomas (154). In man, both the exocrine and endocrine portions of the pancreas are susceptible to injury by common viruses, and viruses have been implicated in the development of diabetes (155, 156). If a viral link to pancreatic cancer does exist, however, it remains to be established.

POSSIBLE MECHANISMS OF CARCINOGENESIS

Wynder et al. (75) have proposed as a working hypothesis that bile may contain carcinogens originating in diet, tobacco or occupational environments and that when this carinogen-containing bile is refluxed into the pancreatic duct, it may cause pancreatic cancer. However, Bates (157) has pointed out that most carcinogens excreted by the liver are converted into water-soluble noncarcinogenic compounds before being excreted in the bile so that reconversion to active carcinogens would be necessary before they could act in the pancreatic ductal system. Another possibility is that the carcinogen becomes carcinogenic only after it is metabolically converted by pancreatic ductal cells. This is purely speculative at the present time, and there is no evidence to support this possibility. There might also be a selective concentration of carcinogens by pancreatic cells so that they act at a ductal site (158).

In this context, when international comparisons are made, the rates of pancreatic cancer in Japanese are among the lowest while the highest rates for cancer of the liver and biliary system are in Japanese males, and fairly high rates also occur in Japanese females. Hence, if the carcinogen is being carried by bile, it does not have the same effect on the biliary tree that it has on the pancreas. In addition, in certain animal species in which pancreatic cancer is also observed, the terminations of the common bile duct and pancreatic duct are quite separate so that a hypothesis involving reflux of bile into the pancreatic duct would seem unlikely to apply at least in these species. Nevertheless, whether this hypothesis could explain part or all of pancreatic cancer etiology in humans remains to be determined.

SUMMARY AND CONCLUSIONS

Data presented in this review indicate that in the United States the incidence of and mortality from pancreatic cancer increased over the past several decades but has tended to level off in recent years. The rates are higher in blacks than in whites and higher in males than in females. Mortality rates increase with age but there appears to be a decline in elderly blacks, possibly on an artifactual basis. There is a suggestion that rates are higher in Jews. No consistent differences by socioeconomic status or by geographic location within the United States have been identified.

The findings suggest that both genetic and environmental factors are playing a significant role in this disease. There is increasing evidence that cigarette smoking may be etiologically related or at the very least it may help to identify a group of patients at increased risk of pancreatic cancer. However, the relative risk estimated for cigarette smoking is much lower than that found for cancer of the lung. The leveling off in incidence and mortality rates for pancreatic cancer in recent years also differs from the time trends observed for lung cancer. However, this could result from differences in site-specific carcinogens and from the fact that the lung is the first organ to be exposed to cigarette smoke in the highest concentrations and prior to the metabolism of any of its components.

A possible role for dietary factors is intriguing but remains unclear. In particular, the possibility that the dietary fats may be implicated in this disease remains to be explored.

Finally, there is strong suggestive evidence that specific chemical exposures may be carcinogenic for the pancreas. Many of these data are from animal studies, but the findings from human studies, although inconclusive, are consistent with these observations.

In summary, a number of potentially valuable clues for clarifying the etiology of pancreatic cancer have been identified. In view of the extremely bleak prognosis and the lack of any significant improvement in therapy for this disease in recent years, there is an urgent need for further studies of etiology in order to develop effective methods for prevention. Despite the significant methodologic problems involved in studying this disease, additional studies designed for testing specific etiologic hypotheses are urgently needed. Any studies to be undertaken should take into consideration the possible multifactoral origin of pancreatic cancer and the potential interrelationships between initiating and promoting agents in the carcinogenic process in this organ. Possible etiologic agents should be investigated in relation to specific cell type and tumor location within the pancreas. The possibility that there may be etiologic differences between pancreatic cancer occurring at younger ages and that occurring at older ages, should also be explored.

REFERENCES

1. National Center for Health Statistics (1968) U.S. Department of Health, Education and Welfare (HSM72-1101).
2. American Cancer Society (1977) 1978 Cancer Facts and Figures. New York.
3. Baylor, S. M., Berg, J. W. (1973) Cross-classification and survival characteristics of 5000 cases of cancer of the pancreas. J. Surg. Oncol. 5, 335–358.
4. Ackerman, L. V., de Regato, J. A. (1962) Cancer, St. Louis: C. V. Mosby Co.
5. Gudjonsson, B., Livstone, E. M., Spiro, H. M. (1978) Cancer of the pancreas: diagnostic accuracy and survival statistics. Cancer 42, 2494–2506.
6. Wood, R. A. B., Moossa, A. R. (1977) The prospective evaluation of tumor-associated antigens for the early diagnosis of pancreatic cancer. Br. J. Surg. 64, 718–720.
7. Reddi, K. K., Holland, J. F. (1976) Elevated serum ribonuclease in patients with pancreatic cancer. Proc. Natl. Acad. Sci. 73, 2308–2310.
8. Dimango, E. F., Malageleda, J. R., Taylor, W. F., Go, V. L. W. (1977) A prospective comparison of current diagnostic tests for pancreatic cancer. N. Eng. J. Med. 297, 737–742.
9. Fitzgerald, P. J., Fortner, J. G., Watson, R. C., Schwartz, M. K., Sherlock, P., Benua, R. S., Cubilla, A. L., Schottenfeld, D., Miller, D., Winawer, S. J., Lightdale, C. J.,

Leidner, S. D., Nisselbaum, J. S., Menendez-Botet, C. J., Poleski, M. H. (1978) The value of diagnostic aids in detecting pancreas cancer. Cancer 41, 868–879.

10. Grieve, D. C. (1973) Adenocarcinoma of the pancreas (a review of 100 cases). J. Roy. Coll. Surg. Edinb. 18, 221–226.
11. Duff, G. L. (1939) The clinical and pathological features of carcinoma of the body and tail of the pancreas. Bull. Johns Hopkins Hosp. 65, 69–96.
12. Richard, L., Jr., Cohn, I., Jr. (1969) Cancer of the pancreas. The American Surgeon 35, 95–103.
13. Sommers, S. C., Murphy, S. A., Warren S. (1954) Pancreatic dust hyperplasia and cancer. Gastroenterology 27, 629–640.
14. Cubilla, A. L., Fitzgerald, P. J. (1976) Morphological lesions associated with human primary invasive nonendocrine pancrease cancer. Cancer Res. 36, 2690–2698.
15. Reber, H. A., Johnson, S. E., Montgomery, C., Carl, W. R. (1976) Pancreatic secretion in hamsters with Pancreatic Cancer. Surgery 82, 34–41.
16. Aoki, K., Ogawa, H. (1978) Cancer of the pancreas: international mortality trends. World Health Stat. Quart. 31, 2–27.
17. Doll, R., Muir C., Waterhouse, J. (1970) Cancer Incidence in Five Continents. Vol. II. Berlin–Heidelberg–New York: Springer–Verlag.
18. Fraumeni, J. F. (1975) Cancers of the pancreas and biliary tract: epidemiological considerations. Cancer Res. 35, 3437–3446.
19. Wynder, E. L., Hirayama, T. (1977) Comparative epidemiology of cancers of the United States and Japan. Prev. Med. 6, 567–594.
20. Haenszel, W., Kurihara, M. (1968) Studies of Japanese migrants. I. Mortality from cancer and other diseases among Japanese in the United States. J. Natl. Cancer Inst. 40, 43–68.
21. Buell, P., Dunn, J. E. (1968) Cancer mortality Among Japanese Issei and Nisei of California. Cancer 18, 656–644.
22. Jablon, S., Angevine, D. M., Matsumoto, Y. S., Ishida, M. (1966) On the significance of cause of death as recorded on death certificates in Hiroshima and Nagasaki, Japan. Nat. Cancer Inst. Monogr. 19, 445–465.
23. Smith, R. L. (1956) Recorded and expected mortality among the Japanese of the United States and Hawaii, with special reference to cancer. J. Natl. Cancer Inst. 17, 459–473.
24. Mancuso, T. F., Sterling, T. D. (1974) Relation of place of birth and migration in cancer mortality in the U.S.—a study of Ohio residents (1959–1967). J. Chron. Dis. 27, 459–474.
25. Burbank, F. (1971) Patterns in cancer mortality in the United States: 1950–1967. National Cancer Institute Monograph 33, May.
26. Greenwald, P., Burnett, W. S., Kirmss, V., Brennan, K., Nasca, P. C. (1976) Cancer Incidence and Mortality in New York State (exclusive of New York City). Bureau of Cancer Control, New York State Department of Health.
27. Klebba, J. A. (1975) Comparability of Mortality Statistics for the Seventh and Eighth Revisions of the International Classification of Diseases, United States. Vital and Health Statistics: Series 2 Data Evaluation and Methods Research, No. 66. United States Department of Health, Education and Welfare DHEW Publication No. (HRA) 76-1304.
28. Krain, L. S. (1972) Cancer Incidence. The crossing of the curves of stomach and pancreatic cancer. Digestion 6, 356–366.
29. Krain, L. S. (1973) Why is pancreatic cancer incidence up; stomach cancer down? Geriatrics 28, 140–145.
30. Krain, L. S. (1970) The rising incidence of carcinoma of the pancreas—real or apparent? J. Surg. Oncol. 2, 115–124.
31. Cutler, S. J., Young, J. L. (eds.) Third National Cancer Survey. Washington, D.C.: U.S. Government Printing Office, National Cancer Institute Monograph 41.

32. Dorn, H. F., Cutler, S. J. (1959) Morbidity from Cancer in the United States: Parts I and II. Public Health Monograph 56, 1–207.

33. Pledger, R. A., Bates, R. R., Saffiotti, V. (1975) Introduction: National Cancer Institute Pancreatic Carcinogenesis Program. Cancer Res. 35, 2226–2227.

34. Arellano, M. G., Linden, G., Dunn, J. E. (1972) Cancer patterns in Alameda County, California. Br. J. Cancer 26, 473–482.

35. Kovi J., Heshmat, M. Y. (1973) Incidence of cancer in Negroes in Washington, D.C., and selected African cities. Am. J. Epidemiol. 96, 401–413.

36. Levin, D. L., Connelly, R. R. (1973) Cancer of the pancreas. Available epidemiologic information and its implications. Cancer 31, 1231–1236.

37. Parkash, O. (1972) On the statistical and clinical evaluation of carcinoma of the pancreas. Digestion 6, 152–164.

38. Moynan, R. W., Neerhour, R. C., Johnson, T. S. (1964) Pancreatic carcinoma in children: case-report and review. J. Pediatrics 65, 711–720.

39. Tsukimoto, I., Watanabe, K., Lin, J. B., Nakajima, T. (1973) Pancreatic carcinoma in children in Japan. Cancer 31, 1203–1207.

40. Taxy, J. B. (1976) Adenocarcinoma of the pancreas in childhood. Cancer 37, 1508–1518.

41. Smith, P. E., Krementz, E. T., Reid, R. J., Bufkin, W. J. (1967) An analysis of 600 with carcinoma of the pancreas. Surg., Gynecol. Obste. 124, 1288–1290.

42. Moldow, R. E., Connelly, R. R. (1968) Epidemiology of pancreatic cancer in Connecticut. Gastroenterology 55, 666–686.

43. Lilienfeld, A. M., Levin, A. L., Kessler, I. I. (1972) Cancer in the United States. Cambridge: Harvard University Press.

44. Cederlof, R., Friberg, L., Hrubec, Z., Lorich, U. (1975) The Relationship of Smoking and Some Social Co-Variables to Mortality and Cancer Morbidity: A Ten Year Follow-up in a Probability Sample of 55,000 Swedish Subjects, Age 18–69. Part I/II. Stockholm: Carolinska Institute.

45. Blot, W. J., Fraumeni, J. F., Stone, B. J. (1978) Geographic correlates of pancreas cancer in the United States. Cancer 42, 373–380.

46. MacMahon, B. (1960) The ethnic distribution of cancer mortality in New York City, 1955. Acto Unio Internat. Contra Cancrum 16, 1716–1724.

47. Newill, V. A. (1961) Distribution of cancer mortality among ethnic subgroups of the white population of New York City, 1953–58. J. Natl. Canc. Inst. 26, 405–417.

48. Seidman, H. (1970) Cancer death rates by site and sex for religions and socioeconomic groups in New York City. Environ. Res. 3, 235–250.

49. Lyon, J. L., Klauber, M. R., Gardner, J. M., Smart, C. R. (1976) Cancer incidence in Mormons and Non-Mormons in Utah. N. Eng. J. Med. 294, 129.

50. Enstrom, J. E. (1978) Cancer and total mortality among active Mormons. Cancer 42, 1943–1951.

51. Phillips, R. L. (1975) Role of life-style and dietary habits in risk of cancer among Seventh-Day Adventists. Cancer Res. 35, 3513–3522.

53. Dorn, H. F. (1959) Some problems arising in prospective and retrospective studies of the etiology of disease. N. Engl. J. Med. 261, 571–579.

53. Cohart, E. M., Muller, C. (1955) Socioeconomic distribution of cancer of the gastrointestinal tract in New Haven. Cancer 8, 379–388.

54. Krain, L. S. (1971) The rising incidence of cancer of the pancreas—further epidemiologic studies. J. Chron. Dis. 23, 685–690.

55. The Registrar-General's Decennial Supplement, England and Wales 1970–72 (1978) Series DS No. 1, Occupational Mortality. London: Her Majesty's Stationery Office.

56. Friedman, J. M., Fialkow, P. J. (1976) Carcinoma of the pancreas in four brothers. Birth Defects 1, XII, 145–150.

57. MacDermott, R. P., Kramer, P. (1973) Adenocarcinoma of the pancreas in four siblings. Gastroenterology 65, 137–139.
58. McKusick, V. A. (1974) Mendelian Inheritance in Man. Catalogs of Autosomal Dominant, Autosomal Recessive and X-Linked Phenotypes. Fourth Ed. Baltimore: The Johns Hopkins Press.
59. Gardner, E. G. (1962) Follow-up study of a family group exhibiting dominant inheritance for a syndrome including intestinal polyps, osteomas, fibromas and epidermal cysts. Am. J. Hum. Genet. 14, 376.
60. Lynch, H. T., Frichot, B. C., Lynch, P., Lynch, J., Guirgis, H. A. (1975) Family studies of malignant melanoma and associated cancer. Surg. Gynecol. Obstet. 141, 517–522.
61. Tomita, T., Vachal, E., Rengachar, S., Watanabe, I. (1978) Occult adenocarcinoma of the pancreas in a patient with Lindau's disease. Digest. Dis. 23, 80–83.
62. Keller, R. T., Logan, G. M. (1977) Adenocarcinoma of the pancreas associated with neurofibromatosis. Cancer 39, 1264–1266.
63. Rashad, M. N. (1977) *In*: Genetics of Human Cancer. Mulvihill, J. J., Miller, R. W., Fraumeni, J. F. (eds.) New York: Raven Press, p. 204.
64. Newell, G. R., Gordon, J. E., Monlezun, A. P., Horwitz, J. S. (1974) ABO blood groups and cancer. J. Natl. Cancer Inst. 52, 1425–1430.
65. Vogel, F. (1970) ABO blood groups and disease. Am. J. Human Genetics 22, 464–475.
66. Terasaki, P. I., Perdue, S. T., Kickey, M. R. (1977) HLA Frequencies in Cancer: A Second Study in Genetics of Human Cancer. Mulvihill, J. J., Miller, R. W., Fraumeni, J. F. Jr., (eds.). New York: Raven Press, pp. 321–328.
67. Sholman, L., Swift, M. (1973) Pancreatic carcinoma and diabetes mellitus in families of ataxis-telangiectasia probands. Am. J. Human Genet. 24, 48A.
68. Rashad, M. N. (1977) *In*: Genetics of Human Cancer. Mulvihill, J. J., Miller, R. W., Fraumeni, J. F. Jr., (eds.). New York: Raven Press, p. 290.
69. Green, R. C., Baggenstoss, A. H., Sprague, R. G., (1958) Diabetes mellitus in association with primary carcinoma of the pancreas. Diabetes 7, 308–311.
70. Bell, E. T. (1957) Carcinoma of the pancreas. I. A clinical and pathologic study of 609 necropsied cases; II. The relation of carcinoma of the pancreas to diabetes mellitus. Am. J. Pathol. 33, 499–522.
71. Jacobson, P. H. (1948) A statistical study of cancer among diabetics. Milbank Mem. Fund. Quart. 26, 90–118.
72. Clark, C. G., Mitchell, P. E. G. (1961) Diabetes mellitus and primary carcinoma of the pancreas. Br. Med. J. 1259–1262.
73. Kessler, I. I. (1970) A genetic relationship between diabetes and cancer. Lancet 218–220.
74. Karmody, A. J., Kyle, J. (1969) The association between carcinoma of the pancreas and diabetes mellitus. Br. J. Surg. 56, 362–364.
75. Wynder, E. L., Mabuchi, K., Maruchi, N., Fortner J. G. (1973) Epidemiology of cancer of the pancreas. J. Natl. Cancer Inst. 50, 645.
76. Hoffman, D., Schmeltz, I., Hecht, S. S., Wynder, E. L. (1976) Chemical studies on tobacco smoke. XXXIX. On the identification of carcinogens, promoters, and carcinogens. *In*: Proceedings, 3rd World Conference on Smoking and Health. I. Modifying the Risk for the Smoker. Washington, D.C. Department of Health, Education and Welfare, p. 125.
77. MMWR (Morbidity and Mortality Weekly Report) (1979) 28, 1–11. Highlights of the Surgeon General's Report on Smoking.
78. Hammond, E. C. (1966) Smoking in relation to the death rates of one million men and women. *In*: Haenszel, W. (ed.). Epidemiological Approaches to the Study of

Cancer and Other Chronic Diseases. U.S. Pub. Health Service, National Cancer Institute Monograph 19, pp. 126–204.

79. Best, E. W. (1966) A Canadian Study of Smoking and Health. Ottawa: Department of National Health and Welfare, pp. 65–86.
80. Kahn, H. A. (1966) Report on 8½ years of observation. *In*: Haenszel, W. (ed.). Epidemiological Approaches to the Study of Cancer and Other Chronic Diseases. U.S. Public Health Service, National Cancer Institute Monograph 19, pp. 1–125.
81. Hirayama, T. (1977) Changing patterns of cancer in Japan with special reference to the decrease in stomach cancer mortality. *In*: Origins of Humans Cancer. Hiatt, H. H., Watson, J. D., Winston, J. A. (eds.). Cold Spring Harbor Laboratory, Vol. 4, pp. 55–75.
82. Weir, J. M., Dunn, J. E., Jr. (1970) Smoking and mortality: a prospective study. Cancer 25, 105–112.
83. Stocks, P. (1970) Cancer mortality in relation to national consumption of cigarettes, solid fuel, tea and coffee. Br. J. Cancer 24, 215–225.
84. Hakulinen, T., Lehtimaki, L., Lehtonen, M., Teppo, L. (1974) Cancer morbidity among two male cohorts with increased alcohol consumption in Finland. J. Natl. Cancer Inst. 52, 1711–1714.
85. Burch, G. E., Ansari, A. (1968) Chronic alcoholism and carcinoma of the pancreas. Arch. Intern. Med. 122, 273–275.
86. Lowenfels, A. B. (1974) Alcohol and cancer. N.Y. State J. Med. Part I, 56–59.
87. Monson, R. R., Lyon, J. L. (1975) Proportionate mortality among alcoholics. Cancer 36, 1077–1079.
88. Comfort, M., Steinberg, A. G. (1952) Pedigree of a family with hereditary chronic relapsing pancreatitis. Gastroenterology 21, 54–63.
89. Gross, J. B., Bambill, E. E., Ulrich, J. A. (1962) Hereditary pancreatitis. Description of a fifth kindred and summary of clinical features. Am. J. Med. 33, 358–364.
90. Whitten, D. M., Feingold, M. Eisenklam, E. J. (1968) Hereditary pancreatitis. Am. J. Dis. Child. 116, 426–428.
91. Davidson, P., Costanza, D., Swieconeck, J. A., Harris, J. B. (1968) Hereditary pancreatitis. A kindred without gross aminoaciduria. Ann. Intern. Med. 68, 88–96.
92. Lapey, A., Kattwinkel, J., DiSant Angese, P. A., Laster, L. (1971) Hereditary pancreatitis (HP) without amino-aciduria: two new kindred. Pediatr. Res. 5, 389.
93. Appel, M. F. (1974) Hereditary pancreatitis: review and presentation of an additional kindred. Arch. Surg. 108, 63–65.
94. Castleman, B., Scully, R., McNeely, B. U. (1972) Case records of the Massachusetts General Hospital, Case 25–1972. N. Engl. J. Med. 286, 1353–1359.
95. Cope, O., Culver, P. G., Mixter, Jr., C. G., Nardi, G. L. (1957) Pancreatitis, a diagnostic clue to hyperparathyroidism. Ann. Surg., 145, 857–863.
96. Leeson, P. M., Fourman, P. (1966) Acute pancreatitis from vitamin-D poisoning in a patient with parathyroid deficiency. Lancet 1185–1186.
97. Greenberger, N. G., Hatch. F. T., Drummey, G. D., Isselbacher, K. J. (1966) Pancreatitis and hyperlipemia: a study of serum lipid alterations in 25 patients with acute pancreatitis. Medicine 45, 161–175.
98. Zamcheck, N., Moore, T. L., Ohar, P., Kupchik, R. (1972) Immunologic diagnosis and prognosis of human digestive tract. N. Engl. J. Med. 286, 83–86.
99. Mikal, S., Campbell, A. J. A. (1950) Carcinoma of the pancreas. Diagnostic and operative criteria based on one hundred consecutive autopsies. Surgery 28, 963–969.
100. Bartholomew, L. G., Gross, J. B., Comfort, M. S. (1958) Carcinoma of the pancreas associated with chronic relapsing pancreatitis. Gastroenterology 35, 473–477.
101. Gambill, E. E. (1972) Pancreatitis associated with pancreatic carcinoma. A study of 26 cases. Mayo Clin. Proc. 46, 174–177.

102. Paulino-Netto, A., Drehling, D. A., Baronofsky, I. D. (1960) The relationship between pancreatic calcification and cancer of the pancreas. Ann. Surg. 151, 530–537.

103. Mikhailichenko, V. A., Bruk, B. B., Rovenskaia, N. M., Tamarkin, M. A. (1974) The relation between chronic pancreatitis and cancer of the pancreas. Vopr. Onkol. 20, 57–61.

104. Ishii, K., Nakamura, K., Takeuchi, T., Hirayama, T. (1973) Chronic calcifying pancreatitis and pancreatic carcinoma in Japan. Digestion 9, 429–437.

105. Slye, M., Holmes, H. F., Wells, H. G. (1935) The comparative pathology of carcinoma of the pancreas, with report of two cases in mice. Am. J. Cancer 23, 81–86.

106. Rowlatt, U. (1967) Spontaneous epithelial tumours of the pancreas of mammals. Br. J. Cancer 21, 82–107.

107. Reddy, J. K., Svoboda, D. J., Rao, M. S. (1974) Susceptibility of an inbred strain of guinea pigs to the induction of pancreatic adenocarcinoma by *N*-methyl-*n*-nitrosourea. J. Natl. Cancer Inst. 52, 991–993.

108. Pour, P., Kruger, F. W., Althoff, J. Cardesa, A., Mohr, U. (1974) Cancer of the pancreas induced in the Syrian golden hamster. Am. J. Pathol. 76, 349–358.

109. Kruger, F. W., Pour, P., Althoff, J. (1974) Induction of pancreas tumors by DI-isobropano-linitrosamine. Naturwissenschaften 61, 328.

110. Rao, M. S., Svoboda, D. J., Reddy, J. K. (1974) The ultrastructural effects of aflatoxin B in the rat pancreas. Virchows. Arch. (Zellpathol.) 17, 149–157.

111. Longnecker, D. S., Crawford, B. G. (1974) Hyperplastic nodules and adenomas of exocrine pancreas in azaserine-treated rats. J. Natl. Cancer Inst. 53, 573–577.

112. Wilson, R. H., McEds, F., Cox, A. J. (1941) The toxicity and carcinogenic activity of A-acetaminogluorene. Cancer Res. 1, 595.

113. Hoch-Ligeti, C. (1949) Primary pancreatic tumors in rats fed *P*-dimethylaminoazogenzene. Br. J. Cancer 3, 285.

114. Gorski, T. (1959) Induction of experimental pancreas carcinoma in mice. Vopr. Onkol. 5, 413.

115. Rosen, V. J., Jr., Castandera, T. J., Jones, D. C., Kimeldorf, D. J. (1961) Islet cell tumors of the pancreas in the irradiated and nonirradiated rat. Lab. Invest., 10, 608.

116. Pour, P., Mohr, U., Cardesa, A., Althoff, J., Kruger, F. W. (1975) Pancreatic neoplasms in an animal model: morphological, biological, and comparative studies. Cancer 36, 379–389.

117. Althoff, J., Pour, P., Malick, L., Wilson, R. B. (1976) Pancreatic neoplasms induced in Syrian golden hamsters. Am. J. Pathol. 83, 517–530.

118. Levitt, M. H., Harris, C. C., Squire, R., Springer, S., Wenk, M., Mollelo, C., Thomas, D., Kingsbury, E., Newkirk, C. (1977) Experimental pancreatic carcinogenesis. Am. J. Pathol. 88, 5–15.

119. Druckrey, H., Ivankovic, S., Bucheler, J., Preussmann, R., Thomas, C. (1968) Erzeugung von Magen- und Pankreas-krebs beim Meerschweinchen durch Methylnitrosoharnstoff und -Urethan. Z. Krebsforsch 71, 167–182. *Cited in*: Pledger, R. A., Bates, R. R., Saffiotti, U. (1975) Introduction: National Cancer Institute Pancreatic Carcinogenesis Program. Cancer Res. 35, 2226–2227.

120. Priester, W. A. (1974a) Pancreatic islet cell tumors in domestic animals. Data from 11 colleges of veterinary medicine in the United States and Canada. Natl. Canc. Inst. 53, 227–229.

121. Soloway, H. B., Sommers, S. C. (1966) Endocrinopathy associated with pancreatic carcinomas. Review of host factors including hyperplasia and gonadotropic activity. Ann. Surg. 164, 300–304.

122. The Registrar General's Decennial Supplement, England and Wales, 1951, Part II, Occupational Mortality. (1958) London: Her Majesty's Stationery Office.

123. Redmond, C. K., Strobino, B. R., Cypress, R. H. (1976) Cancer experience among coke by-product workers. Ann. N.Y. Acad. Sci. 271, 102–115.

124. Turner, H. M., Grace, H. G. (1938) An investigation into cancer mortality among males in certain Sheffield trades. J. Hyg. 38, 90–101.
125. Dorken, H. (1964) Einege Daten bei 280 Patienten mit Pankreaskrebs. Gastroenterologia 102, 47–77.
126. Study Finds Cancer-Woodworking Tie (Anonymous) (1974) Eng. News Rec. 195, 15.
127. Mancuso, T. F., El-Attar, A. A. (1967) Cohort study of workers exposed to betanaphythylamine and benzidine. J. Occup. Med. 9, 277–285.
128. Li, F. P., Fraumeni, J. F., Mantel, N., Miller, R. W. (1969) Cancer mortality among chemists. J. Nat. Cancer. Inst. 43, 1159–1164.
129. Capurro, P. U. (1976) Hydrocarbon exposure and cancer. Lancet, 253–254.
130. Monson, R. R., Fine, L. J. (1978) Cancer mortality and morbidity among rubber workers. J. Nat. Cancer Inst. 61, 1047–1053.
131. Hirayama, T. (1972) Smoking in relation to the death rates of 265,118 men and women in Japan. (1972) A report on five years of follow-ups. Presented at the American Cancer Society's 14th Science Writers Seminar, Clearwater Beach, Florida, March 24–29, 1972.
132. Wynder, E. L. (1975) An epidemiological evaluation of the causes of cancer of the pancreas. Cancer Res. 35, 2228–2233.
133. Wynder, E. L. (1976) Nutrition and cancer. Fed. Proc. 35, 1309–1315.
134. Segi, M., Kurihara, M., Matsuyama, T. (1969) Cancer Mortality of Selected Sites in 24 Countries No. 5, 1964–1965. Sendai, Japanese Department of Public Health, Tohokii University School of Medicine.
135. Food and Agriculture Organization (1969) Good Balance Sheets. New York: United Nations.
136. Wynder, E. L., Reddy, B. S., McCoy, G. D., Weisburger, J. H., Williams, G. M. (1976) Diet and gastrointestinal cancer. Clin. Gastroenterol. 5, 463–482.
137. Priester, W. A. (1974) Data for 11 United States and Canadian colleges of veterinary medicine on pancreatic carcinoma in domestic animals. Cancer Res. 34, 1372–1375.
138. Mihas, A. A., Ceballos, R., Mihas, A., Gibson, R. G. (1978) Zollmger-Ellison Syndrome assoicated with ductal adenocarcinoma of the pancreas. N. Engl. J. Med. 298, 144–146.
139. Howson, C. P., Asal, N. R. (1976) A case-control study of pancreatic carcinoma in Oklahoma City hospitals, 1970–1975. Presentation at Society of Epidemiological Research Meeting, June 1976.
140. Robinette, C. D., Fraumeni, J. F. (1978) Asthma and subsequent mortality in World War II veterans. J. Chron. Dis. 31, 619–624.
141. Fisherman, E. W. (1960) Does the allergic diathesis influence malignancy? J. Allergy 31, 74–78.
142. Mackay, W. D. (1966) The incidence of allergic disorders and cancer. Br. J. Cancer 20, 434–437.
143. Ure, D. M. J. (1969) Negative association between allergy and cancer. Scott. Med. J. 14, 51–54.
144. Gabriel, R., Dudley, B. M., Alexander, W. D. (1972) Lung cancer and allergy. Br. J. Clin. Pract. 26, 202–204.
145. Meers, P. D. (1973) Allergy and cancer. Lancet 1, 884–885.
146. Alderson, M. (1974) Mortality from malignant disease in patients with asthma. Lancet 2, 1475–1477.
147. Dworin, M., Diamond, H. D., Craver, L. F. (1955) Hodgkin's disease and allergy. Cancer 8, 128–131.
148. McKee, W. D., Arnold, C. A., Perlman, M. D. (1967) A double-blind study of the comparative incidence of malignancy and allergy. J. Allergy 39, 294–301.

149. Shapiro, S., Heinonen, O. P., Siskind, V. (1971) Cancer and allergy. Cancer 28, 396–400.
150. Logan, J., Saker, D. (1953) The incidence of allergic disorders in cancer. N. Z. Med. J. 52, 210–212.
151. Angevine, D. M., Jablon, S. (1964) Late radiation effects: neoplasia and other diseases in Japan. Ann. N.Y. Acad. Sci. 114, 823–831.
152. Beebe, G. W., Kato, H., Land, C. E. (1970) Mortality and radiation do October 1950–September 1966. JNIH-ABCC Life Span Study, Hiroshima-Nagasaki, Technical Report 11–70.
153. Upton, A. C. (1978) Radiation. Bull. N.Y. Acad. Med. 54, 428–434.
154. Popken, F. E., Faughn, C. O. (1961) Pancreas passage of Rous sarcoma. J. Natl. Cancer Inst. 26, 305–312.
155. Steinke, J., Taylor, K. W. (1974) Viruses and the etiology of diabetes. Diabetes 23, 631–633.
156. Yoon, J. W., Austin, M., Onodera, T., Louis, A. (1979) Ineffectiveness of topical adenine arabinoside 5′-monophosphate in recurrent herpes labialis. N. Engl. J. Med. 300, 1173–1179.
157. Bates. R. R. (1975) Chemical carcinogenesis and the pancreas. J. Surg. Oncol. 7, 143–149.
158. Morgan, R. G. H., Wormsley, K. G. (1977) Progress report: Cancer of the pancreas. Gut 18, 580–596.

EXOGENOUS SEX HORMONES AND CANCER

VALERIE BERAL, M.B., M.R.C.P.

CONTENTS

INTRODUCTION

In this review of current knowledge on the relationship between exogenous sex hormones and malignant disease in humans, both female hormones (estrogens, progestogens, and estrogen–progestogen combinations) and male hormones (androgens) will be considered. Because therapy with male hormones is comparatively rare, the main emphasis will be on the effects of female hormones.

Many of the sex hormones were first isolated or synthesized before or during the Second World War, but they were not widely used as therapeutic agents until after the war. Initially, the hormones were used for the treatment of a variety of reproductive disorders and as palliative therapy for disseminated carcinoma.

Since the 1960s, the main use of exogenous hormones has been as contraceptive agents. The "combined" oral contraceptive, which contains both estrogen and progestogen, is by far the most commonly used hormonal contraceptive. The "minipill," which contains progestogens only (and is taken orally), is not widely used except in Scandinavia. The injectable contraceptives, such as medroxyprogesterone acetate (DMPA), which contain progestogens only, are also not widely used except in certain developing countries. Unless otherwise specified, in this review the terms "Pill" and "oral contraceptive" refer to the combined estrogen–progestogen contraceptive agents. The combined oral contraceptive is dispensed in packets of 21 tablets, referred to as a cycle of tablets. There are many brands, each containing somewhat different doses and types of semisynthetic estrogens and progestogens. For almost all brands the constituents of each tablet in the cycle are similar, the exception being the sequential oral contraceptives, for which the relative doses of estrogen and progestogen vary within the cycle. Sequential oral contraceptives are not widely used, and indeed have been withdrawn from the market in several countries, but they are important because they have been specifically linked with certain types of cancer.

Another common use of hormonal therapy today is in the treatment of menopausal symptoms. In general, estrogens are used alone, although in recent years the use of estrogen–progestogen combinations has been advocated. The type of estrogen most commonly used is "conjugated" or "natural" estrogen. Synthetic estrogens such as diethylstilbestrol (DES) are rarely used today in the treatment of menopausal symptoms.

With the widespread use of oral contraceptives by women of child-bearing age, and of estrogens by menopausal women, there has been growing concern about the effects of these agents on health. Because women taking these hormones are generally young and healthy, any alteration in their risk of developing various diseases may have serious consequences in the future. This is particularly so for malignant disease, where the latent period is expected to be long.

From the London School of Hygiene and Tropical Medicine, Keppel Street (Gower Street), London WC1E 7HT, England.

Scope and Structure of the Review

As the review is concerned with the relationship of exogenous sex hormones to the development of malignant disease in humans, their use in the treatment of malignant disease will not be discussed. Also, their relation to the development of benign tumors is omitted, with two important exceptions: liver tumors and pituitary tumors. Both of these tumors may have serious effects on women. Benign liver tumors may lead to massive bleeding into the abdominal cavity, which may be fatal; they may undergo malignant transformation. Pituitary tumors may lead to a variety of endocrine and neurological disorders.

Because hormones have widespread effects throughout the body, they may affect the risk of developing cancer at a large number of organ sites. Each site is considered separately, beginning with the reproductive organs and including all sites for which there is some evidence that sex hormones might affect cancer risk. In the discussion of each site, the effects of estrogen therapy alone are considered first, then the effects of progestogens alone, followed by the effects of estrogen–progestogen combinations. Finally, if evidence is available, the effects of androgen therapy are considered. It will become clear that relevant information is frequently unavailable.

Mechanism of Action

Exogenous sex hormones may predispose to the development of malignancy because of some intrinsic carcinogenic property of the hormone itself. It might be expected that synthetic hormones would be more likely to be carcinogenic than naturally occuring hormones, but with present knowledge little is known about the relative carcinogenicity of synthetic and non-synthetic compounds. In general it would seem, however, that most hormones have minimal direct carcinogenic properties (1).

The most important way in which exogenous hormones may affect cancer risk is that by altering the hormonal balance within the body, thereby affecting the metabolism, immune response, and the entire homeostatic mechanism. Considerable evidence suggests that *endogenous* hormones affect cancer risk, especially of the reproductive organs; therefore, it is plausible that *exogenous* hormones should do the same. As with other etiological factors, the risk of developing cancer might be expected to depend on the dose of the hormone used, the duration of exposure, and the precise type of hormone used. It is also reasonable to expect that malignancy would not appear until after a certain lag or latent period. In addition, certain individuals are likely to be more prone than others to develop hormone-induced cancer.

Relevance of Animal Experiments

There is considerable debate about the validity of extrapolating findings from animal experiments to human populations. In general, it is unwise to do so without qualification, mainly because certain animal species seem to be particularly prone to certain tumor types. Nevertheless, as information accumulates about effects on humans, it is interesting to note how closely they parallel the animal findings.

Although this review is concerned with the effects of hormone use in humans, the results of the extensive animal experiments that have been carried out are summarized briefly for each cancer site (1,2). The purpose is twofold: to illustrate that the findings in animals and humans are often similar; and to draw attention to those sites where animal experiments indicate possible increase in cancer risk, and those where no change or a decrease in cancer risk is indicated. The findings from the animal experiments should provide clues for future studies in humans.

Special Methodologic Considerations

As was previously pointed out, exogenous hormones are likely to affect cancer risk by altering the hormonal balance within the body rather than by some intrinsic carcinogenic property of the hormones themselves. Because of this, the effects of hormone use on cancer risk may be complex indeed, and may even vary from one hormonal preparation to another. For example, it is possible that certain estrogen–progestogen combinations in the combined Pill might induce cancer, whereas other combinations might suppress it. Such complex relationships are particularly likely to occur with cancers of the reproductive tract, where endogenous hormonal factors are known to be important determinants of cancer risk. Furthermore, the effects may vary in different groups of women, for example, in nullipara and multipara, or in pre- and postmenopausal women. Finally, endogenous hormonal factors may determine exogenous hormone use: Women with an early menarche may well begin using the Pill at younger ages than women with a late menarche; and women who have children at a young age may not begin taking the Pill until after their first childbirth, whereas women who delay their first birth may begin taking the Pill at an early age. These factors need to be taken into account in studies of the relationship of exogenous hormone use to cancer risk. It is important that factors related to endogenous hormones do not confound the analysis.

Other Reviews

In 1974 the International Agency for Research on Cancer published an extensive review of the carcinogenic effects of sex hormones (1). This and the review by Hertz (2) provide excellent accounts of the findings from animal experiments. The World Health Organization has recently summarized the evidence concerning the risk of neoplasia with steroidal contraceptives (3). The report deals mainly with contraceptive agents, and relatively little is included about the effects of menopausal estrogen therapy or androgens on the development of cancer.

BREAST CANCER

Estrogens

So far, the relatively few reported studies of the relationship of exogenous estrogen use to the development of breast cancer have yielded contradictory results. Three case-control studies have examined the relationship; these are

TABLE 1. Case-Control Studies of Breast Cancer and Exogenous Estrogens

Author and year of publication (reference)	Year(s) of diagnosis of breast cancer	Age range	Number of cases	Relative risk associated with estrogen use
Craig et al., 1974 (4)	1949–1967	30+	134	1.0
Casagrande et al., 1976 (5)	1969–1972	50–64	100	0.8[a]
	1972–1973	50–59	47	3.1[a]
Sartwell et al., 1977 (6)	1969–1972	20–74	284	0.8[b]

[a]Adjusted for age at menopause and age at diagnosis (for cases) or age at interview (for controls). Note: Only women with a natural menopause were included in this study.

[b]Adjusted for age, race, marital status, menopausal status, pregnancy history, and age at first pregnancy.

summarized in Table 1 (4–6). The relative risk estimates vary considerably from study to study. The analyses by Casagrande and his colleagues (5) of breast cancer in women who had a natural menopause are instructive. They demonstrate that simply comparisons of the proportions of cases and controls who have and have not used postmenopausal estrogens may be misleading; that women who develop breast cancer tend to reach their natural menopause at older ages than the controls, and, as a consequence, have different patterns of postmenopausal hormonal use. After adjusting for age at the onset of menopause and age of diagnosis of breast cancer, the investigators noted that the relative risk associated with estrogen use increased from 0.5 to 0.8 in a group of women interviewed in 1969 to 1972 and from 2.2 to 3.1 in another group interviewed in 1973. They concluded that their earlier work which suggested that estrogen use protected against breast cancer was invalid because they had failed to account for the timing of menopause and diagnosis (7). They also point out that other factors linked with breast cancer, such as reproductive history and socioeconomic status, are so closely related to exogenous estrogen use that it is exceedingly difficult to adjust for these potential confounding factors in case-control or cohort studies. The issues that they discuss are fundamental to the interpretation of epidemiologic studies of exogenous hormone use and breast cancer. Moreover, they raise serious doubts about the validity of almost all the studies of breast cancer discussed here [with the exception of the randomized trial of Bibbo et al. (8) described later].

There have been many reports on the follow-up of women treated with estrogens during menopause (8–14). In the large majority of these, little information is provided about the duration of completeness of follow-up. It is, therefore, impossible to estimate the number of expected cases of breast cancer among the women, and no conclusions about the effects of estrogen can be drawn from such studies. Burch et al. (13) and Hoover et al. (14) did attempt to calculate the expected number of breast cancers in their study populations. Both found an excess of breast cancer; Hoover et al. (14) also noted that the excess breast cancer occurred particularly after a long latent period—15 years or more—and with high doses of estrogens. Unfortunately, neither study had included the follow-up of a comparison group of women who had not taken estrogens. Furthermore, the expected rates of breast cancer were calculated from national data on breast cancer incidence and may well not apply to the small groups of women involved in their studies. Thus, their findings are interesting but provide little firm evidence about the effect of estrogen use on breast cancer risk.

The study of Bibbo et al. (8) is certainly the most important one reported so far that is concerned with the effects of estrogen use on breast cancer risk. This study involved the follow-up of 1,361 women over a period of 25 years; about half had been given high doses of diethylstilbestrol (DES) 25 years earlier, and the other half had not. The DES was given for approximately 8 months, during pregnancy, supposedly to prevent fetal wastage. Most important, the women were *randomly* allocated to receive high doses of DES or a placebo. The study therefore can be regarded as a true randomized trial of the long-term effects of DES in a human population. The problems of interpretation described by Casagrande et al. (5) for other studies do not apply here.

An excess incidence of breast cancer was noted among those who had been exposed to DES; 4.6% of those given DES developed breast cancer, compared with 3.1% for those given a placebo. The differences were not statistically significant, but they do suggest that estrogens given in the premenopausal period may well increase the risk of breast cancer. It is possible that estrogens given pre- and postmenopausally have different, even opposite, effects on breast cancer risk. Unfortunately, few studies other than this one and the study of Casagrande and his colleagues distinguish clearly between women who received estrogens before and those who recieved them after menopause.

There have been several case reports of breast cancer developing in men treated with DES and other estrogenic substances. Symmers (15) reported the occurrence of breast cancer in two men, who by feminizing surgical procedures and by hormonal therapy, had altered their secondary sexual characteristics. Both were exposed to very high doses of varying types of estrogen, and both rapidly developed fatal breast cancer in their early 30s. In each instance, this was more than 5 years after hormonal therapy was first begun. In addition, there have been at least 30 reports of breast cancer occurring in men treated with estrogens for prostatic cancer (1,16). Although there has been some debate about the origin of some of these tumors (it has been argued that some are secondary deposits from the cancers of the prostate), there is little doubt that many are primary breast cancers (16,17). If we consider the overall rarity of breast cancer in males, the case reports suggest that a true increase in breast cancer incidence does occur among men treated with estrogens.

Animal experiments show that all estrogens that have been tested have increased the incidence of breast cancer in various species of animals (1). Although this information cannot be extrapolated directly to humans, it does warn us that we should not be complacent about the potential adverse effects of exogenous estrogens on breast cancer risk.

In conclusion, the available evidence hints that estrogens, when given alone, are likely to increase the risk of breast cancer in both men and women. Of course, considerably more information is required before any definite conclusions can be drawn. Furthermore, there are serious methodological and logical problems inherent in any study of the possible relationship of breast cancer and exogenous hormone use by women. Estrogen use is closely related to reproductive history and menopausal status and these factors are known to affect breast cancer risk (18,19). At present it is not clear how these interrelationships can best be disentangled either in the design or the analysis of epidemiologic studies. It is important that these methodological issues be resolved before other investigators repeat the errors of their predecessors.

Progestogens

The relationship of breast cancer to progestogen-only contraceptives or to medroxyprogesterone acetate (DMPA) in humans has not been reported. Considerable concern has been expressed about the induction of breast nodules and breast cancers in beagle dogs following the administration of certain progestogens, particularly DMPA and chlormadinone acetate (1). Clearly, this urgently needs investigation in human populations.

Oral Contraceptives

Findings of reports from five case-control studies, and three cohort studies of the possible relationship between oral contraceptive use and breast cancer (6,20–26) are summarized in Tables 2 and 3. In general, no clear pattern emerges, and one must presently conclude that the effect of oral contraceptives on breast cancer risk is still uncertain. When the characteristics of the women included in the studies are examined in detail, it becomes clear why the findings of the studies are inconclusive. The duration of the Pill use is generally very short: In the case–control studies reported so far, fewer than

TABLE 2. Case-Control Studies of Breast Cancer and Oral Contraceptive Use

Author and year of publication (reference)	Year(s) of diagnosis of breast cancer	Age range	Number of cases	Relative risk associated with oral contraceptive use
Boston Collaborative Drug Surveillance Program, 1973 (20)	1968–1971	20–44	23	0.6
Vessey et al., 1975 (21)	1968–1971	16–45	322	0.9
Paffenbarger et al., 1977 (22)	1970–1972	15–49	452	1.1[a]
Sartwell et al., 1977 (6)	1969–1972	20–74	284	0.9[b]
Kelsey et al., 1978 (23)	1971–1973	20–44	99	1.6[c]

[a]Adjusted for age, race, religion, and age at first childbirth.

[b]Adjusted for age, race, marital status, menopausal status, pregnancy history, and age at first pregnancy.

[c]Adjusted for religion, father's country of birth, pregnancy history, age at first pregnancy, use of douche, and previous breast operation.

TABLE 3. Cohort Studies of Breast Cancer and Oral Contraceptive Use

Author and year of publication (reference)	Age range	Number of cases	Relative risk associated with oral contraceptive use
Royal College of General Practitioners, 1974 (24)	15–49	31	1.1
Ory et al., 1976 (25)	25–49	137	0.6–0.7
Vessey et al., 1976 (26)	25–39	16	0.4

10% of the case or controls had taken the Pill for 5 years or longer. If oral contraceptive use affects breast cancer risk, it seems likely that duration of use—which largely determines the dose of hormones to which a woman is exposed—will be related to the risk. Such a dose–response relationship would only be detectable when a larger proportion of the population had taken the Pill for longer periods of time than have been reported to date.

More important, if the Pill alters breast cancer risk, it is unlikely to do so immediately. It is probable that there would be a delay before its effect becomes evident. Existing information about the effects of exogenous estrogen, limited as it is, suggests that the latent period may be 15 years or longer (14). In the studies reported so far, only those of Vessey et al. (21) and of Paffenbarger et al. (22) specified the length of time since their cases and controls had begun using the Pill. In Vessey's study, 8% had begun taking the Pill more than 8 years before the diagnosis of cancer and in Paffenbarger's, 24% had begun more than 6 years before. Considering that the effects of the Pill on breast cancer risk can only be properly and completely evaluated when a sizeable proportion of the study population began taking the Pill 15 years earlier, we need to wait for about 10 years before such a situation will exist.

The role of confounding factors must be considered carefully when assessing the effects of the Pill on breast cancer. On the one hand, Pill use is influenced by socioeconomic factors and reproductive events such as age at first childbirth, parity, age at menopause, and so on. On the other hand, its use can also influence these factors, and they in turn may affect the risk of breast cancer (18,19). These complex relationships must be taken into account in any analysis of the effect of Pill use on breast cancer risk. Paffenbarger and his colleagues (22) have attempted to do so, and their findings have been interesting, although conflicting. They noted that in young nulliparous women and in those who had used the Pill before their first childbirth (but not in those who had used the Pill after their first childbirth) there were increases in breast cancer risk. These findings may be chance observations—since many statistical tests were performed on one data set—but there is an urgent need for other investigators to carry out similar analyses. Other factors must also be taken into account: Family history of breast cancer is a powerful predictor of breast cancer risk, especially in the young (7); a history of previous breast surgery is as well (7,22,29). Both are likely to influence a woman's choice of contraception and may well confound comparisons of breast cancer risk in women who have and those who have not used the Pill. It is also possible that the Pill might affect the pre- and postmenopausal breast cancer risk in different ways. There is already considerable evidence that the etiology of pre- and postmenopausal breast cancer may differ (4,18,27,28).

Animal experiments have shown that oral contraceptives increase the risk of breast cancer. The two estrogens in oral contraceptives—ethinylestradiol and mestranol—both produce breast cancer in a wide range of animals, when given either alone or in combination with progestogens (1).

Because breast cancer risk is so closely linked with reproductive history and because reproductive history both influences and is influenced by Pill use, the sorting out of the relationship between Pill use and breast cancer will be an extremely difficult task indeed. But, because breast cancer is the most common cancer in women, it is vital that this issue be resolved.

ENDOMETRIAL CANCER

Estrogens

The findings of several case–control studies of the relationship between exogenous estrogen use and the risk of endometrial cancer are summarized in Table 4 (30–39). In general, a clear pattern emerges from these studies: The relative risk of endometrial cancer is increased in women who have used exogenous estrogen, the risk increasing with duration and dose of hormone use. This is particularly notable for studies carried out in 1975 or later. The only exception is the study by Wynder et al. (31). Horwitz and Feinstein (37) claim that their study showed no relationship between exogenous estrogen use and endometrial cancer risk, but this occurred only in comparisons with controls who were specifically chosen with diagnoses of estrogen-related disorders. When controls who were more representative of the general population were chosen, they observed a relative risk of 12.0 associated with exogenous estrogen use. The majority of studies reported a relationship of endometrial cancer with conjugated (natural) estrogen use because this is the type of estrogen that is widely used by menopausal women. But it does appear that other estrogens, including the synthetic diethylstilbestrol, also increase the risk of endometrial cancer (30,34,38,39).

Hulka et al. (40) have criticized the methodology used in the case-control studies. They argue that it is invalid to exclude from the controls women who have had a hysterectomy. Gray et al. (36) have, however, carried out a case-control study choosing controls from women undergoing hysterectomy, and their findings are essentially in agreement with that of other workers. Another criticism is that the incidence of endometrial cancer does not seem to be increasing in the United States. This criticism is not necessarily valid, as it must be remembered that the quality of incidence data is variable, and may change markedly over time. Even in the United Kingdom, where cancer registration is generally more advanced and more complete than in the United States, incomplete coverage may still limit the usefulness of registration data for monitoring disease trends (41). United States data may be similarly misleading. Second, even if estrogen therapy does increase the risk of endometrial cancer, it does not necessarily follow that the incidence of endometrial cancer must be increasing now. Other factors do affect endometrial cancer. It is possible that the incidence of endometrial cancer would have declined dramatically during the last decades for other reasons, and that the widespread use of exogenous estrogens has curbed that decline but has been insufficient to reverse the trend. Finally, two recent studies (39,42) have presented evidence suggesting that the incidence of endometrial cancer has, in fact, increased parallel to increasing estrogen use.

There has also been discussion of the biases inherent in the fact that women who are receiving estrogen therapy may be more likely than those who do not receive estrogen therapy to have endometrial cancer diagnosed. It is argued that this might be so because women receiving exogenous estrogens are especially likely to visit their doctors regularly, to complain of postmenopausal bleeding and to have endometrial biopsies taken. This process could result in overdiagnosis of endometrial cancer in women taking estrogens, only if a sizable proportion of endometrial biopsies yielded false positive results (43); there is little evidence to suggest that this is so. The women's increased contact with the medical profession is perhaps reflected in the observation that women taking estrogens have their endometrial cancers diagnosed at an earlier stage than do those not taking estrogens (35). Early diagnosis should not, however, be confused with diagnostic error, and it should not bias the association between endometrial cancer and estrogen use.

Several authors have reported on the occurrence of endometrial cancer in women who have taken exogenous estrogens and been followed for varying periods of time (8–11,44,45). Unfortunately, the majority of these studies are of little value in elucidating the effects of exogenous estrogen therapy on endometrial cancer risk; the ages of the women and the duration or completeness of follow-up are generally not specified. Thus, it is not possible to determine whether the incidence of endometrial cancer was higher, lower, or the same as would be expected in the general population. The results of the study by Cutler et al. (44), although suffering from some of these deficiencies, are nonetheless interesting. Among twenty-four patients with gonadal dysgenesis treated with stilbestrol for an average of 12.3 years, two (8%) and possibly three (13%) developed endometrial cancer. All these tumors developed in women under the age of 50 years, and in two, an uncommon type of tumor, an adenoacanthoma, was found. The high incidence of endometrial cancer at early ages, and the unusual histological type make it very likely that the malignancies were induced by hormone use. This is especially true given that endometrial cancer rarely occurs spontaneously in women with ovarian dysgenesis.

The cohort studies by Hoover et al. (45) and Bibbo et al. (8) are the only two that permit direct comparison between the incidence of endometrial cancer in groups who were and groups who were not given estrogen therapy. Their findings are contradictory. Hoover et al. reported an increased risk of endometrial cancer in women receiving estrogens, with the relative risk increasing with longer duration of follow-up. On the other hand, the study by

TABLE 4. Case-Control Studies of Endometrial Cancer and the Use of Exogenous Estrogens

Author and year of publication (reference)	Year(s) of diagnosis of endometrial carcinoma	Age range	Number of cases	Relative risk associated with estrogen use: Duration of use	Relative risk associated with estrogen use: Relative risk	Risk related to estrogen dose?
Jensen et al., 1954 (30)	1939–1952	31–80	105	6.5 (average)	1.9	Not specified
Wynder et al., 1966 (31)	1940–1964	All ages	112	Not specified	0.6	Not specified
Smith et al., 1975 (32)	1960–1972	48+	317	Not specified	4.5	Not specified
Ziel and Finkle, 1975 (33)	1940–1974	All ages	94	<5 years	5.6	Not specified
				5–6 years	7.2	
				7+ years	13.9	
Mack et al., 1976 (34)	1971–1975	All ages	63	<1 year	2.8	Yes
				1–4 years	4.5	
				5–6 years	9.3	
				7+ years	8.8	

McDonald et al., 1977 (35)	1945–1974	25+	145	6+ months	2.0	Yes
				3+ years	7.9	
Gray et al., 1977 (36)	1947–1976	All ages	205	<4 years	1.2	Yes
				5–9 years	4.1	Yes
				10+ years	11.6	
Horwitz et al., 1978 (37) (a)	1974–1976	All ages	119	Not specified	6.0 to 12.0[a]	Not specified
(b)	1974–1976	All ages	149	Not specified	1.7 to 2.3[a]	Not specified
Antunes et al., 1979 (38)	1973–1977	All ages	451	<1 year	2.2	Yes
				1–5 years	2.9	
				5+ years	15.0	
Jick et al., 1979 (39)	1975–1977	50–64	67	<9 years	6.6	Yes
				9+ years	20.5	

[a]Depending on choice of control group.

Bibbo and her colleagues, in which women were randomly allocated 25 years before into "diethylstilbestrol" and "nondiethylstilbestrol" groups showed, if anything, an excess of uterine cancers in the untreated group. However, a higher proportion of the "nondiethylstilbestrol" group had used exogenous estrogens for menopausal symptoms. Use of exogenous estrogens at that time might have a more important effect on endometrial cancer risk than its use at premenopausal ages.

Although there are some gaps in the evidence, it does seem that the risk of endometrial cancer is increased with exogenous estrogen use. Moreover, the kind of estrogen used—synthetic (such as diethylstilbestrol) or natural (such as the conjugated estrogens)—seems unrelated to the cancer risk. Thus, it would seem that the pathogenic mechanism is related to estrogenic stimulation rather than some carcinogenic property of specific synthetic or nonsynthetic estrogens. The consistency of the findings from various studies, the very high relative risks reported, and the observations that the risk increases with duration of estrogen use and dose of hormone, all argue strongly in favor of a causal relationship between exogenous estrogens and endometrial cancer. There is, as well, strong biologic evidence to support the association: estrogen use leads to endometrial hyperplasia (46) and endometrial hyperplasia is a recognized precursor of endometrial carcinoma. In addition, estrogen administration leads to endometrial cancer development in many animal species (1).

Progestogens

There have been no reports of the relationship of exogenous progestogen use to the development of endometrial cancer. Progestogens, particularly DMPA, have been used for palliative therapy in women with advanced endometrial cancer. Because it is effective, it has been predicted that progestogens may protect against endometrial cancer; but direct evidence for its protective role is lacking. In fact, animal experiments suggest that the reverse may be true. Rhesus monkeys treated with high doses of DMPA for long periods of time have an increased risk of developing endometrial cancer (47).

Oral Contraceptives

Because endometrial cancer is relatively rare at premenopausal ages, few studies have accumulated sufficient numbers of cases to permit conclusions about the relationship of oral contraceptive use and endometrial carcinoma. There have been four case reports of endometrial cancer in women taking oral contraceptives (48–51). These are summarized in Table 5. Unfortunately, the reports are of limited value in determining whether oral contraceptives have an etiologic relationship with endometrial cancer. Had there been some information about the numbers of cases of endometrial carcinoma occurring at the same time in women who were not using oral contraceptives, it might have been possible to draw some tentative conclusions. Despite these problems, the case reports do indicate that the different sorts of oral contraceptives may well have different effects on endometrial cancer risk. In particular, the sequential

TABLE 5. Case Reports of Endometrial Cancer and Oral Contraceptive Use

Author and year of publication (reference)	Number of cases	Oral contraceptive (OC) use: Type	Oral contraceptive (OC) use: Duration of use (average)
Lyon, 1975 (48)	4	All were using sequential OCs	7 years
Kelley et al., 1976 (49)	3	All were using sequential OCs	7 years
Cohen and Deppe, 1977 (50)	7	5 sequential OCs	11.7 years
		1 combined OCs	5 years
		1 premarin and provera	15 years
Silverberg et al., 1975 (51)	21	13 sequential OCs	
		7 combined OCs	Not specified
		1 type of OC unknown	

pills seem more likely to be associated with endometrial cancer than the combined pills. In the largest series of cases, reported in the World Health Organization (WHO) review (3), of the thirty cases of Pill-associated endometrial cancer, 90% were associated with the use of sequential pills; however, only 11% of oral contraceptive sales were of the sequential type. Furthermore, the cases associated with the use of sequential oral contraceptives tended to be in women who were at an otherwise low risk of endometrial cancer and in long-term users of the hormones.

As sequential contraceptives have, for other reasons, been withdrawn from the market, it might be argued that these observations are no longer of any practical importance. But this is not so for several reasons. First, it is not clear how long the differential endometrial cancer risk persists between users of the sequential and the combined types of oral contraceptives. It is possible that women who have used the sequential Pill might retain a relatively high risk throughout life. Thus, they may require special surveillance for endometrial cancer as they approach older ages when endometrial cancer occurs more frequently. Second, that endometrial cancer may occur in long-term users of estrogen–progestogen combinations is important when considering the use of estrogens by menopausal and postmenopausal women. These findings suggest that it may be simplistic to assume that if menopausal estrogen therapy increases the risk of endometrial cancer, combinations of estrogen and progestogen would not.

One case-control study has reported on the relationship of endometrial cancer and oral contraceptive use, but the numbers were too small for any clear relationship to be found. Kelsey et al. (23) reported thirteen cases of endometrial cancer at ages 20 to 44 years; four (31%) of the cases had used oral contraceptives compared with seven (54%) of the controls.

More time is required before the relationship of oral contraceptive use and endometrial cancer is clarified. In the meantime, it is reassuring to note that animal experiments have, in general, failed to show an increase in endometrial cancer risk following the administration of oral contraceptives.

CANCER OF THE UTERINE CERVIX

Estrogens

Lately there has been concern that young women who were exposed to estrogens in utero may be at an increased risk of developing cervical cancer. There is evidence that the risk of clear cell adenocarcinoma of the cervix is increased (52). Stafl and Mattingly (53,54) suggested that the risk of squamous cell carcinoma, which is more common than adenocarcinoma, may also be increased in women exposed to diethylstilbestrol (DES) in utero, although their findings have been disputed by others (55).

Nevertheless, there is evidence that women who were exposed to DES in utero do have an increased frequency of abnormal cervical cytological smears, indicative of squamous metaplasia. Bibbo and her colleagues (56) reported that mild cervical dysplasia was found in 4.5%, and moderate dysplasia in 1.8% of 229 women exposed to DES in utero, as compared with 2.3% mild dysplasia and 0% moderate dysplasia in 136 women not exposed to DES. The cervical smears were taken by gynecologists and the results recorded by cytologists who did not know whether the women had or had not been exposed to estrogens in utero. Furthermore, Lanier et al. (57) reported that in following up 818 women who had been exposed to DES in pregnancy and whose median age was 22 years, four had developed squamous-cell carcinoma of the cervix. Based on incidence data in the United States (58), only two cases would be expected.

Few studies have been done on the relationship between exogenous estrogen use in adult women and cervical cancer. The study by Bibbo et al. (8), in which 1,361 women had been randomly allocated to receive either diethylstilbestrol or a placebo during pregnancy, is interesting in this respect. After a 25-year follow-up, they noted that cervical cancer had occurred in seven (1.0%) of women exposed to DES, and three (0.4%) of those not exposed.

These findings do suggest that estrogen use by premenopausal women may increase the risk of developing cervical cancer. Moreover, animal experiments have shown that estrogens, given alone to newborn animals or to adults, increase the risk of cervical cancer in several animal species (1). Although it seems likely that sexual activity is a major determinant of cervical cancer in humans, clearly more information needs to be known about the effects of estrogen therapy on the development of cervical cancer.

Progestogens

Two studies suggest that the risk of abnormal cervical cytology or carcinoma in situ of the cervix is increased in women using DMPA (1,59). Another study in Chile found no difference in risk (60). These studies did not, however, take into account possible confounding factors.

Animal experiments have indicated that progestogens, when given alone, do not seem to increase the risk of cervical cancer (1). Data for DMPA are not available, however. It seems important to determine whether DMPA actually does increase the risk of cervical cancer in humans, as cervical cancer is frequent in many developing countries where there is widespread use of DMPA.

Oral Contraceptives

The findings of four case-control studies and four cohort studies that have examined the relationship between oral contraceptive use and cervical cancer are summarized in Tables 6 and 7, respectively (26,61–67). In these studies, "cases" of cervical cancer generally consist of in situ carcinoma or dysplasia; information on invasive cancer is lacking. However, about one tenth of untreated cases of in situ carcinoma may progress to invasive cancer (68), although it may take 10 years on the average for such progression to occur (69).

Studies of the relationship of oral contraceptive use and cervical cancer are beset with methodologic problems. Women who choose different methods of contraception may have differing risks of developing cervical cancer for reasons unrelated to the contraceptive method. Sexual activity, and particularly the number of sexual partners a women has had, is a powerful determinant of her risk of developing cervical cancer (69), and it is plausible that such factors might also influence the type of contraceptive used. Stern et al. (70) showed

TABLE 6. Case-Control Studies of Cervical Cancer and Oral Contraceptive Use

Author and year of publication (reference)	Year(s) of diagnosis of cervical cancer	Age range	Number of cases	Type of cancer	Relative risk associated with oral contraceptive use	
					Duration of use	Relative risk
Worth and Boyes, 1972 (61)	1969–1970	20–24	91	In situ	All	1.7
		25–29	219	In situ	All	1.0
Thomas, 1972 (62)	1965–1969	15–50	324	In situ and dysplasia	All	1.1
Boyce et al., 1977 (63)	1969–1975	15–50	689	In situ	All	1.0
Ory et al., 1977 (64)	1967–1972	15–44	147	In situ	≤1 year	1.3
					1–2 years	2.5
					2–3 years	2.6
					3+ years	4.7
			854	Dysplasia	≤1 year	1.2
					1–2 years	1.6
					2–3 years	1.9
					3+ years	1.6

TABLE 7. Cohort Studies of Cervical Cancer and Oral Contraceptives Use

Author and year of publication (reference)	Age range	Number of cases	Type of cancer	Relative risk associated with oral contraceptive (OC) use: Comparison group	Duration of OC use	Relative risk
Melamed and Flehinger, 1973 (65)	Not specified	30	In situ	Diaphragm users	All	1.5
		34	In situ	IUD users	All	0.8
Vessey et al., 1976 (26)	25–39	19*	In situ	IUD users	All	1.0
Peritz et al., 1977 (66)	18–58	35	In situ	Users of other methods of contraception	<2 years	2.4[b]
					2–4 years	3.0[b]
					4+ years	4.1[b]

[a]Total number of cases in OC and IUD users.
[b]Adjusted for age, education, marital status, number of Pap smears, and religion.

that women who chose to take the Pill during the early 1960s were more likely than IUD users to have an abnormal cervical smear, even before they began using the Pill. They also pointed out that, with the adverse publicity about the effects of oral contraceptives, this pattern was reversing for women who first chose to take the Pill during the late 1960s. Another problem with these studies relates to the fact that cervical dysplasia and carcinoma in situ are usually asymptomatic and detected by a routine Pap smear. The probability that an abnormal smear will be found varies considerably with the number of Pap smears a woman has: the more smears she has had in the past, the lower the probability of an abnormal one being found (69). Oral contraceptive use influences the number of Pap smears a woman has; in general, women taking the Pill tend to have more Pap smears than those who use other methods of contraception (24).

None of the studies reported thus far has taken into account all of the factors that might confound the relationship between oral contraceptive use and cervical cancer. The case-control studies of Thomas (62) and Boyce et al. (63) did record information on sexual activity but not on the number of previous Pap smears. On the other hand, the case-control studies of Ory et al. (64) and the cohort study of Peritz et al. (66) did account for the number of Pap smears, but neither study included detailed information on sexual activity. The case-control study of Worth et al. (61) and the cohort study by Vessey et al. (26) took neither into account.

In general, however, the findings from the studies do suggest that oral contraceptive use, particularly long-term use, may increase the risk of cervical cancer development. Most persuasive in this respect are the studies by Ory et al. (64) and Peritz et al. (66), both of which demonstrated a clear increase in the relative risk of cervical cancer with increasing duration of oral contraceptive use. Such findings cannot be readily ascribed to the indirect effects of confounding factors; it is unlikely that duration of oral contraceptive use is related to other factors that influence cervical cancer risk. Close inspection of the data from the case-control studies of Worth et al. (61) and Boyce et al (63), reveals an excess of long-duration oral contraceptive users among the cases. The differences are small and not statistically significant, but they are consistent with the observations of Ory et al. and Peritz et al. The only case-control study whose findings conflict with the others is the Thomas study (62). However, his cases were diagnosed between 1965 and 1969 and the average duration of oral contraceptive use was 20 months. His study may well have been performed too soon after the Pill was introduced to detect any effect that might have resulted from its use.

The cohort study by Stern et al. (67) was designed to answer the question: does oral contraceptive use influence the rate progression of cervical dysplasia to in situ carcinoma? Beginning with 300 women with dysplastic cervical lesions and 300 with normal cervical smears, Stern showed that, after 86 months, 30% of Pill users with dysplasia had progressed to in situ cancer, whereas 5% of those not using the Pill had shown a similar progression. Thus, oral contraceptives may accelerate the rate at which dysplasia progresses to in situ carcinoma of the cervix.

In conclusion, available evidence suggests that oral contraceptive use, especially over a long period of time, may increase the risk of cervical cancer. This relationship, which needs to be confirmed by carefully designed studies taking into account women's sexual activity as well as their contraceptive use, is generally consistent with the findings from animal experiments (1).

CHORIOCARCINOMA

Estrogens

It is unknown whether estrogens, when administered alone, may affect the development of choriocarcinoma or promote malignant change in a hydatidiform mole.

Progestogens

As with estrogens, it is unknown whether progestogens affect the development of choriocarcinoma or promote malignant change in a hydatidiform mole. In light of the evidence that oral contraceptives may promote malignant change in hydatidiform moles, discussed in the following section, it seems important to determine whether the same is true for progesterone-only contraceptives, especially DMPA. There are several reasons for concern about the role of progestogens in the induction of malignant change in the trophoblast. First, under normal conditions the survival of the trophoblast seems attributable to progesterone (71). Second, DMPA is widely used in developing countries, where the incidence of choriocarcinoma is relatively high (72). Progestogens are also the preferred form of hormonal contraception in the immediate post partum period because, in contrast to oral contraceptives, they appear not to suppress breast-milk production (73,74).

Oral Contraceptives

Stone and his colleagues (75) reported that the use of oral contraceptives by women after the evacuation of a hydatidiform mole appeared to have adverse effects on the subsequent development of trophoblastic tumors. Only 9% of the 464 women who were not taking oral contraceptives required subsequent cytotoxic drug therapy, whereas 25% of the 65 women taking oral contraceptives required the therapy. Moreover the study noted that oral contraceptive use delayed the fall in human chorionic gonadotropin (HCG) excretion in women who did not require cytotoxic drug therapy.

No information is available on whether hydatidiform mole or choriocarcinoma are more common in women who had used oral contraceptives or other hormones in the past. Clearly, this is an important question that needs to be answered, and it is particularly relevant for developing countries.

VAGINAL CANCER

Estrogens

In 1970, Herbst and Scully (76) reported that, between 1966 and 1969, seven girls aged 15 to 22 years with adenocarcinoma of the vagina had been seen at the Vincent Memorial Hospital, Boston. Because vaginal cancer is exceedingly rare and usually occurs in women over 50 years of age, Herbst and his colleagues set out to find an explanation for this unexpected cluster of vaginal cancer cases. In 1971, they reported the findings of a case-control study involving eight girls with vaginal cancer and 32 matched controls. They found that the mothers of seven out of the eight girls had taken DES during pregnancy, whereas none of the mothers of the thirty-two controls had taken this hormone (77). Since then, more than 100 cases of adenocarcinoma of the vagina in young women have been reported in the United States (52). About three-quarters of the women are known to have been exposed to estrogens in utero. The type of estrogen used was usually DES, but the occurrence of vaginal cancer has also been reported following in utero exposure to chemically related synthetic estrogens such as dienestrol and hexestrol, as well as exposure to estrone, a natural estrogen, and to progestational agents (52,78). All the women with adenocarcinoma of the vagina who were exposed to natural estrogens or progestational agents in utero, were also exposed to synthetic estrogens at the same time. As natural estrogens were rarely given alone as therapy during pregnancy (79,80), it is unwise to conclude at present that it is only synthetic estrogens that may predispose to the development of vaginal cancer. Animal experiments have indicated that newborns exposed to either synthetic or natural estrogens may develop vaginal cancer in later life (1).

The risk of developing vaginal (or cervical, see Cancer of the Uterine Cervix) adenocarcinoma after in utero exposure to estrogens is still not known with any precision. From the available evidence, Herbst and his colleagues (52) concluded that the peak incidence is between the ages of 14 to 19 years. They speculated that the onset of puberty may be related to tumor induction. They also estimated that the cumulative risk of developing the malignancy is between 0.14 and 1.4 per 1,000 women exposed to estrogens. That the risk is of this magnitude is supported by three follow-up studies of women exposed to estrogens in utero: in one study (57) 818 women were followed, in another (81) 110, and in the third (56) 229. None of those studies identified a woman with vaginal cancer.

Finally, despite the considerable evidence indicating that vaginal cancer in young women can arise as a consequence of estrogen exposure in utero, there have been no reports suggesting that estrogen use in later life may predispose to the development of vaginal cancer. Nor do estrogens appear to induce vaginal cancer when given to adult animals either orally or by injection or subcutaneous implantation (1). When implanted intravaginally, however, vaginal cancers have been induced with the three estrogens—stilbestrol, estrone and estradiol—that have been tested (1).

Progestogens

There have been no reports suggesting that exposure to progestogens alone, either while in utero, or in later life, may affect the risk of vaginal cancer in humans. No animal experiments have been reported which investigated the potential carcinogenic effects of in utero exposure to progestogens alone.

Oral Contraceptives

No reports have appeared suggesting that oral contraceptive use may affect the risk of vaginal cancer. Nor is there any evidence that animals exposed to high doses of oral contraceptives develop vaginal cancer (1). The effects of oral contraceptive use during pregnancy, i.e., of in utero exposure to oral contraceptives, has not yet been investigated. Nor have any experiments been reported where animals were exposed to oral contraceptives in utero or soon after birth (1).

OVARIAN CANCER

Estrogens

One report has suggested that women who have taken conjugated estrogens or DES may have an increased risk of developing ovarian cancer (82). However, in three other studies no association was found (83–85). There are certain methodological problems, in the study that noted a positive association between estrogen use and ovarian cancer: The findings were based on small numbers—eight cases observed and three expected; the expected number of cases was calculated from U.S. cancer registry data and only women with at least one ovary were considered to be at risk of developing ovarian cancer. Annegers et al. (85) pointed out that the U.S. cancer incidence figures included women with no ovaries, and that, as a result, the expected number of cases of ovarian cancer in the study population was underestimated. Moreover, the study population included white women only, but the expected number of cases was calculated from rates in the general U.S. population, including both white and nonwhite women, after 1950. White women have higher rates of ovarian cancer than nonwhites (86), a finding that would further tend to underestimate the expected number of cases in the study population. Although these errors would lead to relatively small changes in the "expected" number of cases (87), because of the small numbers involved, it may substantially reduce the estimated relative risk. Finally, it is not clear whether the authors distinguished between women who received estrogens for menopausal symptoms, and those who recieved the therapy for conditions that may be linked to ovarian cancer or for other reasons.

Animal experiments have indicated that estrogens may increase the risk of ovarian cancer (1). Thus, such a relationship in humans is plausible, but the evidence must at this stage be regarded as uncertain.

Progestogens

There have been no suggestions that the use of progestogenic substances may increase or decrease the risk of ovarian cancer in humans. In animal experiments certain progestogens, such as progesterone, norethisterone, and norethisterone acetate, were found to increase the risk of ovarian cancer, but the majority of progestogens tested did not (1).

Oral Contraceptives

One case-control study, by Newhouse and her colleagues (88), has examined the relationship between oral contraceptive use and ovarian cancer. It suggested that oral contraceptive use reduced the risk of ovarian cancer, and that the apparent protection was greater the longer the duration of Pill use and was independent of parity (89). This finding is consistent with what is known about the pathogenesis of ovarian cancer, since it is likely that the cyclic stimulation of the ovary associated with ovulation enhances the development of ovarian cancer (90,91). The Pill, which suppresses ovulation, may therefore, for physiological reasons, reduce ovarian cancer risk. However it is difficult to determine whether it also has some direct carcinogenic effect on the ovaries. If, for example, the Pill is taken by postmenopausal women, whose ovaries do not undergo cyclical changes, it might well have a different effect on ovarian cancer risk than it has when taken by premenopausal women.

The combined Pill has been shown to have no apparent effect on the risk of ovarian cancer in various animal species (1). As the pattern of ovulation is not the same in humans as in animals, this observation is probably of little relevance for humans. Nevertheless, it may indicate that oral contraceptives have no intrinsic carcinogenic effect on the ovaries.

MALIGNANT MELANOMA

Estrogens

Data from a prospective study in Walnut Creek, California, have suggested that the incidence of malignant melanoma may be increased among women using estrogens for menopausal symptoms (92). But this observation was based on a small number of cases and needs to be confirmed elsewhere.

Follow-up studies of women with ovarian dysgenesis have indicated that there may be an increased risk of malignant melanoma among them (93). The usual treatment of this condition includes the administration of high doses of estrogens to induce female secondary sexual characteristics. The high rate of endometrial cancer in women with ovarian dysgenesis has been attributed to estrogen use (44), and it is possible that the melanomas are also attributable to estrogen use. That estrogen use should increase the incidence of malignant melanoma is biologically plausible, as it has been shown in animals that estrogen is an important stimulant of melanogenesis (94).

Progestogens

The possibility that progestogens, when taken alone, alter the risk of malignant melanoma has not been investigated.

Oral Contraceptives

The findings from a study in Walnut Creek, California, suggest that oral contraceptive use may be associated with an increased risk of malignant melanoma. In that study risk increased with increasing duration of oral contraceptive use (92). Moreover, a small case-control study also indicated that oral contraceptive use was associated with an increased risk of malignant melanoma, the overall relative risk being estimated at 1.8 (92). Because the number of cases was small, and no information was available about exposure to sunlight, it is difficult to exclude the possibility that the association is indirect, as women who take oral contraceptives may be particularly likely to be exposed to sunlight.

Harlap (95) reported that babies born to mothers who had taken oral contraceptives had a twofold increase in pigmented skin lesions when compared with controls. In this context, in following 818 girls exposed to estrogens in utero, Lanier and her colleagues (57) noted that one girl had developed an "amelanotic melanoma" during the follow-up period.

With animal experiments indicating that estrogen-progestogen combinations are more powerful stimulants of melanogenesis than estrogens alone (94), these findings are a cause for some concern. There is clearly a need to know more about the effects of oral contraceptive use on melanoma risk, not only for women using the Pill, but also for their children.

HEPATIC TUMORS

Benign Hepatic Tumors

Estrogens. Occasional reports have appeared of hepatic tumors occurring in women who have taken exogenous estrogens (96), but they have been considerably less frequent than those relating to oral contraceptive use (See Below). Animal experiments have demonstrated that estrogens when given alone rarely lead to an increased incidence of hepatic tumors (1,97).

Progestogens. There have been no reports of hepatic tumors occurring in women who have been exposed to progestogens alone. On the other hand, animal experiments indicate that the administration of certain (but not all) progestogens may lead to an increased incidence of benign hepatic tumors (1). It thus seems important that the role of progestogens in the development of benign hepatic tumors in humans be investigated more fully.

Oral Contraceptives. In 1973 Baum (98) suggested that oral contraceptive use might predispose to the development of benign hepatic adenomas. She noted that seven cases of benign liver adenoma had occurred in the Ann Arbor region of Michigan during the previous 5 years, although the tumor was generally regarded as being very rare. Moreover, all the tumors were in young women taking oral contraceptives. After her findings were published, there followed numerous reports of similar instances of benign liver tumors occurring in women using oral contraceptives. By 1978 more than 200 cases had been reported, the large majority from the United States (2,99–101). Two case-control studies have been carried out (102,103) both showing very large relative risks of benign liver disease in women using oral contraceptives, with the risk increasing with increasing duration of Pill use. These will be discussed in detail later.

There appears to be some uncertainty about the nomenclature of these benign liver tumors. Three types of tumors have been described in association with oral contraceptives: hepatocellular adenoma, focal nodular hyperplasia, and hamartoma (99). It is not clear, however, whether these represent different histological types, or different names given to tumors of similar appearance. Vana (99) noted that the prevalence of oral contraceptive use was high in association with each reported tumor type: in 87% of 82 reported cases of hepatocellular adenoma; in 84% of 51 reported cases of focal nodular hyperplasia; and in 52% of 25 reported cases of hamartoma. (These percentages are based on those cases for whom the history of oral contraceptive use was known.)

There is general agreement that the tumors are highly vascular. Between 10% and 25% are diagnosed when the tumor ruptures and bleeds into the intraabdominal cavity (102,103); others present as abdominal masses with pain or are found incidentally. In recent years, an increasing proportion of these tumors are being found incidentally; focul nodular hyperplasia is particularly liable to be diagnosed in this way (96). The tumors are generally single but may also be multiple (102,104).

Although the tumors are "benign," there is a considerable mortality associated with them. About 10% are fatal, usually as a result of massive intraperitoneal hemorrhage (99,102,103). Rupture of the tumors seems to be associated with the onset of menstruation (99), suggesting that the blood vessels of the tumors are under hormonal control.

Two case-control studies have reported on the relative risk of benign liver tumors in women taking oral contraceptives (102,103). Both noted an excess of oral contraceptive use among those with hepatic tumors, with the relative risk increasing markedly with increasing duration of oral contraceptive use. A study in California by Edmondson et al. (102) reported a 25-fold increase in risk associated with oral contraceptive use for 9 years or more; whereas the CDC/AFIP study (100) found a 500-fold increase in risk associated with oral contraceptive use of 8 years or longer. The greater risk noted in the CDC/AFIP study may be explained by the fact that the cases included in that study were diagnosed more recently than those in the California study; alternatively, the method of selection of controls may account for the difference. In the CDC/AFIP study, neighborhood controls were chosen by sampling from neighboring households, whereas in the California study the controls were friends of the case. The latter method of selecting controls may result in "overmatching," because a woman is more likely to have more habits similar to her friend than to other women living in the same area. This would lead to an underestimation of the relative risk.

The size of the attributable risk of hepatocellular adenoma in women under 30 years of age taking oral contraceptives is estimated to be 3 per 100,000 women per year, regardless of length of oral contraceptive use (3). It is probably greater for older women, although no risk estimates are available. These estimates are based on U.S. data; the risks might be lower in the United Kingdom. Neither of the two large cohort studies in the United Kingdom (which together include about 200,000 women-years of observation) of women taking oral contraceptives has yet recorded a single case of liver-cell adenoma; six cases might have been expected, based on U.S. data (105). Although this might be a chance finding, it is possible that the risks are lower in the United Kingdom than in the United States. Other forms of liver disease, particularly cirrhosis, are more common in the United States than in the United Kingdom (106). This may well be related to the greater consumption of alcohol by women in the United States. It might also be that other factors such as alcohol consumption predispose the liver to adverse effects of oral contraceptives.

Animal experiments have yielded conflicting findings about the development of benign tumors after oral contraceptive administration. In 1966, Bosner reported to the Committee on Safety of Medicines that oral contraceptives, and particularly the long term use of mestranol-containing compounds, might increase the risk of hepatic tumors in animals; but her findings were not confirmed in further studies reported by the Committee in 1972 (97). It is ironic that less than a year after the Committee concluded that there was no evidence to support previous work incriminating oral contraceptives in the development of hepatic tumors, there followed increasing numbers of reports of hepatic tumors occurring in women who had taken oral contraceptives for long periods of time (98).

Androgens

Reports of benign hepatomas occurring in patients treated with androgens are surprisingly common, considering the rarity of androgen use in the population. In 1960, Kintzen and Silny (107) reported vascular liver infiltration following treatment of a patient with fluoxymesterone. In 1972, Bernstein and his colleagues (108) reported multiple vascular hepatomas in a male with Fanconi's anemia who had been treated with oxymetholine. Since then there have been several reports of hepatic nodules occurring after androgen therapy

(109), but those reports are less frequent than those of hepatic carcinoma following androgen therapy. Westby and his colleagues (11) examined 60 patients who were receiving long-term therapy with methyltestosterone for a variety of medical indications. The majority had abnormal liver scans and one patient was found to have an asymptomatic adenoma.

Animal experiments have indicated that androgens increase the risk of developing benign liver tumors (1).

Malignant Hepatic Tumors

Estrogens. Malignant liver tumors developing after long-term therapy with estrogens have been sporadically reported (101,111). One of the reports was of liver cell carcinoma in a 30-year-old woman "treated for infertility with varying doses of drugs with estrogenic activity" (111). The only drug specifically mentioned was clomisphene.

In the light of frequent reports of liver cell carcinoma following oral contraceptive or androgen therapy (discussed below) and the widespread use of postmenopausal estrogens, it is curious that there have been so few reports even if the relationship were coincidental. It is therefore tempting to conclude that estrogen therapy is unlikely to predispose to hepatic carcinomas. Moreover, animal experiments indicate that when estrogen is given alone it uncommonly causes an increase in hepatoma development (1).

Progestogens. No case reports have appeared of malignant liver tumors occurring in association with progestogen therapy, either in the form of the progestogen-only oral contraceptives or as an injectable contraceptive. If we consider the relative rarity of use of these hormones in Western countries, this is not unexpected. However, the lack of such reports does not necessarily mean that an association does not exist. Animal experiments suggest that progestational substances may well be carcinogenic to the liver (1).

As injectable contraceptives are widely used in developing countries where liver tumors are more common than in the developed countries, it seems important to determine whether progestational substances do increase the risk of hepatic malignancies.

Oral Contraceptives. Since the suggestion by Baum and her colleagues (98) of the possible relationship of benign liver tumors to oral contraceptive use, several reports have appeared of hepatocellular carcinoma in women taking oral contraceptives (101,112–120). In general, the cases tend to have occurred in young women, with relatively short durations of oral contraceptive use. This would seem to argue against a causal relationship, particularly as benign liver tumors associated with oral contraceptive use tend to occur after 5 or more years of Pill use (102,103). Thus it is possible that the reported associations are coincidental. However, Davies and his colleagues (114) reported malignant transformation in a benign tumor where the histological changes resembled those associated with Pill use. Moreover, the tumors are generally atypical. It might be expected that the large majority would develop in the presence of preexisting cirrhosis, but this is rarely the case; also the majority of tumors are not associated with elevations of serum α-fetoprotein.

In the report by Vana (99) of liver tumors occurring in women under the age of 45 years, 54% of women with malignant liver tumors were oral contraceptive users (excluding those whose history of oral contraceptive use was unknown). Although this proportion was less than the 78% of oral contraceptive users noted for women with benign tumors, the percentage is likely to be greater than would be expected among women of a similar age in the United States, particularly as the women with malignant liver tumors were considerably older than those with benign liver tumors (121). In addition, their average duration of oral contraceptive use was longer than for women with benign tumors.

It would therefore seem possible that oral contraceptive use predisposes to the development of hepatocellular carcinoma. Indeed, results from animal experiments, although somewhat contradictory, seem to support such an association (1). Clearly, case-control studies in human populations need to be carried out so that the relationship can be examined in detail.

Androgens. Eight cases of malignant hepatoma following androgen therapy have been reported. Johnson and his colleagues (122) reported four patients treated with androgenic or anabolic steroids for periods varying from 2 to 7 years who developed malignant disease of the liver. They included a 2.5 year-old girl treated with oxmetholone for 46 months for aplastic anemia; a 17-year-old female treated for 28 months with oxymetholone for aplastic anemia; a 27-year-old male treated with methyltestosterone for 40 months and testosterone enanthate for 10 months for Fanconi's anemia, and a 21-year-old male treated with methandienone for 89 months for Fanconi's syndrome. Guy and Anslander (123) reported another case of hepatocellular carcinoma in a 38-year-old male with Fanconi's syndrome, but because of the short duration of treatment with anabolic steroids they suggested that the carcinoma was a complication of Fanconi's syndrome, rather than of the anabolic steroid therapy. Since then, there have been three further case reports of hepatocellular carcinoma associated with androgen therapy for paroxysmal nocturnal hematuria, hypopituitarism, and cryptorchidism, respectively (124). Antony (125) has criticized these reports by suggesting that histological evidence of carcinoma is generally lacking and that the relatively benign course of the disease and normal α-fetoprotein estimations in these cases indicate that they may not be malignant. Although these criticisms are valid, it is possible that the hepatocellular carcinomas are indeed atypical, and that the associations found with the more usual forms of hepatocellular adenoma do not apply in these circumstances.

Considering the relative rarity of the use of androgens (compared, for example, with the widespread use of estrogens and oral contraceptives), the frequency of the case reports of malignant liver tumors after androgen therapy should not be ignored. Case control studies and further prospective studies of the type described by Westaby and his colleagues (110), are required to evaluate the risk of the development of liver tumors in patients receiving androgen therapy.

PITUITARY TUMORS

Estrogens

So far there have been no reports suggesting that the use of exogenous estrogens may affect the risk of pituitary tumors in humans. In contrast, animal studies indicate that almost all estrogenic substances which have been tested may induce pituitary hypertrophy or pituitary adenomas (1).

Progestogens

No reports have appeared suggesting that the use of exogenous progestogens may affect the risk of pituitary tumors in humans. Animal experiments indicate that some, but not all, progestogens when given alone may induce pituitary tumors (1). No information was available for DMPA or dimethisterone.

Oral Contraceptives

Clinicians have for some time been impressed by the apparent increase in the incidence of pituitary adenoma among women of childbearing age (126,127). Recently their suspicions have been confirmed. Annegers and his colleagues (128) at the Mayo Clinic reported that the mean annual incidence of pituitary tumors in Olmstead county, Minnesota, increased from 1.7 per 100,000 women aged 15–44 in 1935–1969, to 7.1 per 100,000 women in 1970–1977. At the same time the incidence rate in men and in women aged 45 years and older remained relatively stable.

The reason for the fourfold increase in incidence of pituitary tumors in young women remains elusive. Several authors have suggested that oral contraceptive use by young women is responsible for the increased incidence. Chang and his colleagues in California (126) reported the findings relating to 35 women who were thought to have pituitary adenoma. At operation, 13 of these were found to have macroscopic pituitary adenomas and 12 to have microscopic tumors; 89% of those with macroscopic tumors and 71% of those with microscopic tumors had used oral contraceptives in the past. These proportions are higher than the proportion of women aged 15–44 in California who have ever used oral contraceptives (129). Gomez and his colleagues in Canada (130) reported 17 pituitary tumors among women with galactorrhea or hyperprolactinemia. In 7 (i.e., 41%) of these, the galactorrhea was precipitated by oral contraceptive use. Unfortunately they do not state the proportion of women who had ever used oral contraceptives. Finally, Sherman and his colleagues in Ohio (127) reported that 74% of women with histologically verified pituitary adenomas had taken oral contraceptives in the past. These studies indicate that the proportion of women who have used oral contraceptives is indeed high among women with pituitary tumors, and, further, that the proportion is probably greater than would be expected among women of a similar age in the general population. However, Annegers and his colleagues (128) argue that oral contraceptive use cannot explain the recent increase in pituitary adenoma. Referring to a case-control study that they have performed but that has not yet been published, they quote a relative risk of 0.5 (with 95%

confidence limits of 0.1–2.2) for pituitary tumors associated with oral contraceptive use. They suggest instead that improvements in diagnostic techniques and advances in the investigation of infertility may explain the increase in pituitary adenomas in young women.

In the light of the findings of other authors, the low relative risk of pituitary tumors associated with oral contraceptive use found by the group from the Mayo Clinic is somewhat surprising. Of course, since it is the only case–control study of pituitary adenoma and oral contraceptive use reported so far, the study is extremely important. Unfortunately, it is not possible to comment on it at this stage, because details of the study have not yet been published. However, a case-control approach is a particularly difficult method for investigating the relationship between oral contraceptive use and pituitary adenoma because extraneous factors, such as the presence of infertility or subfertility, are closely related to pituitary tumors and also influence the choice of contraceptive method. In addition, pituitary tumors may appear in the immediate postpartum period (127,130), when it is unlikely that a woman would be using any form of contraception. Unless care is taken to match or adjust for such factors, spurious associations may well be found. In general, the relationship between oral contraceptive use and pituitary tumors is best investigated in a prospective study, but as yet no prospective studies have reported on the occurrence of pituitary tumors. The annual incidence of pituitary adenoma in women of childbearing age is estimated to be 7.1 per 100,000 women (128); thus, the cohort studies in progress should eventually accumulate sufficient numbers of cases to examine this question.

At this stage it is not possible to draw firm conclusions. However, the circumstantial evidence that oral contraceptive use may increase the risk of pituitary adenoma cannot be ignored. It is well recognized that oral contraceptive use alters pituitary function markedly and that it increases prolactin production (131). Also, post-Pill amenorrhea with or without galactorrhea is frequently reported and is the most frequent presenting syndrome of secondary amenorrhea (132). Its temporal relationship with cessation of oral contraceptive use makes the syndrome unlikely to be a chance association (133). Of those with post-Pill galactorrhea and amenorrhea, between 15% (132) to 32% (134) are associated with a pituitary adenoma. Thus, the links between the Pill use, prolactin hypersecretion, amenorrhea, galactorrhea, and pituitary tumors, are biologically plausible and are commonly observed clinically. Furthermore, animal studies have indicated that the majority of estrogen–progestogen combinations tested have induced pituitary tumors (1). More definitive studies are still required to elucidate the nature of this relationship in humans.

CONCLUSIONS

The effect of exogenous hormones on the development of cancer is a controversial issue. New information on this subject is accumulating week by week. By the time this review is published, several of the findings described here may already have been superseded by more up-to-date and reliable observations.

A large expansion in the use of female hormones occurred during the mid-1960s. Assuming a lag of 15 years or more before any carcinoengenic effects of these hormones would become apparent (as available evidence suggests), the related cancers would not occur until 1980 or later. Studies conducted during the next decade may well detect cancer risks that were not yet apparent in the surveys reported here. Thus, the next 10 years will be particularly important in evaluating the risk of cancer associated with hormone use.

ACKNOWLEDGMENTS

I am grateful to Nicola Robinson for helping in the collection of literature for this report; to Patricia Fraser, Clair Chilvers, and Paul Fine for their useful comments in the preparation of the manuscript; and to Audrone Hodgson for typing it.

REFERENCES

1. IARC Working Group on the Evaluation of Carcinogenic Risk of Chemicals to Man (1974) Sex Hormones. International Agency for Research on Cancer, Lyon.
2. Hertz, R. (1968) Experimental and clinical aspects of the carcinogenic potential of steriod contraceptives. Int. J. Fert. 13, 273–286.
3. World Health Organization (1978) Steroid Contraception and the Risk of Neoplasia. Technical Report Series 619, World Health Organization, Geneva.
4. Craig, T. J., Comstock, G. W., and Geiser, P. B. (1974) Epidemiologic comparison of breast cancer patients with early and late onset of malignancy and general population controls. J. Natl. Cancer Inst. 53, 1577–1581.
5. Casagrande, J., Gerkins, V., Henderson, B. E., Mack, T., Pike, M. C. (1976) Brief communication: Exogenous estrogens and breast cancer in women with natural menopause. J. Natl. Cancer Inst. 56, 839–841.
6. Sartwell, P. E., Arthes, F. G., Tonascia, J. A. (1977) Exogenous hormones, reproductive history, and breast cancer. J. Natl. Cancer Inst. 59, 1589–1592.
7. Henderson, B. E., Powell, D., Rosario, I., Keys, C., Hanish, R., Young, M., Casagrande, J., Gerkins, V., Pike, M.C. (1974) An epidemiologic study of breast cancer. J. Natl. Cancer Inst. 53, 609–614.
8. Bibbo, M., Haenszel, W. M., Wied, G. L., Hubby, M., Herbst, A. L. (1978) A twenty-five year follow-up study of women exposed to diethylstilbestrol during pregnancy. N. Engl. J. Med. 298, 763–767.
9. Wallach, S., Henneman, P. H. (1959) Prolonged estrogen therapy in postmenopausal women. J. Am. Med. Assoc. 171, 1637–1642.
10. Wilson, R. A. (1962) The roles of estrogen and progesterone in breast and genital cancer. J. Am. Med. Assoc. 182, 327–331.
11. Leis, H. P. Jr. (1966) Endocrine prophylaxis of breast cancer with cyclic estrogen and progesterone. Int. Surg. 45, 496–503.
12. Burch, J. C., Byrd, B. F., Jr. (1971) Effects of long-term administration of estrogen on the occurrence of mammary cancer in women. Annals Surg. 174, 414–418.
13. Burch, J. C., Byrd, B. F., Jr., Vaughn, W. K. (1974) The effects of long-term estrogen on hysterectomized women. Am. J. Obstet. Gynecol. 118, 778–782.
14. Hoover, R., Gray, L. A., Cole, P., MacMahon, B. (1976) Menopausal estrogens and breast cancer. N. Eng. J. Med. 295, 401–405.
15. Symmers, W. St. C. (1968) Carcinoma of breast in trans-sexual individuals after surgical and hormonal interference with primary and secondary sex characteristics. Br. Med. J. 2, 83–85.

16. O'Grady, W. P., McDivitt, R. W. (1969) Breast cancer in a man treated with diethylstilbestrol. Arch. Pathol. 88, 162–165.
17. Benson, W. R. (1957) Carcinoma of the prostate with metastases to breasts and testis. Cancer 10, 1235–1245.
18. Lilienfeld, A. M. (1956) The relationship of cancer of the female breast to artificial menopause and marital status. Cancer 9, 927–934.
19. MacMahon, B., Cole, P. and Brown J. (1973) Etiology of human breast cancer: a review. J. Natl. Cancer Inst. 50, 21–42.
20. Boston Collaborative Drug Surveillance Program (1973) Oral contraceptives and venous thromboembolic disease surgically confirmed, gall-bladder disease, and breast tumors. Lancet 1, 1399–1401.
21. Vessey, M. P., Doll, R., Jones, K. (1975) Oral contraceptives and breast cancer: Progress report of an epidemiological study. Lancet 1, 941–944.
22. Paffenbarger, R. S. Jr., Fasal, E., Simmons, M. E., Kampert, J. B. (1977) Cancer risk as related to use of oral contraceptives during fertile years. Cancer 39, 1887–1891.
23. Kelsey, J. L., Holford, T. R., White, C., Mayer, E. S., Kilty, S. E., Acheson, R. M. (1978) Oral contraceptives and breast disease: an epidemiological study. Am. J. Epidemiol. 107, 236–244.
24. Royal College of General Practitioners (1974) Oral Contraception and Health. London: Pitman Medical.
25. Ory, H., Cole, P., MacMahon, B., Hoover, R. (1976) Oral contraceptives and reduced risk of benign breast diseases. N. Engl. J. Med. 294, 419–422.
26. Vessey, M. P., Doll, R., Peto, R., Johnson, B., Wiggins, P. (1976) A long-term follow-up study of women using different methods of contraceptive—an interim report. J. Biosoc. Sci. 8, 373–427.
27. DeWaard, F. (1969) The epidemiology of breast cancer: review and prospects. Int. J. Cancer 4, 577–586.
28. Hems, G. (1970) Epidemiological characteristics of breast cancer in middle and late age. Br. J. Cancer 24, 226–234.
29. Fasal, E. and Paffenbarger, R. S., Jr. (1975) Oral contraceptives as related to cancer and benign lesions of the breast. J. Natl. Cancer Inst. 55, 767–773.
30. Jensen, E. K., Denmark, V., Ostergaard, E. (1954) Clinical studies concerning the relationship of estrogens to the development of cancer of the corpus uteri. Am. J. Obstet. Gynecol. 67, 1094–1102.
31. Wynder, E. L., Escher, G. C., Mantel, N. (1966) An epidemiological investigation of cancer of the endometrium. Cancer 19, 489–520.
32. Smith, D. C., Prentice, R., Thompson, D. J., Herrmann, W. L. (1975) Association of exogenous estrogen and endometrial carcinoma. N. Engl. J. Med. 293, 1164–1167.
33. Zeil, H. K., Finkle, W. D. (1975) Increased risk of endometrial carcinoma among users of conjugated estrogens. N. Engl. J. Med. 293, 1167–1170.
34. Mack, T., Pike, M., Henderson, B. D., Pfeffer, R. I., Gerkins, V. R., Arthur, M., Brown, S. (1976) Estrogens and endometrial cancer in a retirement community. N. Engl. J. Med. 294, 1262–1267.
35. McDonald, T. W., Annegers, J. F., O'Fallon, W. M., Dockerty, M. B., Malkasian, G. A., Kurland, L. T. (1977) Exogenous estrogen and endometrial carcinoma: Case-control and incidence study. Am. J. Obstet. Gynecol. 127, 572–580.
36. Gray, L. A., Christopherson, W. M., Hoover, R. N. (1977) Estrogens and endometrial carcinoma. Obstet. Gynecol. 49, 385–389.
37. Horwitz, R., Feinstein, A. (1978) Alternative analytic methods for case-control studies of estrogens and endometrial cancer. N. Engl. J. Med. 299, 1089–1094.
38. Antunes, C. M. F., Stolley, P. D., Rosenshein, N. B., Daveis, J. L., Tonascia, J. A., Brown, C., Burnett, L., Rutledge, A., Pokempner, M., Garcia, R. Endometrial cancer and estrogen use. N. Engl. J. Med. 300, 9–13.
39. Jick, H., Watkins, R. N., Hunter, J. R., Dinan, B. J., Madsen, S., Rothman, K. J.,

Walker, A. M. (1979) Replacement estrogens and endometrial cancer. N. Engl. J. Med. 300, 218–222.

40. Hulka, B. A., Hogue, C. J. R., Greenberg, B. G. (1978) Methodologic issues in epidemiologic studies of endometrial cancer and exogenous estrogen. Am. J. Epidemiol. 107, 267–276.

41. Fraser, P., Beral, V., Chilvers, C. (1978) Monitoring disease in England and Wales: methods applicable to routine data-collecting systems. J. Epidemiol. Comm. Health 32, 294–302.

42. Weiss, N., Szekely, D. R., Austin, D. F. (1976) Increasing incidence of endometrial cancer in the U.S. N. Engl. J. Med. 294, 1259–1262.

43. Hutchinson, G. B., Rothman, K. J. (1978) Correcting a bias? N. Engl. Med. J. 299, 1129–1130.

44. Cutler, B. S., Forbes, A. P., Scully, R. E. (1972) Endometrial carcinoma after stilbestrol therapy in gonadal dysgenesis. N. Engl. J. Med. 287, 628–631.

45. Hoover, R., Fraumeni, J. F., Everson, R., Myers, M. H. (1974) Cancer of the uterine corpus after hormonal treatment for breast cancer. Lancet 1, 885–887.

46. Gusberg, S. B. (1976) The individual at high risk for endometrial carcinoma. Am. J. Obstet. Gynecol. 126, 535–542.

47. Upjohn Company (1979) Evidence submitted to the FDA.

48. Lynon, F. (1975) The development of adenocarcinoma of the endometrium in young women receiving long-term sequential oral contraceptives. Am. J. Obstet. Gynecol. 123, 299–301.

49. Kelley, H. W., Miles, P. A., Buster, J. E., Scragg, W. H. (1976) Adenocarcinoma of the endometrium in women taking sequential oral contraceptives. Obstet. Gynecol. 47, 200–202.

50. Cohen, C. J., Deppe, G. (1977) Endometrial carcinoma and oral contraceptive agents. Obstet. Gynecol. 49, 390–392.

51. Silverberg, S. G., Makowski, E. L. (1975) Endometrial carcinoma in young women taking oral contraceptive agents. Obstet. Gynecol. 46, 503–506.

52. Herbst, A. L., Cole, P., Colton, T., Robboy, S. J., Scully, R. E. (1977) Age-incidence and risk of diethylstilbestrol-related clear cell adenocarcinoma of the vagina and cervix. Am. J. Obstet. Gynecol. 128, 43–50.

53. Stafl, A., Mattingly, R. F. (1974) Vaginal adenosis: a precancerous lesion? Am. J. Obstet. Gynecol. 120, 666–677.

54. Mattingly, R. F., Stafl, A. (1976) Cancer risk in diethylstilbestrol exposed offspring. Am. J. Obstet. Gynecol. 126, 543–548.

55. Robboy, S. J., Prat, J., Welch, W. R., Barnes, A. B. (1977) Squamous cell neoplasia controversy in the female exposed to diethylstilbestrol. Human Pathol. 8, 483–485.

56. Bibbo, M., Gill, W. B., Azizi, F., Blough, R., Fang, V. S., Rosenfield, R. L., Schumacher, G. F. B., Sleeper, K., Sonek, M. G., Wied, G. L. (1977) Follow-up study of male and female offspring of DES-exposed mothers. Obstet. Gynecol. 49, 1–8.

57. Lanier, A. P., Noller, K. L., Decker, D. G., Elveback, L. R., Kurland, L. T. (1973) Cancer and stilbestrol: a follow-up of 1,719 persons exposed to estrogens in utero and born 1943–1959. Mayo Clinic Proceedings 48, 793–799.

58. Cramer, D. W. (1974) The role of cervical cytology in the declining morbidity and mortality of cervical cancer. Cancer 34, 2018–2027.

59. Powell, L. C., Seymour, R. G. (1971) Effects of depo-medroxyprogesterone acetate as a contraceptive agent. Am. J. Obstet. Gynecol. 110, 36–41.

60. Dabancens, A., Prado, R., Larraguibel, R., Zanartu, J. (1974) Intraepithelial cervical neoplasia in women using intrauterine devices and long-acting injectable progestrogens as contraceptives. Am. J. Obstet. Gynecol. 119, 1052–1056.

61. Worth, A. J., Boyes, D. A. (1972) A case control study into the possible effects of birth control pills on pre-clinical carcinoma of the cervix. J. Obstet. Gynaec. Brt. Commonwealth 79, 673–679.

62. Thomas, D. B. (1972) Relationship of oral contraceptives to cervical carcinogenesis. Obstet. Gynecol. 40, 508–518.
63. Boyce, J. G., Lu, T., Nelson, J. H., Fruchtner, R. G. (1977) Oral contraceptives and cervical carcinoma. Am. J. Obstet. Gynecol. 128, 761–766.
64. Ory, H. W., Conger, S. B., Niab, Z., Tyler, C. W., Hatcher, R. A. (1977) Preliminary analysis of oral contraceptives use and risk of developing pre-malignant lesions of the uterine cervix. *In*: Pharmacology of Steriod Contraceptive Drugs. Garrattini, S. Berendes, H. W. (eds.), New York: Raven Press.
65. Melamed, M. R., Flehinger, B. J. (1973) Early incidence rates of precancerous cervical lesions in women using contraceptives. Gynecol. Oncol. 1, 290–298.
66. Peritz, E., Ramcharan, S., Frank, J., Brown, W. L., Huang, S., Ray, R. (1977) The incidence of cervical cancer and duration of oral contraceptive use. Am. J. Epidemiol. 106, 462–469.
67. Stern, E., Forsythe, A. B., Youkeles, L., Coffelt, C. F. (1977) Steriod contraceptive use and cervical dysplasia: increased risk of progression. Science 196, 1460–1462.
68. Kinlen, L. J., Spriggs, A. I. (1978) Women with positive cervical smears but without surgical intervention. Lancet 2, 463–465.
69. Cervical Cancer Screening Programs (1976) Can. Med. Assoc. J. 114, 1003–1033.
70. Stern, E., Clark, V. A., Coffelt, G. F. (1970) Contraceptives and dysplasia: higher rate for pill choosers. Science 169, 497–498.
71. Jollie, W. P. (1960) The persistence of trophoblast on extrauterine tissues in the rat. Am. J. Anat. 106, 109–115.
72. Leading Article, Brit. Med. J. (1975) 3, 606–607.
73. Guiloff, E., Ibarra-Polo, A., Zanartu, J., Toscanini, C., Mischler, T. V. and Gomez-Rogers, C. (1974) Effects of contraception on lactation. Am. J. Obstet. Gynecol. 118, 42–45.
74. Parks, A. S., Thompson, A. M., Potts, M., Herbertson, M. A. (1977) (eds.) Fertility regulation during human lactation. J. Biosoc. Sci. Suppl. 4, Cambridge: Galton Foundation.
75. Stone, M., Dent, J., Kardana, A., Bagshawe, K. D. (1976) Relationship of oral contraception to development of trophoblastic tumour after evacuation of a hydatidiform mole. Br. J. Obstet. Gynaecol. 83, 913–916.
76. Herbst, A. L., Scully, R. E. (1970) Adenocarcinoma of the vagina in adolescence. Cancer 25, 745–757.
77. Herbst, A. I., Ulfelder, H., Poskanzer, D. C. (1971) Adenocarcinoma of the vagina: Association of maternal stilbestrol therapy with tumor appearance in young women. N. Engl. J. Med. 284, 878–881.
78. Greenwald, P., Barlow, J. J., Nasca, P. C., Burnett, W. S. (1971) Vaginal cancer after maternal treatment with synthetic estrogens. N. Engl. J. Med. 285, 390–392.
79. Heinonen, P. O. (1973) Diethylstilbestrol in pregnancy: frequency of exposure and usage patterns. Cancer 31, 573–577.
80. Kinlen, L. J., Badaracco, M. A., Moffett, J., Vessey, M. P. (1974) A survey of the use of estrogens during pregnancy in the United Kingdom and of the genito-urinary cancer mortality and incidence rates in young people in England and Wales. J. Obstet. Gynaecol. Br. Commonwealth 81, 849–855.
81. Herbst, A. L., Poskanzer, D. C., Robboy, S. J., Friedlander, L., Scully, R. E. (1975) Prenatal exposure to stilbestrol: a prospective comparison of exposed female offspring with unexposed controls. N. Engl. J. Med. 292, 334–339.
82. Hoover, R., Gray, L. A., Fraumeni, J. F. (1977) Stilboestrol (diethystilbestrol) and the risk of ovarian cancer. Lancet 2, 533–535.
83. West, R. O. (1966) Epidemiologic study of malignancies of the ovaries. Cancer 19, 1001–1007.
84. Wynder, E. L., Dodo, H., Barber, H. R. K. (1969) Epidemiology of cancer of the ovary. Cancer 23, 352–370.

85. Annegers, J. F., O'Fallon, W., Kurland, L. T. (1977) Exogenous oestrogens and ovarian cancer. Lancet 2, 869–870.

86. Weiss, N. S., Young, J. L., Roth, G. J. (1977) Marital status and incidence of ovarian cancer: the U.S. Third National Cancer Survey, 1969–71. J. Nat'l. Cancer Inst. 58, 913–915.

87. Hoover, R., Fraumeni, J. F., Gray, L. A. (1978) Exogenous estrogens and ovarian cancer (Letter). Lancet 1, 325–326.

88. Newhouse, M. L., Pearson, R. M., Fullerton, J. M., Boesen, E. A. M., Shannon, H. (1977) A case-control study of carcinoma of the ovary. Br. J. Prev. Soc. Med. 31, 148–153.

89. Newhouse, M. L. (1978) Personal Communication.

90. Fathalla, M. F. (1972) Factors in the causation and incidence of ovarian cancer. Obstet. Gynecol. Survey 27, 751–768.

91. Beral, V., Fraser, P., Chilvers, C. (1978) Does pregnancy protect against ovarian cancer? Lancet 1, 1083–1087.

92. Beral, V., Ramcharan, S., Faris, R. (1977) Malignant melanoma and oral contraceptive use among women in California. Br. J. Cancer 36, 804–808.

93. Mulvihill, J. J. (1975) Congenital and genetic diseases. *In*: Persons at High Risk of Cancer. Fraumeni, J. F. Jr. (ed.), New York: Academic Press, pp. 3–35.

94. Snell, R. S., Bischitz, P. G. (1960) The effect of large doses of estrogen and estrogen and progesterone on melanin pigmentation. J. Invest. Dermatol. 35, 73–82.

95. Harlap, S. (1978) Pigmented skin lesions in babies born to underweight former oral contraceptive users. Lancet 2, 39.

96. Christopherson, W. M. (1975) Liver tumors and the pill (Letter). Brit. Med. J. 4, 756.

97. Committee on Safety of Medicines (1972) Carcinogenicity Tests of Oral Contraceptives. London: HMSO.

98. Baum, J. K., Holtz, F., Bookstein, J. J., Klein, E. W. (1973) Possible association between benign hepatomas and oral contraceptives. Lancet 2, 926–929.

99. Vana, J., Murphy, G. P., Aronoff, B. L., Baker, H. W. (1977) Primary liver tumors and oral contraceptives: results of a survey. J. Am. Med. Assoc. 238, 2154–2158.

100. Mahboubi, E., Shubik, P. (1977) Epidemiological Relationship between steriod hormones and liver lesions. J. Toxicol. Environ. Health 3, 207–218.

101. Christopherson, W. M., Mays, E. T., Barrows, G. (1978) Hepatocellular carcinoma in young women on oral contraceptives (Letter). Lancet 2, 38–39.

102. Edmondson, H. A., Henderson, B., Benton, B. (1976) Liver-cell adenomas associated with use of oral contraceptives. N. Engl. J. Med. 294, 470–472.

103. Center for Disease Control (1977) Increased risk of hepatocellular adenoma in women with long-term use of oral contraceptives. Morbidity and Mortality Weekly Report 26, 293–294.

104. Model, D. G., Fox. J. A., Jones, R. W. (1975) Multiple hepatic adenomas associated with an oral contraceptive. Lancet 1, 865.

105. Vessey, M. P., Kay, C. R., Baldwin, J. A., Clarke, J. A., Macleod, I. B. (1977) Oral contraceptives and benign liver tumours. Br. Med. J. 1, 1064–1065.

106. World Health Organization (1974) World Health Statistics Annual. Geneva.

107. Kintzen, W., Silny, J. (1960) Peliosis hepatis after administration of fluoxymesterone. Can. Med. Assoc. J. 83, 860–862.

108. Bernstein, M. S., Hunter, R. L., Yachnin, S. (1971) Hepatoma and peliosis hepatis developing in a patient with Franconi's anemia. N. Engl. Med. J. 284, 1135–1136.

109. Lesna, M., Spencer, I., Walker, W. (1976) Liver nodules and androgens (Letter). Lancet 1, 1124.

110. Westaby, D., Ogle, S. J., Paradinas, F. J., Randell, J. B., Murray-Lyon, I. M. (1977) Liver damage from long-term methyltestosterone. Lancet 2, 261–263.

111. Thalassinos, N. C., Lymberatos, C., Hadjioannou, J., Gardikas, C. (1974) Liver-cell carcinoma after long-term oestrogen-like drugs (Letter). Lancet 1, 270.

112. Hermann, R. E., David, T. E. (1973) Spontaneous rupture of the liver caused by hepatomas. Surgery 74, 715–719.

113. Meyer, P., Liviolsk, V. A., Cornog, J. L. (1974) Hepatoblastoma associated with an oral contraceptive (Letter). Lancet 2, 1387.

114. Davis, M., Portmann, B., Searle, M., Wright, R., Williams, R. (1975) Histological evidence of carcinoma in a hepatic tumor associated with oral contraceptives. Br. Med. J. 4, 496–498.

115. Glassberg, A. B., Rosenbaum, E. H. (1976) Oral contraceptives and malignant hepatoma (Letter). Lancet 1, 479.

116. Tigano, F., Ferlazzo, B., Barrile, A. (1976) Oral contraceptives and malignant hepatoma (Letter). Lancet 2, 196.

117. O'Sullivan, J. P., Rosswick, R. P. (1976) Oral contraceptives and malignant hepatic tumours (Letter). Lancet 1, 1124–1125.

118. Schmidt, G. (1977) Hepatocellular carcinoma. Med. J. Aust. 1, 215–217.

119. Trias, R., Ruis, X., Autonell, J., Algaba, F. (1978) Hepatocarcinoma and oral contraceptives (Letter). Lancet 1, 821.

120. Menzies-Gow, N. (1978) Hepatocellular carcinoma associated with oral contraceptives. Br. J. Surg. 65, 316–317.

121. Westhoff, C. F. (1977) Trends in contraceptive practice: 1965–1973. Family Planning Perspectives 8, 54–57.

122. Johnson, F. L., Feagler, J. R., Lerner, K. G., Majerus, P. W., Siegel, M., Hartmann, J. R., Thomas, E. D. (1972) Association of androgenic-anabolic steroid therapy with development of hepatocellular carcinoma. Lancet 2, 1273–1276.

123. Guy, J. T., Auslander, M. O. (1973) Androgenic steroids and hepatocellular carcinoma (Letter). Lancet 1, 148.

124. Farrell, G. C., Joshua, D. E., Uren, R. F., Baird, P. J., Perkins, K. W., Kronenberg, H. (1975) Androgen-induced hepatoma. Lancet 1:430–431.

125. Anthony, P. P. (1975) Hepatoma associated with androgenic steriods (Letter). Lancet 1, 685–686.

126. Chang, R. J., Keye, W. R., Young, J. R., Wilson, C. B., Jaffe, R. B., (1977) Detection, evaluation, and treatment of pituitary microadenomas in patients with galactorrhea and amenorrhea. Am. J. Obstet. Gynecol. 128, 356–363.

127. Sherman, B. M., Harris, C. E., Schlechte, J., Duello, T. M., Halmi, N. S., Van Gilder, J., Chapler, F. K., Granner, D. K. (1978) Pathogenesis of prolactin-secreting pituitary adenomas. Lancet 2, 1019–1021.

128. Annegers, J. F., Coulman, C. B., Abboud, C. F., Laws, E. R., Kurland, L. T. (1978) Pituitary adenoma in Olmsted County, Minnesota, 1975–1977. A report of an increasing incidence of diagnosis in women of childbearing age. Mayo Clinic Proceedings 53, 641–643.

129. Phillips, N. R. (1974) Socioeconomic characteristics and methods of fertility control of female subscribers to the Kaiser Foundation Health Plan in the Walnut Creek Service Area, 1968. *In*: The Walnut Creek Contraceptive Drug Study. Ramcharan, S., (ed.) Bethesda: United States Department of Health, Education and Welfare, Vol. 1, pp. 21–73.

130. Gomez, F., Reyes, F. I., Faiman, C. (1977) Menopuerperal galactorrhea and hyperprolactinemia. Am. J. Med. 62, 648–660.

131. Mishell, D. R., Kletzky, O. A., Brenner, P. F., Roy, S., Nicoloff, J. (1977). The effect of contraceptive steriods on hypothalamic-pituitary function. Am. J. Obstet. Gynecol. 128, 60–74.

132. Shearman, R. P., Fraser, I. S. (1977) Impact of new diagnostic methods on the differential diagnosis and treatment of secondary amenorrhoea. Lancet 1, 1195–1197.

133. Shearman, R. P. (1971) Prolonged secondary amenorrhozea after oral contraceptive therapy. Lancet 2, 64–66.

134. Van Campenhout, J., Blanchet, P., Beauregard, H., Papas, S. (1977) Amenorrhea following the use of oral contraceptives. Fertility and Sterility 28, 728–732.

EPIDEMIOLOGIC AND RELATED STUDIES OF BREAST CANCER ETIOLOGY

DAVID B. THOMAS, M.D., Dr. P.H.

CONTENTS

INTRODUCTION

Breast cancer is a major health problem for women in many of the more developed countries of the world. In Western Europe and North America, one-fifth of all deaths from cancer, and one twenty-fifth of all deaths, are attributed to breast cancer (1). Roughly a quarter of a million women in the world die from the neoplasms each year (1). Based on incidence data from the New York State Cancer Registry, it has been estimated that a woman's lifetime probability of developing breast cancer is 7.2% (2).

Breast cancer may currently be the subject of more epidemiologic and related clinical and laboratory studies of etiology than any other type of neoplasm. This research activity probably stems in part from its major importance, but also from the considerable number of leads about the etiology of breast cancer that have been identified in recent years. A number of reviews of the results of epidemiologic and related studies which have provided these leads have been published during the 1970s (3–13). Some of these papers are insufficiently complete or critical to provide a balanced assessment of current etiologic hypotheses. Others, although comprehensive and thoughtful, are already out of date because of the extraordinarily large number of studies that have been completed in the past few years.

This review will attempt to provide a critical review of findings from the more recent epidemiologic and related studies of breast cancer etiology, and to evaluate current etiologic hypotheses in view of these findings. In addition, contemporary lines of investigation and the rationale for them will be described.

INCIDENCE AND MORTALITY RATES

Studies based on incidence or mortality rates provide information on geographic variations in rates of occurrence, changes in rates over time, or differences in rates among people characterized by various personal attributes. These so-called descriptive studies can provide clues to disease etiology. In addition, etiologic hypotheses based on other types of studies can be ruled out if inconsistent with patterns of incidence or mortality.

Geographic Variations

Figure 1, from Segi (14), shows incidence rates of female breast cancer in 80 populations. The ratio of highest to lowest rates is almost 8 to 1. Highest rates are in white populations of some Western countries, and lowest rates are in non-Caucasian peoples. However, large differences in rates among various countries are seen for whites, blacks, Chinese, and Spanish-speaking peoples, suggesting that environmental rather than genetic factors are primarily responsible for the observed international variation in rates, and hence for the disease itself.

From the University of Washington and the Fred Hutchinson Cancer Research Center, Seattle, Washington 98104.

FEMALE

1	HAWAII:	CAUCASIAN	80.3
	CANADA,	BRIT.COL.	80.0
	BAY AREA:	WHITE	79.9
	ALAMEDA:	WHITE	76.1
	N'MEXICO:	OTHER WHITE	73.8
	CONNECTICUT		71.4
	SUISSE,	GENEVA	70.6
	HAWAII:	HAWAIIAN	66.2
	DETROIT:	WHITE	65.7
10	CANADA,	MANITOBA	64.2
	CANADA,	SASKATCH.	62.8
	IOWA		61.6
	ISRAEL:	BORN EUR.AMER.	60.8
	CANADA,	MAR.PROV.	58.6
	BAY AREA:	BLACK	57.9
	CANADA,	ALBERTA	57.4
	NEW YORK STATE		57.2
	CANADA,	QUEBEC	56.9
	UTAH		=
20	ALAMEDA:	BLACK	56.5
	ISRAEL:	ALL JEWS	55.5
	UK,	OXFORD	54.5
	HAWAII:	CHINESE	54.2
	EL PASO:	OTHER WHITE	53.8
	ISRAEL:	BORN ISRAEL	53.6
	UK,	BIRMINGHAM	53.0
	N'ZEALAND:	NON-MAORI	52.5
	SWEDEN		52.4
	EL PASO:	SPANISH	52.3
30	UK,	SOUTH WEST	52.1
	N'ZEALAND:	MAORI	=
	UK,	SMCR 1963-66	51.4
	DETROIT:	BLACK	51.0
	UK,	LIVERPOOL	50.8
	F. R. G.,	SAARLAND	50.6
	UK,	AYRSHIRE	50.1
	NORWAY,	URBAN	49.6
	UK,	SHEFFIELD	=
	ICELAND		49.5
40	DENMARK		49.1
	F. R. G.,	HAMBURG	48.4
	UK,	SMCR 1967-71	48.0
	BRAZIL,	SAO PAULO	47.3
	NORWAY		44.4
	HAWAII:	JAPANESE	44.2
	BAY AREA:	CHINESE	44.0
	CANADA,	N'FNDLAND	43.8
	BRAZIL,	RECIFE	41.9
	NORWAY,	RURAL	40.0
50	MALTA		39.6
	JAMAICA,	KINGSTON	=
	G. D. R.		33.4
	FINLAND		32.9
	N'MEXICO:	SPANISH	32.4
	POLAND,	WARSAW,CITY	31.5
	SPAIN,	ZARAGOZA	30.6
	ROMANIA,	TIMIS	29.3
	HUNGARY,	VAS	28.3
	YUGOSLAV.,	SLOVENIA	=
60	CUBA		28.0
	COLOMBIA,	CALI	27.8
	ISRAEL:	BORN AFR.ASIA	26.7
	N'MEXICO:	AMER.INDIAN	26.2
	SINGAPORE:	INDIAN	25.5
	PUERTO RICO		25.4
	POLAND,	KATOWICE	23.2
	HAWAII:	FILIPINO	21.5
	INDIA,	BOMBAY	20.1
	HUNGARY,	SZABOLCS	19.8
70	POLAND,	CRACOW	19.6
	SINGAPORE:	CHINESE	19.4
	POLAND,	CIESZYN ETC	18.5
	SINGAPORE:	MALAY	17.6
	JAPAN,	OKAYAMA	16.6
	NIGERIA,	IBADAN	15.3
	POLAND,	WARSAW,RURAL	=
	BULAWAYO,	AFRICAN	13.8
	JAPAN,	MIYAGI	13.0
	JAPAN,	OSAKA	12.1
80	ISRAEL;	NON-JEWS	11.0

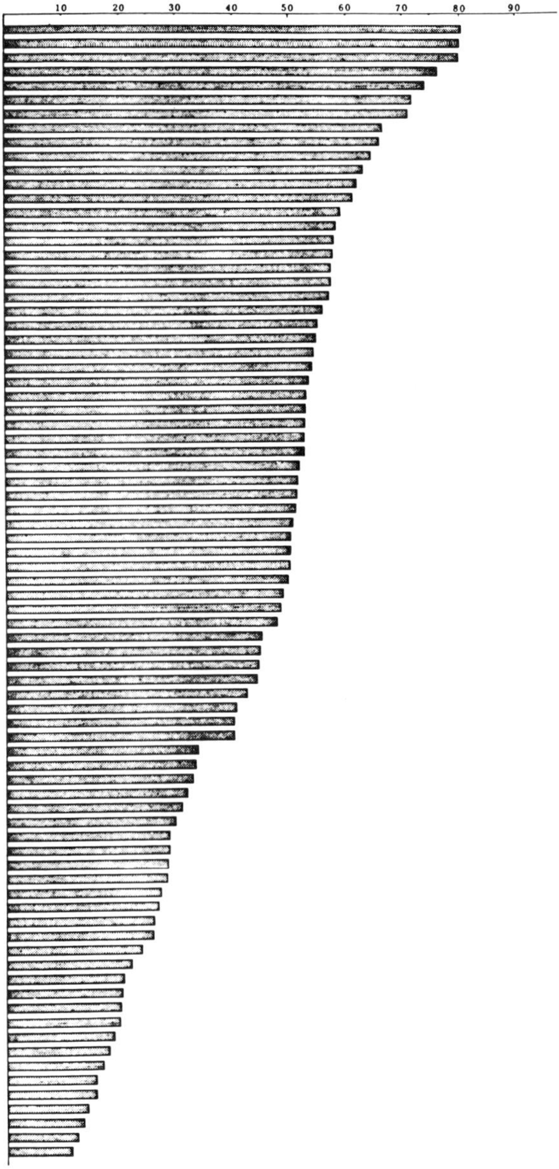

FIGURE 1. Graphic presentation of breast cancer incidence by site and by area and population (14).

TABLE 1. Average Age-Adjusted Female Breast Cancer Mortality Rates from 1950–1969 for U.S. Counties by Geographic Region, Income Level, and Population of County[a]

		Geographic region			
Income level	Population	Northeast	South	Central	West
Low	<10,000	24.1	16.2	20.3	20.9
	10,000–24,000	23.6	16.7	23.3	19.5
	25,000–99,000	25.1	17.8	23.4	21.7
	100,000–249,000	26.2	20.6	25.7	22.0
	250,000+	28.1	22.9	26.4	23.6
High	<10,000	25.2	18.0	22.0	20.7
	10,000–24,000	25.3	18.6	23.2	21.6
	25,000–99,000	26.9	19.1	24.9	21.6
	100,000–249,000	27.3	21.4	26.3	24.4
	250,000+	30.2	25.1	28.6	26.8

Source: Blot, W. J., Fraumeni, J. F., Stone, B. J., Geographic patterns of breast cancer in the United States, J. Nat. Cancer Inst. 59, 1407–1411, 1977.

[a]Deaths per 100,000 person-years.

This contention is supported by studies of mortality within a single country. Table 1, from Blot et al. (15), shows that breast cancer mortality rates for white women in the United States from 1950–1969 were highest in the Northeast and lowest in the South. Rates also showed an urban–rural gradient, with highest levels in urban counties with large populations, and lowest levels in the most sparsely populated counties. These patterns are observed for both relatively affluent and poorer counties.

Although rates of breast cancer tend to be higher in urban than rural areas, differences in the degree of urbanization do not explain the variability in breast cancer incidence among countries. For example, there are higher incidence rates in Norway than in Poland or Hungary in both urban and rural populations (12).

As described in detail in a subsequent section, a number of variables related to childbearing have been implicated as risk factors for breast cancer. However, two pieces of evidence from descriptive studies suggest that the large international differences in rates cannot be explained by variations in these factors. The ratio of breast cancer mortality rates in the United States to those in Japan is approximately the same for males as for females (16); and age-specific rates for single women in ten countries, most of whom had not borne children, showed the same variation by country, social class, and time, as did comparable rates for all women in these countries, most of whom had been married (17).

Variations of Personal Attributes

Sex is by far the personal characteristic that best distinguishes persons at high risk of breast cancer. Incidence rates for women are approximately 100 times those for men; results from the Third National Cancer Survey showed annual

United States rates in 1969–1971 to be 0.7 and 73.8 cases per 100,000 persons for men and women, respectively (18).

As shown in Figure 1, incidence rates within geographic areas differ among various races and ethnic groups. In Hawaii, for example, incidence rates for Caucasians, Hawaiians, Chinese, Japanese, and Filipinos per 100,000 women are, respectively, 80.3, 66.2, 54.2, 44.2, and 21.5; in Israel, such rates for Jewish women born in America or Europe, Israel, and Africa or Asia, are 60.8, 53.6, and 26.7, respectively, and the comparable rate for non-Jews is 11.0. Also, breast cancer death rates for both Mormons in Utah and California (19), and for Seventh Day Adventists in California (20), are lower than for all U.S. white women. As will be discussed, many of these differences are the subject of more detailed studies.

Breast cancer occurs more frequently in women of higher socioeconomic status, as measured in the United States by educational level (21) and income (22) and in the United Kingdom by social class (3). In western India, the relatively more prosperous Parsis have more breast cancer than Hindus, Muslims, Christians, and Jews (23). Relationships between breast cancer and various indices of socioeconomic status, however, provide little specific etiologic information regarding mammary carcinoma. Such indices are statistically related to breast cancer only because they are also associated with one or more reproductive or other factors of more direct etiologic importance. For example, the relationship between breast cancer and education has been accounted for by the fact that education is related to marital status and parity (24,25), as well as to age at first pregnancy (25). Compared to women of other Indian communities, the high-risk Parsis tend to marry less frequently, to marry and have their first child at a later age, and also to have fewer children (23). The main value in identifying socioeconomic variables associated with breast cancer is that such variables can aid in defining groups of women at high risk of breast cancer who should be studied in the search for more specific etiological factors.

As early as 1713 it was recognized that nuns have more breast cancer than lay women (26), and this observation has been well documented in subsequent studies (27,28). Single women are at higher risk of breast cancer than married women. This has been observed in such diverse regions of the world as Australia (29), India (23,25), Israel (30), the United States (31), and Japan (25).

The excess risk in single women tends to be confined to women in their postmenopausal years (23,27,28,29,31). As will be described below, artificial menopause reduces the risk of postmenopausal breast cancer, and it has been shown that at least part of the excess risk in single women is due to their less frequently having artificial menopause than married women (31). This explanation, however, cannot account for the excess risk among nuns prior to the advent of modern surgery. Data from an international collaborative case-control study conducted in seven cities of North and South America, Europe, and Asia (32) suggest that much of the excess risk in unmarried women can be explained by the fact that most single women are nulliparous, and have not been subjected to the apparent protective effect of an early pregnancy, a phenomenon that will be discussed later. This collaborative study also showed that the observed inverse relationship between age at first marriage and risk of breast cancer can be explained by the correlation between the ages of first marriage and first confinement. The absence of a relationship between age at first marriage and breast cancer has subsequently been confirmed by an independent study (33).

As shown in Figure 2, from Bjarnason, et al. (34), incidence rates increase markedly with age between the usual ages of menarche and menopause, and then decline slightly, nearly level off, or increase more slowly, with age in areas of low, intermediate, and high breast cancer incidence rates, respectively. Differences in rates are thus greater for post- than premenopausal women. Figure 3 shows that age-incidence curves nearly identical to those for women in countries with varying rates of breast cancer were observed for women in Iceland at different time periods. Between the first and last of these time periods, 1911–1929 and 1950–1972, respectively, overall breast cancer incidence rates increased over tenfold (34). In both the United States and Japan, breast cancer mortality rates in men, although much lower than those for women, appear to increase steadily with age with no break in the curve at middle age (16).

Shapes of age-incidence curves for female breast cancer have been the subject of considerable study and speculation. DeWaard (35) noted that the fre-

FIGURE 2. Age-specific incidence of breast cancer in Connecticut, Finland, and Miyagi Prefecture, Japan (34).

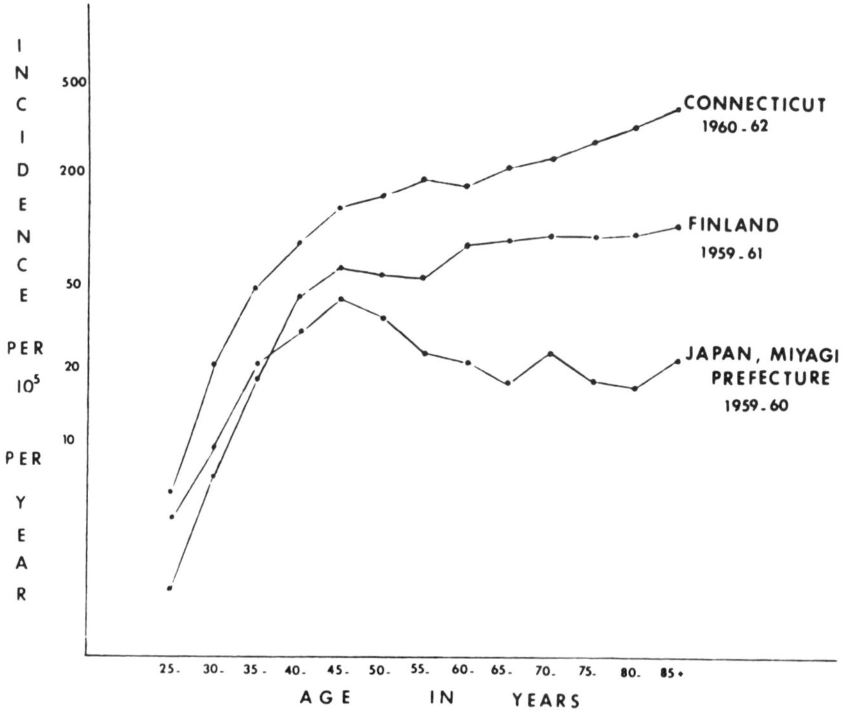

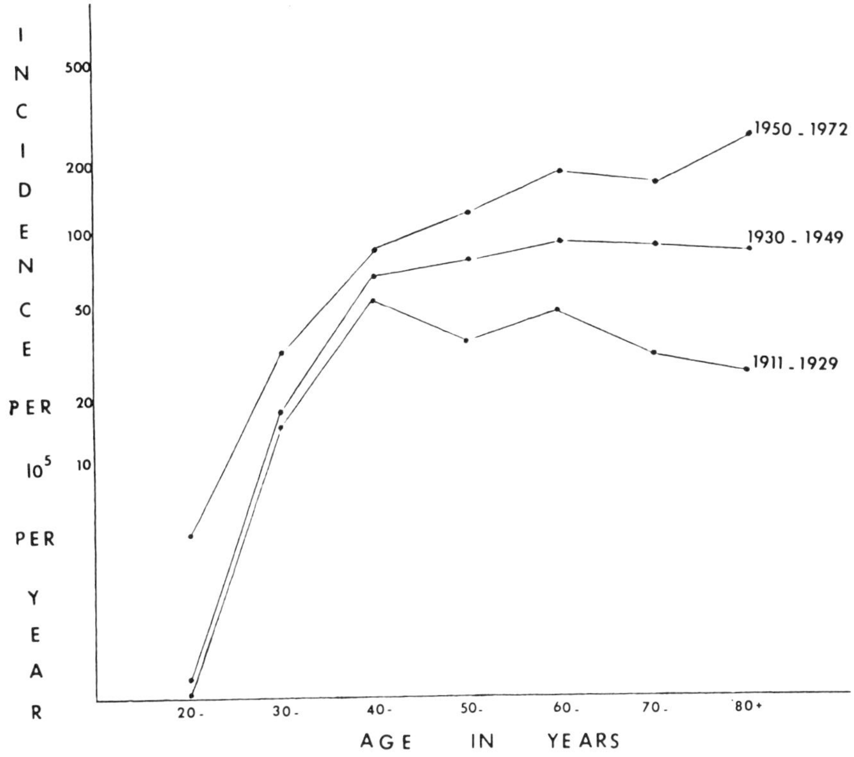

FIGURE 3. Age-specific incidence of breast cancer in Ireland for three time periods (34).

quency distribution of breast cancer cases in Amsterdam by age was bimodal, and hypothesized that this distribution and the age-incidence curve, represent two populations of breast cancer cases: premenopausal disease in which ovarian hormones play an etiologic role, and postmenopausal disease which is related to an imbalance in adrenal estrogens. He also hypothesized (36) that the type of possible ovarian origin is predominant in low rate populations such as Japan, and that the excess in high rate countries is due to factors such as nutrition and obesity that influence the occurrence of the postmenopausal type. Studies to be discussed in a subsequent section were initiated to test these hypotheses.

At variance with DeWaard's interpretation of age-incidence curves is a model proposed by DeLisi (37) which shows that two distinct types of breast cancer with overlapping age distributions need not be hypothesized to explain the shapes of age-incidence curves. DeLisi suggests that the curves can be explained on the basis of a single disease type to which varying portions of people in different populations are susceptible, and which progresses through a number of different developmental stages at a rate which declines at menopause. The nature of the susceptibility, which would have to vary among different populations, and in the same population over time, is unclear.

Lee et al. (38) have noted that, in both high and low rate populations, before menopause the age-incidence curve decreases in steepness, running concave and downward when log age is plotted vs. log incidence. After menopause, it is a straight line. They conjecture that this pre-menopausal decline in the rate of change with age is consistent with an exponential decay with time of a precursor lesion that has its origin early in life. No explanation is offered for the observation that this decline does not continue after menopause, and they note that this is surprising in view of observations by others that early menopause reduces the risk of breast cancer.

Changes in the age-incidence curve in Iceland over time (Figure 3) were shown to be due to an increasing incidence of breast cancer in successive cohorts. Moreover, the shapes of the curves for different cohorts were similar, and resemble those for Connecticut during the years 1935–1951, when incidence rates changed little. These observations were interpreted as indicating that the risk of a woman developing breast cancer is determined before the age at which appreciable numbers of cases become manifest. It was hypothesized that the factors responsible for this risk are either confined to young females or that only young women are susceptible to them. A subsequent study (39) showed that these factors do not include age at menarche, age at birth of first child, or parity, all three of which, as will be discussed below, are risk factors for breast cancer. These observations are consistent with the conclusion that the international differences are not due to factors related to childbearing, and suggest that they may be related to unknown factors that are operative early in life.

Time Trends

Table 2 is derived from a recent summary of temporal trends in mortality rates of breast cancer (1). Of the 19 countries represented, in only two was there a decline in age-adjusted rates between 1950–1951 and 1966–1967, and the magnitude of the decline was sufficiently small to be compatible with possible changes in classification practices. In most countries with rates of over 19 deaths per 100,000 women in 1950–1951 the increase by 1966–1967 was small; the crude average increase in these countries was less than one death per 100,000 women. By contrast, countries with rates below 19 deaths per 100,000 women tended to show larger increases, the crude average increase for these countries being 2.8 cases per 100,000 women. Norway and Japan are the only two countries in this latter group in which large increases did not occur.

Compatible with the findings from Iceland, Table 2 also indicates that relatively large increases in age-adjusted mortality rates in four different countries represent, at least in part, increasing rates in successive birth cohorts of women. A similar observation was made from incidence data for Japanese in Hawaii (40). Cohort effects were not noted in four countries with small increases in age-adjusted rates. However, more recent data from Japan, the one country in this latter group with low rates in 1950–1951, indicate that an in-

TABLE 2. Age-Adjusted Female Breast Cancer Mortality Rates in 1950–1951 and 1960–1967 in 19 Countries

	Deaths per 100,000 women			Percent	Cohort
Country	1950–1951	1966–1967	Increase	increase	effect
1. Denmark	24.36	24.62	0.26	1.07	No
2. Netherlands	23.28	26.75	3.47	14.91	Yes
3. England and Wales	23.19	24.58	1.39	5.99	No
4. New Zealand	22.80	23.11	0.31	1.36	
5. Canada	22.10	23.47	1.37	6.20	
6. Scotland	22.01	22.80	0.79	3.59	
7. United States (white)	21.30	21.99	0.69	2.89	No
8. Switzerland	21.24	22.15	0.91	4.28	
9. Northern Ireland	19.93	20.67	0.74	3.71	
10. Australia	19.37	19.15	−0.22	−1.14	
11. Ireland	17.50	21.03	3.53	20.17	Yes
12. Norway	17.32	16.78	−0.54	−3.12	
13. Israel	16.89	21.48	4.59	27.18	Yes
14. Sweden	15.83	18.00	2.17	13.71	
15. France	12.73	16.98	4.25	33.39	Yes
16. Italy	12.27	16.09	3.82	31.13	
17. Finland	10.73	14.65	3.92	36.53	
18. Chile	7.66	9.73	2.07	27.02	
19. Japan	3.97	3.99	0.02	0.50	No

Source: Logan, W. P. D., Cancer of the female breast. International Mortality Trends, Bull. World Health Org. 28,232–251, 1975.

crease in rates is also now occurring in that country. The increase seems to be largely confined to younger women, who would be members of more recent birth cohorts (41).

From 1960 through 1969, there was a slow, steady increase in incidence rates of breast cancer in whites in Alameda County, California (42), and a similar increase through 1971 in Connecticut (42, 43), and in some age groups in Birmingham and the South Metropolitan regions of England (43). These increases in incidence rates are evidence that the small increases in mortality rates in the countries with high mortality rates in 1950–1951 are not due to decreased survival. Data more recent than that presented in Table 2 also suggest that the small increases in mortality rates in these countries in part also reflect cohort-specific changes in rates. Cohort analyses of mortality rates for the United States, England, and Wales, and of incidence rates from Connecticut, Birmingham, and the South Metropolitan regions of England up to 1971 (43) show that in these areas there have been both cross-sectional and cohort–specific increases in rates. Unlike Iceland, but similar to findings based on mortality rates in Canada (44, 45), and incidence rates in Saskatchewan (45), the small cohort-specific increases seem to correspond in part to decreases in fertility in succeeding cohorts. The reasons for the cross-sectional increases in rates are unknown. Small changes in reporting and classification could play a role.

In the United States, breast cancer incidence and mortality rates are higher for whites than nonwhite women. The difference in incidence has diminished slightly over time, due to a greater temporal increase in rates for nonwhites, which could be due, at least, in part to improved diagnosis and reporting (46).

Migrant Studies

Further evidence that environmental factors are primarily responsible for geographic differences in breast cancer rates has been obtained from studies of immigrants. In Table 3, the breast cancer death rates for 13 countries of origin are listed in order of increasing breast cancer death rates (21). The first 11 countries have rates that are lower than the rate for the United States white population, which is 22.3 per 100,000. The rates are also higher for the migrants from all these 11 countries than for their respective country of origin. Rates for 8 of these 11 migrant groups are intermediate between those in the country of origin and the rates for the United States whites. Three of these 11 migrant groups actually have higher rates than the United States whites, although the difference is only appreciable in the Irish immigrants. Migrants from the United Kingdom, one of the two countries with higher breast cancer rates than the United States whites, have rates that are similar to the United States. These may reflect errors in death certification or inadequate enumerato have even higher rates than resident Canadians. The general pattern for migrants is that they tend to develop breast cancer at a rate comparable to that of the country of adoption, as opposed to that of their country of origin. The two major exceptions to this are the Irish and Canadian immigrants, and data for these groups are of questionable validity because rates for 14 out of 15 different types of cancer in the Irish, and for 11 out of 15 in Canadians, were found to be higher for the migrants than in either the country of origin or the United States. Data may reflect errors in death certification or inadequate enumeration of these migrants in the United States census.

Although many immigrants to the United States came from rural areas and settled in cities, the change in their rates cannot be explained simply by the move from an urban to a rural environment. In all but one category (Italians in rural areas), the death rates among immigrants from all of the first 11 countries in Table 3 to both urban and rural areas of the United States are higher than in the respective country of origin.

Exclusive of Mexico, the only country in Table 3 with a predominantly non-European population, there is no relationship between death rates in the country of origin, and rates among immigrants from that country. This observation, too, seems incompatible with the idea of a genetic basis for the geographic differences in rates.

More detailed studies of Chinese, Japanese, and Latin Americans have provided additional information regarding breast cancer (47–50). Table 4 shows ratios of incidence and mortality rates in various populations of women in these three groups relative to rates in U.S. white women. For all three ethnic groups, rates are lowest for women in their native countries and rates in migrants are intermediate in magnitude between those for women in the native countries and white women in the United States. In addition, rates for Chi-

TABLE 3. Age-Adjusted Breast Cancer Death Rates for Migrants in Urban and Rural Counties in the United States, 1956–1961, and for Residents of the Countries of Origin, 1960[a]

U.S. White Rates = 22.3

		Migrants		
Country of origin	Country of origin	Total in United States	Metropolitan counties (urban)	Nonmetropolitan counties (rural)
Mexico	4.0	13.4	14.4	10.4
Poland	7.1	20.3	20.8	14.5
Yugoslavia	7.3	15.5	16.0	12.1
Hungary	12.5	23.0	23.5	20.1
Czechoslovakia	13.9	21.9	21.8	24.9
Finland	14.1	20.3	19.5	25.7
Italy	15.0	19.5	20.0	14.6
Austria	16.9	25.5	26.5	17.5
Norway	17.4	18.6	18.6	19.0
Sweden	20.3	21.7	20.8	26.0
Ireland	20.7	33.1	32.5	38.3
Canada	24.2	27.3	28.2	24.4
United Kingdom	24.4	22.2	22.6	20.1

Source: Lilienfeld, A. M., Levin, M. L., Kessler, I. I., Cancer in the United States, Cambridge, Harvard University Press, 1972.

[a]Death rates per 100,000 females.

nese women are greater in highly urbanized Singapore and Hong Kong than in less urbanized Taiwan.

The fact that the rates were lower for the Chinese, Japanese, and Latin Americans than for U.S. whites (or European migrants) can be explained by differences in culture as adequately as by differences in genetic makeup. Migrants to the United States from these ethnic groups tend more strongly to adhere to cultural patterns that are similar to those of their country of origin than migrants from Europe or Canada. Supportive of this explanation is the observation that both Polish and Japanese migrants came to the United States primarily during the last two decades of the nineteenth and the first three decades of the twentieth century, and both came from rural areas of countries that have lower breast cancer rates than the United States (49); yet, by 1950, breast cancer mortality rates among Polish immigrants had nearly reached the level for United States white women (51), whereas rates among Japanese immigrants, although higher than in Japan, had not reached the level for United States white women even by the early 1970s (49).

Rates for the descendants of Japanese and Mexican migrants who were born in the United States are higher than rates for their predecessors who migrated. This finding suggests that exposure to Western culture at an early age increases the risk of breast cancer more than exposure later in life, an interpretation consistent with the increase in rates in successive cohorts in Iceland during a period of industrial development (34). The lower mortality rate for

TABLE 4. Age-Standardized Ratios of Mortality and Incidence Rates of Female Breast Cancer in Various Chinese, Japanese, and Latin American Populations Relative to Rates in U.S. White Women

Ethnicity	Population	Years	Mortality ratio[a]	Incidence ratio[b]
Chinese	Taiwan	1950–1960	0.19	
	Singapore	1959–1962	0.35	0.25
	Hong Kong	1961–1964	0.42	
	United States			
	migrants	1959–1962	0.61	
	U.S. born	1959–1962	0.34	
	British Columbia	1960–1962	0.96	
	Hawaii	1968–1972		0.79
	San Francisco Bay Area	1969–1973		0.55
Japanese	Japan			
	total	1958–1959	0.16	
	Miyagi Prefecture	1968–1971		0.18
	Hawaii	1968–1972		0.65
	San Francisco Bay Area	1969–1973		0.59
	California			
	migrants	1956–1962	0.24	
	U.S. born	1956–1962	0.28	
Latin America	Cali, Columbia	1967–1971		0.32
	Cuba	1968–1972		0.33
	Puerto Rico	1968–1972		0.31
	New Mexico Spanish	1969–1972		0.38
	L.A. County Mexican			
	migrant	1972–1973		0.40
	U.S. born	1972–1973		0.83

[a]Mortality ratios for Chinese from reference 48 and for Japanese from reference 49.

[b]Incidence ratios from reference 47, calculated from reference 50.

Chinese born in the United States than for migrants is probably a chance phenomenon.

The fact that the rates were lower in second generation Orientals than in U.S. whites suggests that some factor inherent in non-Western cultures that is maintained by descendants of migrants from such cultures appears to offer a degree of protection against breast cancer. This factor is at least partially specific for breast cancer. Rates in Japanese migrants of some other forms of cancer that occur less frequently in Japan than in the United States, such as cancers of the colon and pancreas, more rapidly approached U.S. white rates with the passage of time than did rates of breast cancer (52).

SUMMARY

In summary, a number of conclusions regarding the etiology of breast cancer can be drawn from the results of analyses of mortality and incidence data. Variations in rates among women of the same race residing in different countries or different parts of the same country, higher rates in urban than rural areas, low rates in certain religious groups, variations by socioeconomic status, and the apparent increase in rates in women who migrate from countries with low rates to countries with higher rates, all indicate that environmental rather than genetic factors are largely responsible for the marked differences in rates among various countries, and must play a large role in the etiology of breast cancer. The factors responsible for the international variation are not related to childbearing practices, as evidenced by the observation that the ratio of Japanese to U.S. rates is nearly as large for men as for women, and the finding that international variations in rates are as great for single women as for all women. The possibility that these factors are largely operative early in a woman's life is suggested by the fact that Japanese and Latin American migrants to the United States have relatively low breast cancer rates whereas their descendants who are born in America have rates closer to rates for native-born U.S. whites. The observation that rates are higher in succeeding cohorts of women in countries such as Iceland in which there has been a marked increase in rates also appears to support this view. The factors responsible for the low rates in Oriental and Latin American countries appear to be well ingrained in the cultural patterns of people from these areas and also appear to be somewhat specific for breast cancer, because rates in second generation migrants from these countries to the United States are not as high as rates for U.S. whites or migrants from European countries, and because rates of breast cancer in Oriental migrants and their descendants increase with time more slowly than do rates of some other neoplasms such as cancers of the colon and pancreas.

Although international variations in rates cannot be explained by childbearing practices, such practices can play a role in the etiology of breast cancer, as evidenced by the high rates of breast cancer in nuns and in single women, relative to married women, and the observation in countries with recent small increases in breast cancer rates of a correspondence between cohort-specific decreases in fertility and cohort-specific increases in breast cancer. Hormonal factors unrelated to childbearing are implicated by the higher rates in women than men, and by the shape of the age-incidence curve for women, which rises rapidly from the usual ages of menarche to menopause and then rises less rapidly after menopause.

These observations and conclusions from analyses of incidence and mortality data have stimulated more detailed investigations of specific risk factors.

SPECIFIC RISK FACTORS

Radiation

Ionizing radiation is the only known cause of breast cancer. The evidence for this causal relationship is overwhelming. Increased rates of breast cancers have been documented in women who received multiple fluoroscopic examinations of the chest (53–57), women treated with radiation for such benign conditions as acute postpartum mastitis (58–60), acne (61), chronic mastitis (60), and fibroadenomatosis (60), and women exposed to atomic bombs in Japan (62,63). A clear increase in risk of breast cancer with increasing dosage of radition to the breast has been documented in studies of atomic bomb survivors (62,63), women treated for postpartum mastitis (59), and women receiving multiple fluoroscopies (57). The dose response curve tends to be linear within the range of dosages studied (57,59,63). However, there is some evidence for a leveling off of the curve at the highest doses (59,63). In studies of women with unilateral exposure, the tumors tended to occur in the irradiated breast (54,55,58–60). In women with multiple fluoroscopies, the tumors tended to occur in the medial aspects of the breast, where dosage was highest and where breast tumors develop less frequently (53,54).

The latent period between radiation exposure and development of breast cancer is at least 8 years (54), and the excess risk persists for over 30 years (57, 59). There is some evidence that the latent period is inversely related to the dosage (59,60). Some studies have shown that women who are irradiated early in their childbearing years are at greater risk of breast cancer than women irradiated later in life (57,60,63), although one study of women treated with x-rays for postpartum mastitis did not show a greater risk in women under or over 30 years old at the time of treatment (59). In one study, early pregnancy, which may reduce the risk of breast cancer, was not found to protect against radiation-induced disease (59). This same study showed that the risk of breast cancer did not differ in those who received equal cumulative doses in 1 to 2 or in 3 to 4 separate treatments, which suggests that fractionation of breast irradiation does not reduce the risk, and that the effects of radiation are cumulative.

The proportion of all current breast cancers that are attributable to the kinds of radiation exposure that were the subject of the above studies is unknown, but must be extremely small. These studies thus provide information of only marginal value in elucidating the causes of most breast cancers currently occurring in the general population.

The findings from these investigations are, however, extremely important in assessing the potential risk of mammography, and have generated considerable controversy (64–67). The basic issue is the applicability of findings based on moderate to high levels of exposure (from tens to hundreds of rads) to the generally lower levels experienced by women who receive mammographic examinations (less than one to about three rads). The dose-response curves based on studies of women treated for postpartum mastitis (59), atomic bomb survivors (63), and women who received multiple fluoroscopic examinations of the chest (57) all are consistent with a linear increase in risk with increasing dosage. If this is true for the low levels of radiation to which women are subjected during mammography, then such women would be at increased risk of breast cancer. Thus, if mammography becomes widely practiced, even a small increase in risk could result in large numbers of additional cases of breast cancer. On the other hand, there could be a threshold level of exposure below which there is no increase in risk of breast cancer, or the risk of breast cancer could be greater than estimated by extrapolating existing dose-response curves to low dosage levels.

Additional information on the risk of breast cancer in women exposed to low levels of radiation is needed before the risk of mammography can be adequately assessed. This information should include: (a) estimates of breast cancer risk at various (low) doses: (b) analyses to determine whether the effects of multiple exposures are indeed cumulative; and (c) determinations of the risk due to radiation for women with or without various known risk factors for breast cancer. It has been suggested that women with characteristics indicative of a high risk be singled out for inclusion in screening programs, and this would only be wise if such women were not more susceptible than others to the carcinogenic effects of radiation.

Considerable effort has been expended to assess the potential risks and benefits of screening for breast cancer using x-rays, and opinions vary widely on this issue (68–71). These opinions, are based on assumptions about the effects of the low doses of radiation used in screening x-rays, and additional information will be necessary before the truth is known. At present, it appears that screening women under 50 is of no benefit (72) and, as already mentioned, that their risk of radiation-induced breast cancer may be greater than that of older women. The magnitude of the risk : benefit ratio for older women is currently conjectural, although a reduction in mortality of 54% seven years after initial screening in women over age 50 in one randomized trial strongly suggests that the benefit may be considerable (72).

Menstrual Factors

A number of case-control studies have shown mean age at menarche to be slightly younger for women with breast cancer than for unaffected individuals, although the observed differences have tended to be small (25,73–78). Other studies have shown no relationship between age at menarche and breast cancer (31,79–82). The international collaborative case-control study of breast cancer in seven countries of the world with varying incidence rates of breast cancer showed risk of this condition to be inversely related to age at menarche, although this was not noted consistently in all seven study areas (83). Prospective studies in Iceland (39), New York (84), and the Isle of Guernsey (85,86) have also shown a clear inverse relationship between breast cancer risk and age at menarche. Early menarche may have a greater influence on the risk of breast cancer during the premenopausal (87,88) and perimenopausal (89) years than in the years following menopause, although the opposite was noted in one study (78). The facts currently available regarding age at menarche are thus inconclusive. Early menarche probably adversely influences a woman's risk of breast cancer, but this effect is very likely less important than the influence of other factors.

A more striking relationship is seen between risk of breast cancer and age at either natural or artificial menopause. With few exceptions (31), most investigators have noted that post–menopausal women with breast cancer went through menopause at a later age than normal women (3,25,73,74,76,78, 79–81,83,84,88–90). Table 5 summarizes data from two studies (88,90) that demonstrate a direct relationship between age at natural menopause and risk of breast cancer. These two studies, plus another (78), showed an apparent protective effect of an early menopause for postmenopausal breast cancer arising in women of all ages, but especially for women over 70. It appears that

TABLE 5. Estimates from Two Studies of Relative Risks[a] of Breast Cancer in Women with Natural Menopause at Various Ages

Age at menopause	First author of study report	
	Trichopoulos (90)	Stavraky (88)[b]
<45	0.73	0.58
45–49	0.93	1.01
50–54	1.07	1.00
≥55	1.48	1.35

[a]Risks relative to risk in women having natural menopause between 45 and 54 years of age.

[b]Values calculated from data provided in the reference.

the increased risk associated with a late menopause may also be greater for older than younger women (90).

A number of studies have shown a lower frequency of artificial menopause among breast cancer cases than comparable controls (23,31,73,75,76,79,90, 91). In some reports, the mean age at which artificial menopause was induced was older for cases than controls (31,79). Artificial menopause thus appears to be protective, but only if ovarian function is disrupted; hysterectomy without oophorectomy does not alter the risk (91,92). The degree of protection is greater for women with bilateral oophorectomy than for those with unilateral oophorectomy or menopause induced by pelvic radiation (91,92). Presumably some women in the latter group retain partial ovarian function, as do those from whom only one ovary is removed.

As with natural menopause, the degree of protection afforded by oophorectomy has been shown in three independent studies to be inversely related to the age at disruption of ovarian function (90–92). In two of these studies (91, 92), it was estimated that women who had had an oophorectomy by about age 40 have approximately a 75% reduction in their risk of breast cancer, a finding roughly in agreement with the data in Table 6 from the third study (90). A comparison of Tables 5 and 6 shows that for any age at menopause, the degree of protection is about the same for artificial and natural menopause. As with natural menopause, the protective effect of oophorectomy is a

TABLE 6. Relative Risk of Breast Cancer by Age at Oophorectomy

Age at oophorectomy	Relative risk[a]
<35	0.36
35–39	0.68
40–44	0.65
45–49	0.73
≥50	0.98

Source: Trichopoulas, D., et al., Menopause and breast cancer, J. Natl. Cancer Inst. 48,605.

[a]Risks relative to risk in women having natural menopause between 45 and 54 years of age.

long-term one. It has been estimated to last at least 30 years and, like early natural menopause, to be greater for elderly than recently postmenopausal women (90). A reduction in breast cancer risk has also been noted in spayed female dogs, and the amount of reduction is inversely related to the age of the dog at surgery (93).

Support for the idea that premenopausal oophorectomy protects against breast cancer is also provided by the observation that women who have had both ovaries removed are less likely to show histologic evidence of severe large-duct hyperplasia in their breasts than do women whose ovaries are intact (94).

As stated previously, in New York State the greater frequency of induced menopause in married women has been shown to account for at least part of the lower rates of post-menopausal breast cancer as compared to single women (31). However, castration prior to the usual age of menopause is relatively rare even in countries such as the United States where hysterectomies are common; therefore, the impact of oophorectomy on the overall risk of breast cancer must be small.

In spite of this fact, studies of the relationship of artificial as well as natural menopause to breast cancer have provided important information regarding mammary carcinogenesis. It can be concluded from such studies that early disruption of ovarian function, whether by artificial or natural means, provides a degree of protection against breast cancer that lasts for decades. This in turn implies that ovarian activity during the later reproductive years is somehow related to the genesis of postmenopausal breast cancer.

A relationship between the total lifetime years of menstrual activity and risk of breast cancer has been reported (24,73,79,88). Years of menstrual activity is a function of age at menarche, age at menopause, and duration of time spent in a pregnant or lactating state. As will be discussed subsequently, lactation does not appear to be associated with breast cancer; the association between breast cancer and age at menarche is also relatively weak; and the role of parity is uncertain. Thus, age at menopause is probably the primary component of this relationship.

The relationship between breast cancer and a number of other aspects of menstrual activity has been investigated. Two studies revealed no association between risk of breast cancer and menstrual irregularity (24,80), but two others provided data suggesting an increased risk associated with this problem (78,89), although one showed this only in peri- and postmenopausal women (89). An early study by Wynder et al. (25) showed no association between length of cycle and breast cancer, but a later study by the same investigator (89) showed an increased risk in women reporting long cycles. Results of a study in Finland (81) suggest that women with irregular or short cycles are at reduced risk of breast cancer. Studies have not shown a relationship of breast cancer risk to pain during menstruation (25) or amount of duration of flow (25). Most studies have also failed to show an association between risk of breast cancer and prior history of swelling or tenderness of the breasts during menstruation (24,25,86), although at least one study did show such an association (75). Breast size has not been found to be related to breast cancer risk

(25,81). The inconsistencies or generally negative nature of these findings suggests that these factors are of little importance in the etiology of breast cancer, although more data on menstrual irregularity and cycle length would be desirable.

Parity and Age at Birth of First Child

The higher risk of breast cancer in single as opposed to married women is undoubtedly related at least in part to childbearing practices. Married women who have never been pregnant are at higher risk of breast cancer than married women who have borne children (29,74,80); and many studies, although not all (41), have shown risks in single women and childless married women to be similar. Two aspects of childbearing have received considerable attention in recent years. These are parity, and age at birth of first child.

In 1970, MacMahon et al. (95) reported that analysis of data from their international collaborative case-control study showed that risk of breast cancer increased with age at which a woman delivered her first child. This relationship persisted after controlling for parity, a factor strongly related to age at first child. These findings were followed by a number of additional studies (76,78,81,88,89,96,97). Results from the international study and subsequent case-control studies are summarized in Table 7, and results from three prospective studies (39,84,86) are shown in Table 8. All three prospective studies, and all but one of the case-control studies (78), show the relative risk of breast cancer to increase with age at first birth. The one exception was a study done in Canada that utilized cases admitted to selected hospitals and neighborhood controls (78). In the study done in Baltimore (96), both hospital and neighborhood controls were utilized, and the apparent relationship of breast cancer risk to age at first birth was stronger and more consistent when cases were compared to hospital than neighborhood controls. This suggests that the neighborhood controls used in the Canadian study may have been selected in a way that obscured the relationship between age at first birth and breast cancer. The alternative explanation that the results of all of the other studies are spurious seems untenable in view of the consistency of the results among so many studies of varied design.

Most studies show that women who have their first child when in their thirties are actually at higher risk of breast cancer than nulliparous women (39,84,86,89,95,97).

The apparent protective effect of an early first pregnancy was found in the international study (95) to diminish with increasing age, but to be evident in most centers even for women in their 70s. Others have noted no protective effect in women over age 55 (23), over age 43 (97), or in postmenopausal women (89). It thus appears that the protective effect is greatest for relatively younger women, and diminishes with the passage of time. However, one study did show the protective effect only in postmenopausal women (88).

The relationship of breast cancer risk to total number of children is less clear than the relationship to age at first birth. Many of the studies summarized in Tables 7 and 8 showed an association between risk and parity, but a number did not. In the international study (95), after taking into account the

TABLE 7. Summary of Results from Case-Control Studies Showing Relative Risks of Breast Cancer in Relation to Age at Birth of First Child

Sources of cases	Sources of controls	Location (reference)	Menopausal status	Unadjusted relationship to parity	Controlled for parity	Age at first birth <20	20–24	25–29	30–34	35+	Nulli-parous
Hospital[a]	Hospital	Boston (95)	All	Yes	Yes	1.00	1.72	2.38	2.81	3.66	3.13
		Glamorgan (95)	All	Yes	Yes	1.00	1.29	1.76	1.92	3.26	2.63
		Athens (95)	All	Yes	Yes	1.00	1.39	1.55	2.08	2.49	1.96
		Slovania (95)	All	Yes	Yes	1.00	.91	1.16	1.38	1.46	1.23
		Sao Paulo (95)	All	Yes	Yes	1.00	1.33	1.92	1.71	3.57	2.04
		Taipei (95)	All	Yes	Yes	1.00	.83	.69	1.65	1.96	1.85
		Tokyo (95)	All	Yes	Yes	1.00	1.88	3.00	3.85	5.31	3.85
Hospital	Hospital	Ontario (88)	Pre-	No	Yes[c]	1.00	1.27	0.90	0.93		—
			Post-	No	Yes[c]	1.00	1.17	1.39	2.91		—
Hospital	Hospital	New York (89)[b]	Pre-	No	No	1.0	1.7	2.6	3.2		1.5
			Peri-	No	No	1.0	1.6	3.0	3.5		3.2
			Post-	No	No	1.0	1.0	1.1	1.1		1.4
Hospital	Screening Clinic	Finland (81)	All	Yes	Yes[c]	1.0		1.3	1.8	2.0	—
Hospital	Fracture Clinic	Ireland (76)	All	No	No	1.00		0.81	1.11	1.73	—
Hospital	Hospital	Baltimore (96)	All	Yes	No	1.00	1.02	1.43	1.48	1.67	2. 33
	Neighborhood	Baltimore (96)	All	Yes	No	1.00	1.03	0.94	1.60	1.46	1.48
Hospital	Neighborhood	Canada (78)	All	No	No	1.0	1.0		0.7		0.9
Population	Population	Washington Co. (97)	All	Yes	No	1.00	1.16		2.09		1.95

[a] Attempted to obtain all cases in indefined populations.
[b] Ages at first birth are <22, 22–25, 26–30, 31–40.
[c] Relative risks shown are unadjusted for parity, but adjustment did not alter trends shown.

TABLE 8. Summary of Results from Prospective Studies Showing Relative Risks of Breast Cancer in Relation to Age at Birth of First Child

Location (reference)	Study population	Age at first birth					Nulliparous
		<20	20–24	25–29	30–34	35+	
Iceland (39)	Cervical cancer screenees	1.00	1.63	2.61	2.53	4.12	3.76
New York (84)	Prepaid health plan	1.00	1.50	1.68	2.00		1.63
Guernsey (86)	General population	1.00		2.54	3.59		2.88

strong relationship between age at first birth and parity, the association of breast cancer with parity tended to disappear. However, the risk in women having more than one birth before age 25 was found to be somewhat lower than the risk in women having one child before that age. Also, in women whose first birth occurred after age 35, additional births were associated with an increased risk.

Table 9 summarizes results from one case-control study (81), and two of the prospective studies shown in Table 8 (39,84), plus a third one from Japan (41). All show that the risk of breast cancer appears to increase with age at first pregnancy or marriage; but, for each age at first pregnancy or marriage, the risk seems to decline with increasing numbers of children. It would be of interest to see the results of other studies shown in Tables 7 and 8 presented in this manner. A trend similar to that shown in Table 9 was observed for

TABLE 9. Relative Risks[a] of Breast Cancer by Age at First Pregnancy and Parity

Location (reference)	Age at first pregnancy[b]	Number of pregnancies[c]			
		1	2	3–4	≥5
Iceland (39)	<20	1.00		0.70	0.56
	20–24	1.53		1.07	0.86
	25–29	2.27		1.60	1.28
	30–34	2.20		1.40	1.12
	≥35	2.91		2.04	1.63
Finland (81)	<25	1. 00		0.74	
	≥25	1.52		0.82	
New York (84)	<20	1.00		0.83	
	20–29	1.88		1.11	
	≥30	2.11		1.85	
Japan (41)	<25	1.00	0.32	0.32	
	≥25	1.26	0.67	0.47	

[a]Values calculated from published reports.
[b]Age at first marriage for Japanese data.
[c]Number of children for Japanese data.

women whose first pregnancy was under age 25 in Sao Paolo, the one area in the international collaborative study (98) from which data have been so presented. On balance, it thus appears that high parity is associated with a lowered risk of breast cancer, at least in women first pregnant at a relatively young age, and probably in other women as well.

The relationship between early first birth and reduced risk of breast cancer could be due to either a direct protective effect of an early first birth, or due to a third factor which both reduces fertility (and hence delays pregnancy), and increases the risk of breast cancer. Data from two case-control studies were analyzed by Lilienfeld et al. (33), to determine which interpretation is correct. As shown in Table 10, a reduced risk associated with an early first pregnancy is evident for those whose first birth occurred less than two years after marriage, as well as for those who first give birth more than two years after marriage, which suggests that it is an early first birth per se, and not lowered fertility, which reduces the risk of breast cancer. This interpretation is supported by the observation that only full-term births are associated with an altered risk (5). Studies have shown either no relationship between breast cancer and a history of spontaneous abortions (25, 80) or a slight increase in risk (5,81,88).

On the other hand, Table 10 also shows that, for most categories of age at first birth, the relative risk is greater for those whose first birth was later than two years subsequent to marriage. This supports the hypothesis that there is a third factor that both delays pregnancy and increases the risk of breast cancer.

Thus, the presently available evidence suggests that an early first birth per se does confer a degree of protection against breast cancer. However, the suggestion that ovulatory failure predisposes to the development of breast cancer and also to late or no pregnancies (99–101) is not refuted. Additional studies to investigate further the determinants of an early first birth are currently underway.

TABLE 10. Relative Risks of Breast Cancer in Parous Women by Age at First Birth and Interval from First Marriage to First Birth[a]

Study	Sources of subjects: Cases	Sources of subjects: Controls	Age at diagnosis	Years between first marriage and first birth	Age at birth of first child: <20	20–24	25–29	30–34
1	Population-based registry	Population sample	≥40	≤2	0.30	0.60	0.76	0.86
				>2	0.76	0.72	0.82	0.77
2	Single hospital	Hospitalized patients without cancer	≥40	≤2	0.40	0.66	1.08	1.22
				>2	0.12	0.77	1.14	1.45
			>40	≤2	0.57	1.26	1.20	2.75
				>2		1.93	3.27	

Source: Lilienfeld, A. M., et al., Marital and reproductive experience in a community-wide epidemiological study of breast cancer, Johns Hopkins Med. J. 136, 157–162.

[a]Risks relative to risk in nulliparous women.

Lactation

There was considerable reason for earlier investigators to suspect that breast feeding might protect against breast cancer. Low rates of breast cancer are generally observed in those parts of the world in which breast feeding is both more common and more prolonged than in Western countries with higher rates of breast cancer (25). Also, because premenopausal oophorectomy reduces the risk of breast cancer, it seems reasonable to suspect that lactation, which suppresses ovarian function, may also do so.

Table 11 summarizes the results of nine studies from which sufficient data were published so that relative risks of breast cancer in women with varying duration of lactation could be calculated (25,32,75,79,81,102–105). A "protective effect" of lactation is apparent primarily from those studies in which the relationship between lactation and parity was not taken into account. Where the apparent effect of lactation was adjusted for parity, little association between lactation and breast cancer is evident. After controlling for parity, a slight protective effect of breast feeding for more than five years is noted in Sao Paolo and Taipei, but not in Tokyo, although the magnitude of the effect is small. It is noteworthy that the study by Kamoi (104) showed a protective effect, but this totally disappeared after controlling for parity. It thus appears that the risk of breast cancer is altered little by breast feeding. This conclusion

TABLE 11. Results of Case-Control Studies of Lactation and Breast Cancer

First author (reference)	Population	Duration of lactation	Relative risks controlled for parity[a]	
			No	Yes
MacMahon (103)	United States	≥1 week		1.05
Kaplan (75)	United States	≥2 weeks	0.75	0.81
Soini (81)	Finland	≥6 months	0.9	
Anderson (102)	South African	≥10 months	0.51	
Abramson (105)	Israel	≥1 year		1.00
Kamoi (104)	Japan	≥3 years	0.60	1.20
Levin (79)	United States	≥3 years	0.46	
Wynder (25)	White United States	≥3 years	1.10	
	Black United States	≥3 years	0.59	
	Britain	≥3 years	0.38	
	India	≥3 years	0.31	
	Japan	≥3 years	0.38	
MacMahon (32)	Boston	≥3 years		1.10
	Glamorgan	≥3 years		0.96
	Athens	≥3 years		0.94
	Slovenia	≥3 years		1.08
Wynder (25)	India	≥5 years	0.45	
	Japan	≥5 years	0.37	
MacMahon (32)	Sao Paulo	≥5 years		0.78
	Taipei	≥5 years		0.82
	Tokyo	≥5 years		0.99

[a]Risks in women who breast fed relative to those who did not.

is supported by the observation that, although breast feeding has declined markedly in the United States in recent decades (106), incidence rates of breast cancer have not increased by a corresponding amount.

There are, however, unanswered questions regarding the relationship of lactation to risk of breast cancer that could be answered by reanalysis of existing data sets. In particular:

1. What is the effect of age at first lactation (as opposed to age at first pregnancy or birth) on the risk of breast cancer?
2. Conversely, does the association between age at first birth and breast cancer remain after controlling for age at first lactation?

Even though risk of breast cancer appears to be minimally effected by usual breast feeding practices, unilateral suckling may influence the development of mammary neoplasms. In 1952, Segi et al. (107) reported that women with breast cancer and a history of unilateral "hypolactation" tended to have their tumors on the side that had previously not lactated sufficiently. The belief that the cancer was not related to some inherent defect in the breast which caused the hypolactation is supported by the recent observation from Hong Kong (108) that women who habitually breast feed only from the right breast tend to develop breast cancer in their left breasts. This tendency was noted only for women over age 55. It is unknown whether the suckled breast is protected, whether the unsuckled one is at increased risk, or whether unilateral nursing merely influences the side in which a tumor develops without altering the woman's overall risk of breast cancer. To determine which of these possibilities is correct, data are needed on the incidence of breast cancer in women who habitually suckled from one breast.

Height and Weight

In 1960, Wynder et al. (25) noted that women with breast cancer tended to be more obese than matched hospital controls. Four years later, DeWaard (109) reported a similar observation for postmenopausal but not premenopausal women; on the basis of this and other observations he hypothesized that the etiologies of pre- and postmenopausal breast cancer are different and that some adrenocortical estrogen disturbance may play a role in postmenopausal disease. Although this hypothesis has subsequently been modified, the observations on which it is based led to many more studies of body dimensions and breast cancer, the results of which are summarized in Table 12.

The striking thing about these studies is the inconclusiveness of the results. A number of recent case-control studies have found no association between breast cancer and height (76,81,89,110), weight (81,89,110,111) or Quetelet Index (wt/ht^2) (81,88,89,110,112,113); these studies include controls of varying types, as do those that do show a relationship between breast cancer and height (41,78,87,98,111–116), weight (41,78,87,98,112, 114–116), or Quetelet Index (41,87,98,111,116).

One case-control study (78) showed premenopausal patients to be lighter and shorter than control subjects, a finding at variance with all other investi-

TABLE 12. Relationship of Height and Weight to Risk of Breast Cancer

First author (reference)	Location of study	Source of subjects		Menopausal status	Relationship of breast cancer to:		
		Cases	Controls		Height	Weight	Ht/wt^2
Valaoras (111)	Athens	Hospital[a]	Hospital	All	+	0	+
Mirra (98)	Sao Paulo	Hospital[a]	Hospital	Pre-	0	0	0
				Post-	+	++	+
Ravnihar (114)	Slovenia	Hospital[a]	Hospital	All	+	+	
Lin (115)	Taiwan	Hospital[a]	Hospital	All	+	++	
				Pre-		+	
				Post-		++	
Stavrasky (88)	Ontario	Hospital	Hospital	Pre-			0
				Post-			0
DeWaard (112,113)	Holland	Population	Population	Pre-	+	+	0
				Post-	++	++	0
Herity (76)	Ireland	Hospital	Fracture clinic	All	0		
Soini (81)	Finland	Hospital	Breast cancer screenees	All	0	0	0
Adami (110)	Sweden	Population	Population	Pre-	0	0	0
				Post-	0	0	0
Staszewski (87)	Poland	Hospital	Hospital	Pre-	++	0	0
				Post-	+	++	+
Wynder (89)	New York	Hospital	Hospital	Pre-	0	0	0
				Peri-	0	0	0
				Post-	0	0	0
Choi (78)	Canada	Hospital	Neighborhood	Pre-	−	—	
				Post-	+	++	
Hirayama (41)	Japan	Hospital	Hospital	Pre-		+	+
				Post-		++	++
Hirayama (41)[b]	Japan	Screening Program	Screening Program	All	++	++	
DeWaard (116)[c]	Holland	General Practice	General Practice	All	++	++	+

[a]Attempt made to study all cases in a defined population.
[b]Prevalence study.
[c]Prospective study.
0 = no association between variable and breast cancer.
\+ = increased risk with increasing value of variable, magnitude small or not statistically significant.
++ = increased risk with increasing value of variable, magnitude large or statistically significant.
− = decreased risk with increasing value of variable, magnitude small or not statistically significant.
— = decreased risk with increasing value of variable, magnitude large or statistically significant.

gations. This is the same study that failed to show an association between breast cancer risk and age at birth of first child (Table 7), and, as discussed previously, may have resulted in spurious findings.

In spite of the apparent inconsistencies in Table 12, a few tentative generalizations can be made. First, if there is a relationship between weight and breast cancer, it is strongest for postmenopausal disease, and may not exist for premenopausal breast cancer. Second, the relationship of height to breast cancer, if any, is probably not as strong as the relationship of weight to breast cancer, and existing data are too inconsistent to judge whether this relationship is stronger for pre- or postmenopausal disease. Third, the generally nonexistent association between weight corrected for height (Quetelet Index) indicates that obesity per se is not a risk factor for breast cancer. Fourth, total body size may be a risk factor, as indicated by the observation from several studies that the influences of height and weight on risk of breast cancer are independent (41,112,116), and by the finding of DeWaard et al. (112) that risk is related to body surface area, an index of overall body size. Additional data are obviously needed before these tentative conclusions can be accepted as truths. However, the observation that from 1950 to 1975 there was more than a doubling of the overall mortality rate from breast cancer in Japan, and that during this period Japanese became taller and heavier, is consistent with these conclusions (117). DeWaard et al. (113) have estimated that about one half of the differences in breast cancer incidence between Holland and Japan can be "attributed" to differences in body weight and height.

Statistical relationships between indices of body size and breast cancer do not, however, indicate that large body size per se is a cause of breast cancer. Some other factor related to body size could instead be causally related to breast cancer. The obvious suspect is nutrition prior to cessation of body growth. The potential role of specific dietary factors in the genesis of breast cancer is discussed in the next section.

Good nutritional status results in an early menarche and also a relatively large body size (118). Age at menarche and body size are thus inversely correlated, and an early age at menarche may be associated with an increased risk of breast cancer. However, this is an unlikely explanation for the relationship between body size and breast cancer. Age at menarche is a weak risk factor, and appears to be more strongly associated with premenopausal breast cancer. In addition, in one study (87) the association between breast cancer and both height and weight persisted after controlling for age at menarche.

Compared to women of normal weight, obese women with breast cancer tend to have tumors with less favorable prognostic characteristics. These include axillary metastases (113,119), clinical stage, infiltrative tumor margins, vascular involvement, and low nuclear grade (119). These observations could simply indicate that tumors are detected later in obese women. However, they could also suggest that tumors that develop in obese women are more aggressive, a finding that implies that obesity is related to promotion of tumor growth. The latter interpretation is supported by the observation that 15-year disease-free and survival rates were less favorable for relatively heavy than lighter patients without axillary metastases (120).

Other explanations for the association between body size and breast cancer are discussed in the section on endogenous hormones.

Diet

Incidence and mortality rates of breast cancer in various countries have been shown to be correlated with indices of sugar (121), fat (121–123), and animal protein (122,123) consumption. Mortality rates in 12 districts of Japan have also been found to be correlated with consumption of animal fat, especially pork (41), and increases in rates from 1955 to 1975 in these districts have been associated with increases in animal fat consumption. Results from correlation studies such as these can provide clues to etiology, but must be interpreted with caution. Women who consume diets rich in animal products are generally well off economically and may be characterized by other factors of more direct etiologic importance. The most recent correlation study of international rates (123) supports this contention. It was found that breast cancer rates were more highly correlated with Gross National Product (GNP) than fat consumption, and that the strength of the correlation between fat consumption and breast cancer markedly diminished after controlling for GNP. Also, in the study of rates in 12 districts in Japan, the increase in rates were found to also be correlated with daily consumption of AF2 (2-(2-furyl)-3-(5-nitro-2-furyl) acrylamide), a mutagenic chemical that was widely used as a food additive in Japan from 1965 to 1975, and that has caused breast tumors in experimental rats. Moreover, the correlation between rates in these 12 districts and pork consumption is not consistent with the relatively high breast cancer rates in Israeli Jews (50). In addition, breast cancer mortality rates are only slightly lower for Seventh-Day Adventists, many of whom are vegetarians, than for non-Adventists in California (124).

Nonetheless, dietary factors may well be responsible for the marked international differences in rates of breast cancer. The international collaborative case-control study (32,95), and studies of breast cancer rates in males (16) and single women (17) all indicate that these differences cannot be explained by factors related to childbearing or menses. The increase in rates among migrants from low to high risk countries and in the women of Iceland and Japan, are also consistent with dietary factors playing a role. In Japan, for example, between 1950 and 1975 there has been a 15-fold increase in milk consumption, a 7.5-fold increase in consumption of meat, poultry, and eggs, and a 6-fold increase in fat intake (117); during the same time period mortality from breast cancer more than doubled.

Two case-control studies of breast cancer and diet from which results are available (124,125) provide data showing greater consumption of fats by cases than controls. Preliminary results from a study of Seventh-Day Adventists show an association between breast cancer and consumption of fried foods and use of hard (more saturated) fat for frying (124). A study in Canada also showed a relationship between both pre- and postmenopausal breast cancer and total fat consumption (125). Preliminary results from a prospective study in Japan suggest an association between breast cancer and meat intake, and a prevalence study done in conjunction with an adult health survey in Hiroshima showed breast cancer to be related to consumption of meat, eggs, butter, and cheese (41). Other case-control studies of diet and breast cancer are currently being conducted in Japan and Hawaii (126), and Israel (127). A study is also being made of the dietary practices of daughters of cases and controls among the Seventh-Day Adventists in Southern California (127).

Data from animal experiments support the idea that dietary fats increase the risk of breast cancer. A high fat diet was found to enhance breast tumor formation in rats given the mammary carcinogen 7,12-dimethylbenz(a)anthracene (DMBA) (128).

All of the studies cited relating breast cancer to fats and meats are based on recent food consumption or dietary habits as adults. The results may thus be interpreted at least three ways:

1. The results are spurious, and simply a consequence of some unrecognized association between dietary habits and other risk factors for breast cancer. The consistency of the results among the various correlation, case-control, prevalence, and prospective studies does not support this interpretation.
2. The results suggest that intake of animal products as an adult influences the risk of breast cancer.
3. Dietary practices as an adult are correlated with such practices earlier in life and thus are supportive of the hypothesis that the types of foods eaten early in life influence subsequent risk of breast cancer.

The influence of nutrition on age at menarche and the observation that premenopausal breast cancer is related to fat intake (125), as well as to age at menarche, support the validity of the last interpretation. It is also supported by cohort analyses of the data from Iceland (34) and by observations that Japanese and Mexican migrants have low breast cancer rates whereas their daughters have higher rates. On the other hand, the second interpretation is supported by the larger international differences in postmenopausal breast cancer than in premenopausal disease, and by the association between (recent) dietary practices and breast cancer in the postmenopausal years. Both interpretations could be correct.

Two mechanisms by which a high fat diet could alter the risk of breast cancer have been suggested. One, based on rat experiments (129), is that the increased risk may result from an alteration in levels of circulating prolactin. The other (130) is based on observations in humans and experiments with bacteria in vitro, and is particularly attractive because it is consistent with the hypothesis that endogenous estrogens alter the risk of breast cancer. A high fat diet increases the amount of biliary steroids (cholesterol and bile-salt degradation products) in feces, and also renders the intraintestinal environment more favorable to the growth of anaerobic lecithinase-negative clostridia. In vitro, these organisms can produce estrone, estradiol, and 18-methoxyestradiol from cholesterone, a bacterial metabolite of cholesterol that is present in human feces. This finding suggests that dietary fat may influence the development of breast cancer by affecting the production of these hormones in the gut and thereby altering their levels in the body. Studies are currently underway to investigate further the influence of diet on the metabolic products of bacteria in the large bowel.

It is also possible that dietary fats or substances used in the preservation of animal products are metabolized to carcinogens, or that additives to animal products are themselves carcinogenic, such as AF2 in Japan (41).

ENDOGENOUS HORMONES

The relationship of breast cancer risk to ages at menarche, menopause, oophorectomy, and time of birth of first child, as well as to nulliparity, the decline in the slope of the age-incidence curve at menopause, and the one hundred times greater risk of breast cancer in women than men, all suggest that endogenous hormones play a role in the genesis of mammary carcinomas. Despite this, extensive endocrinologic studies of breast cancer patients during the past two decades have provided no clear understanding of the etiologic role of any hormone. Differences in levels of specific hormones in blood and urine from cases and controls tend to be small and inconsistently observed by different investigators. The low sensitivity of some hormone assay methods that have been used may be a partial explanation for this. Another could be that hormonal aberrations that lead to breast cancer probably occur years prior to the development of clinically apparent disease, and may not be present when the disease is recognized. Also, the tumor itself, or the body's reaction to it, could alter normal hormonal patterns and either obliterate prior hormonal abnormalities of interest or result in the development of abnormalities that are of no value in elucidating etiology.

More recently, collaborative efforts between endocrinologists and epidemiologists have provided findings that do seem likely to further our understanding of the etiology of breast cancer. These findings, and the contemporary causal hypothesis for which they serve as a basis, will be reviewed in this section.

Androgens

Dehydroepiandrosterone, its sulfate, and androstenedione are secreted by the adrenal cortex and measurable in plasma. Their principle metabolites are androsterone, and etiocholanolone. These metabolites, and dehydroepiandrosterone sulfate are the principle 17-ketosteroids excreted in the urine. Measurements of these urinary metabolites are probably rough indicators of the excretion rate of their precursors (131).

A number of studies of the relationship of breast cancer to levels of these substances in plasma and urine have been conducted. In the early 1960s, Bulbrook et al. reported that women with advanced breast disease who responded poorly to adrenalectomy were distinguishable from women whose response was favorable by their urinary levels of 17-ketosteroids. In particular, those with low levels of etiocholanolone relative to levels of 17-hydroxysteroids responded poorly (132). These and other findings, although not consistently confirmed by other studies, led the investigators to hypothesize that low levels of etiocholanolone and other urinary androgen metabolites might be related to the development of breast cancer, in addition to its clinical progression. To test this hypothesis, a long term prospective study on the Isle of Guernsey was undertaken (133). Beginning in 1961, approximately 5000 women without breast cancer were recruited, 24-hour urine specimens were collected from them, and then they were followed over time for development of breast cancer. The urine specimens were frozen and stored. Subsequently, measurements of dehydroepiandrosterone, androsterone, and etiocholanolone, and total 17-hydroxycorticosteroids were performed on the urine from women who developed breast cancer, and from a sample of women who did not. It was found that women with low levels of androsterone and etiocholanolone had elevated risks of breast cancer. This relationship was evident for all ages of women studied and was predictive of breast cancer occurring up to 9 years later. Urinary levels of androsterone and etiocholanolone were highly correlated, although etiocholanolone was slightly the better predictor of subsequent breast cancer.

More recent analyses of data from the Guernsey study (85) showed that risk of breast cancer was related to etiocholanolone level, age at menarche, family history of breast cancer, and age at birth of first child, and that these factors exerted independent additive effects (on a logistic scale). Thus, although low urinary levels of androgen metabolites are predictive of breast cancer, they cannot explain the mechanism by which the other factors that were considered influence the risk.

As an alternative to long-term prospective studies of androgens and breast cancer, a number of investigators have compared levels of various androgen metabolites in individuals at high and low risk of breast cancer. Higher ratios of androsterone to etiocholanolone were found in urine from normal Japanese than in normal British women (134). In other reports urinary levels of etiocholanolone and androsterone, and plasma levels at dehydroepiandrosterone sulfate and androsterone sulfate were lower in sisters of breast cancer cases than controls (135); and 20- to 40-year old women with benign breast disease, but not older women, were found to have low plasma levels of dehydroepiandrosterone sulfate and total 17-ketosteroids, and low urinary levels of 17-ketosteroids (136). However, another study showed no difference in urinary levels of etiocholanolone in normal women and women with benign breast conditions (137).

It thus appears that at least some women at increased risk of breast cancer excrete low levels of androsterone and etiocholanolone, and possibly are characterized by subnormal adrenal production of their precursors. However, additional studies in high-risk women are needed to confirm the results of those so far obtained, and to provide a clearer picture of the types of hormonal aberrations associated with specific high risk characteristics.

Estrogens

There are three estrogens of primary importance, the production and excretion of which are complicated processes that have been reviewed in relation to breast cancer by Lipsett (131). Briefly, androstenedione is produced in the ovaries and adrenal gland, and gives rise to estrone and testosterone. Both testosterone and estrone can in turn be converted into estradiol, as can various nonhormonal steroids. The conversion of testosterone to estradiol and androstenedione to estrone takes place in the ovary, and also peripherally in the liver and fat. In the liver, and probably elsewhere, estrone is metabolized to estriol and 2-hydroxyestrone (as well as to estradiol). Almost all of the estriol is immediately conjugated and little measurable free estriol is found in the blood. The other two estrogens, estradiol and estrone, are also ultimately conjugated; all three are excreted largely as conjugates in the urine. The estrogen found in highest concentrations in the blood is estradiol. Estriol is the estrogen found in highest concentration in the urine. Thus, urinary levels of estrogens do not directly reflect plasma levels. Production of all three major estrogens varies with the menstrual cycle and decreases at menopause, after which time the ovaries produce little or no estrogens. Plasma estrone levels have also been shown to have diurnal variation.

As with the androgens, results of early studies that compared levels of plasma estrogen or urinary estrogen metabolites in cases of breast cancer and controls were generally inconsistent and unrevealing. In 1969, however, Lemon (138) reviewed the results of recent studies of estrogens conducted by himself and others and formulated a specific hypothesis for the role of estrogens in the etiology of breast cancer. He noted that:

1. Estriol was a weak estrogen with no known carcinogenic activity in animal models.
2. The estrogenic effect (uterine growth) of estradiol and estrone could be inhibited by estriol, indicating that estriol could compete with other estrogens at estrogen receptor sites.
3. Caucasian women with breast cancer tended to excrete low levels of estriol relative to the other more active estrogens (the estriol quotient or urinary estriol excretion ratio).
4. The estriol quotient was increased during pregnancy, which could explain the reduced risk of breast cancer in parous women.
5. The estriol excretion quotient was low in women with benign breast conditions, who tend to be at increased risk of breast cancer.
6. Some women with infertility (who may be at increased risk of breast cancer) secreted subnormal amounts of estriol, presumably because many had anovulatory menstrual cycles and hence no luteal phase (during which relatively more estriol is excreted than during the follicular phase).

Based on these observations, Lemon (138) hypothesized that estriol exerted an antineoplastic action on the breast by competing with more active estrogens. The reduced risk of breast cancer associated with parity was hypothesized to be due to the production of large amounts of estriol from the fetoplacenta during pregnancy which block the carcinogenic effects of other estrogens.

Based largely on the observation that breast cancer risk was related more to age at birth of first child than to total number of children, this hypothesis was modified by Cole and MacMahon (139). They suggested that the levels of estriol in relation to the other estrogens between the ages of puberty and about 25 years of age was the important determinant of a woman's lifetime risk of breast cancer.

To test this hypothesis, MacMahon and Cole, and later others, compared the estriol excretion quotient in women in various populations at different risks of breast cancer (140–144). Results from these studies are summarized in Table 13. In all studies shown, the proportion of urinary estrogen that was found to be estriol was highest in women from low risk populations and lowest in women from high risk populations; women from populations at intermediate risk had intermediate values. As one would expect if this hypothesis is valid, this inverse relationship between the estriol excretion ratio and breast cancer risk in the population was strongest for women in their teens and twenties, and weaker for women in their thirties. This relationship was not observed by Bulbrook et al. (144) in menopausal or postmenopausal women, although a negative correlation was found between amounts of estriol excretion in normal 50- to 59-year-old Israeli women from four different ethnic groups and rates of breast cancer in these groups (145). Additional support for the hypothesis comes from the observation by Cole et al. (146) that urinary estriol excretion ratios were higher during both the follicular and luteal phases in young parous women than in either older parous women or young nulliparous women. This finding suggests that the protective effect of an early first birth might be mediated through some alteration by an early pregnancy in estrogen production, metabolism, or excretion, and studies are currently underway to more clearly delineate the endocrinologic consequences of an early first pregnancy.

Although this hypothesis seems attractive, there are several reasons to doubt its validity:

1. Estriol has now been shown to produce mammary cancer in experimental mice (147), thus, if it does compete with other estrogens at receptor cell sites, it has to be less carcinogenic than estrone or estradiol.
2. Urinary levels of various estrogens do not reflect plasma levels, and plasma levels of estriol are so low that it is unlikely that this estrogen could effectively compete with others (131,148).
3. Women with high and low urinary estriol excretion ratios were found not to differ in their production rates (the amount entering the blood) of free, unconjugated, biologically active estriol or other estrogens, or in their metabolic clearance rates of these estrogens (149). Thus, differences in estriol excretion ratios may be attributed to differences in final pathways of estrogen metabolism. These observations explain why observed differences in plasma levels of estrogens in women from high and low risk groups have not been impressive (144).

We must thus reject the hypothesis that estriol competes with other, more carcinogenic estrogens at the cellular level to reduce the risk of breast cancer. The inverse associations of urinary estriol excretion ratios to rates of breast cancer in various populations (Table 13), and to age at first pregnancy (146) must be indirect ones.

These associations are nonetheless important leads that suggest that a common endocrinologic mechanism might explain both the international differences in rates and the influence of age at first birth on risk of breast cancer, even though differences in age at first birth cannot explain the international variation in rates. This hypothetical endocrinologic mechanism is probably not an explanation for the increased risk in relatives of breast cancer patients; estriol excretion ratios have not been found to differ in daughters of women with breast cancer and controls (150,151). Studies to attempt to identify envi-

TABLE 13. Urinary Estriol Excretion Ratios[a] and Proportions[b] in Normal Women from Populations with Varying Incidence Rates of Breast Cancer

Fist author (reference)	Age	Population	Relative incidence	Phase of menstrual cycle: Follicular	Phase of menstrual cycle: Luteal
MacMahon (140)[a]	15–19	Asian	Low	1.49	1.76
		North American	High	0.49	0.78
	35–39	Asian	Low	1.00	1.55
		North American	High	1.07	1.06
Briggs (141)[b]	Premenopausal	Indian	Low	0.54	0.60
		African	Intermediate	0.52	0.44
		European	High	0.47	0.39
MacMahon, Dickinson (142,143)[b]	15–19	Asian	Low	0.59	0.63
		Hawaiian-Oriental	Intermediate	0.48	0.52
		Hawaiian-Caucasian	High	0.37	0.40
		North American	High	0.40	0.44
	20–24	Asian	Low	0.53	0.57
		Hawaiian-Oriental	Intermediate	0.46	0.50
		Hawaiian-Caucasian	High	0.37	0.43
		North American	High	0.39	0.43
	30–39	Asian	Low	0.51	0.55
		Hawaiian-Oriental	Intermediate	0.46	0.52
		Hawaiian-Caucasian	High	0.43	0.49
		North American	High	0.38	0.45

Bulbrook (144)[a]	Adolescent	Japanese	Low	1.24
		British	High	0.97
	Premenopausal	Japanese	Low	1.20
		British	High	0.96
	Menopausal	Japanese	Low	0.46
		British	High	0.88
	Postmenopausal	Japanese	Low	0.65
		British	High	0.64

[a]Numbers are values of estriol/estrone + estradiol (estriol excretion ratio).
[b]Numbers are values of estriol/estrone + estradiol + estriol (estriol excretion proportion).

ronmental and other factors that may be related to breast cancer and influence the distal metabolism of estrogens and hence the estriol excretion ratio should be conducted. Additional attempts to identify various endocrinologic features that are correlated with this ratio might also be fruitful.

The findings described in the section on androgens are probably not inconsistent with the findings related to estrogens. Each set of observations very likely provides a view of a different portion of the endocrinologic etiology of breast cancer, and there are a number of additional investigations that might clarify the roles of both of these classes of hormones. These should certainly include additional studies of the interrelationship between androgens and estrogens. It is known, for example, that most estrone is derived from the peripheral metabolism of androstenedione (152). Furthermore, the rate of this reaction is increased in both postmenopausal and ovulatory and nonovulatory premenopausal obese women (153–156). Although obesity per se may not be an important risk factor for breast cancer, specific dietary constituents such as fats or other unknown factors that may be correlated with obesity may be risk factors. Studies to identify dietary and other factors that may influence the conversion of androstenedione to estrone should be conducted.

Androstenediol, a metabolite of dehydroepiandrosterone, has been found to compete with estrogens at estrogen receptor sites (157). Thus, like estriol, high levels of this androgen may reduce cancer risk by impeding the carcinogenic effects of endogenous estrogens. Studies to identify factors that influence the metabolism of dehydroepiandrosterone to androstenediol may therefore also be rewarding.

Progesterone

Progesterone is produced primarily during the luteal phase of the menstrual cycle by the corpus luteum of the ovary. Following stimulation by estrogens produced during the follicular phase, this hormone causes alveolar cell growth and proliferation in the breast. Little progesterone is produced during anovulatory cycles because of inadequate corpus luteum formation.

Sherman and Korenman (158) have hypothesized that the development of breast cancer is related to inadequate corpus luteum formation, and hence to estrogenic stimulation in the absence of sufficient cyclic progesterone. This suggestion is based on the following observations:

1. Early age at menarche is a risk factor, and early menstrual cycles tend to be anovulatory.
2. Delayed first pregnancy increases risk; if this is due to relative infertility, then menstrual cycles in women with a later first child would tend to be anovulatory.
3. Obesity, which may be a risk factor, is often accompanied by anovulatory cycles.
4. Subnormal androgen excretion, which has been related to subsequent risk of breast cancer, could result from inadequate corpus luteum formation.
5. The estriol excretion ratio would tend to be increased during anovulatory cycles.

In support of this hypothesis, studies based on luteal plasma progesterone levels (159) and endometrial biopsies (99) have shown breast cancer cases to more frequently have anovulatory cycles than controls.

However, anovulatory cycles in women with breast cancer could result from their disease rather than be a cause of it; and, as shown in Table 10 (33), the effect of a delayed first pregnancy on risk of breast cancer does not seem to be solely due to relative infertility. In addition, obesity may not be a risk factor (Table 12). Also, in one study, low-risk Japanese and high-risk British women were found to have similar levels of plasma progesterone and urinary pregnanediol (144). In another study (150), daughters of breast cancer patients were found to actually have somewhat higher levels of plasma progesterone and urinary pregnanediol than controls. Although these findings do not support the hypothesis of Sherman and Korenman (158), insufficient information is currently available to make a final judgment of its validity. Ongoing studies of breast cancer in women with menstrual irregularities and infertility may provide the needed facts.

Prolactin

Prolactin is secreted by the pituitary gland and acts on the estrogen-primed breast to stimulate and maintain lactation. In nonlactating premenopausal women there is a marked diurnal variation in prolactin release and highest plasma levels are found during sleep (160). Large amounts of prolactin are released during nursing and the absence of a relationship between lactation and breast cancer thus does not support the idea that prolactin is involved in the genesis of breast cancer. This is also true of observations that neither basal plasma prolactin levels (161–165), nor levels in response to provocative tests such as the thyrotropin-releasing hormone stimulation test (164), have been found to differ appreciably in breast cancer cases and controls. One study has revealed no difference in plasma prolactin levels drawn between 9:00 and 9:30 A.M. from normal pre- and postmenopausal Bantu, Caucasian, and Japanese women (166), although the time of the blood drawing may not have been optimal.

Prolactin may, however, play a role in the increased risk of breast cancer in family members of women with this disease. Compared to women without a family history of breast cancer, women on the Isle of Guernsey whose mothers were affected had higher luteal phase plasma prolactin levels at 7:00 P.M., a time when a minor increase in prolactin was noted, but not between 3:00 and 6:00 A.M., when a more massive daily surge of prolactin occurs (167). In a study in Los Angeles, blood was drawn between 8:00 and 10:00 A.M. from daughters of breast cancer patients and controls; it was found that the daughters of the cases had higher plasma levels of prolactin, as well as estradiol and estrone, on days 6 and 11 of the menstrual cycle, but not on day 22 (150).

The implications of these findings for breast cancer etiology are conjectural, although additional studies of prolactin might serve to clarify the mechanism by which breast cancer risk is increased in family members of cases. Blood specimens collected in conjunction with such studies should be obtained at a time of day when the diurnal variation in plasma prolactin levels is least likely to interfere with comparisons of high and low risk individuals.

Thyroid

The relationship between thyroid hormones and breast cancer, if any, is not well understood; it very likely involves interactions with other hormones. Hypothyroidism is associated with an increase in etiocholanolone production (168). Hyperthyroidism is accompanied by production of relatively more 2-hydroxyestrone and less estradiol from estrone (169).

Studies have generally shown thyroid function to be normal in women with breast cancer (170,171). In one study (164,172), thyroid function tests and levels of prolactin were normal in women with breast cancer, but levels of thyroid stimulating hormone (TSH) were elevated, and there was an elevated TSH response to stimulation by thyrotrophin-releasing hormone (TRH). These observations led the investigators to hypothesize that women at increased risk of breast cancer tend to have slight hypothyroidism of thyroid gland origin, and that their epithelial cells may be abnormally sensitized to prolactin. Further studies are needed to confirm or refute these observations.

Results of studies of breast cancer in relation to thyroid function states and disease are inconsistent. Associations have been reported between breast cancer risk and hyperthyroidism (173), thyroid cancer (174), and Hashimoto's thyroiditis (175). A decreased risk of breast cancer has been associated with hypothyroidism in some reports (176,177). Other studies have shown no such associations (178–180). The inconsistency of these results and the interrelationships between thyroid and other hormones suggest that an association between thyroid and breast cancer is likely to be an indirect one, and that other lines of investigation are likely to prove more rewarding.

One recent study report proported to show an increase in breast cancer associated with use of thyroid supplements for hypothyroidism (181). However, this study suffered from several methodologic errors and reanalysis of the original data showed no association (182). An independent investigation has also shown no relationship of hormone use to risk of breast cancer (183).

Hormone Receptors

Unfortunately, most studies of estrogen receptors are directed toward improvement of therapy; few provide data of value in elucidating etiology (184). It has been shown that reported percentages of primary carcinomas that contain estrogen receptors vary from about 50 to 85%, depending on the sensitivity of the assay methods used, and that this percentage is higher in post- than premenopausal women and tends to increase with age (184). The prevalence of androgen receptors has been shown not to increase with age (185). The presence of estrogen receptors is not related to the histologic type of the tumor or the extent of disease at diagnosis but may be related to the degree of dedifferentiation (184).

Studies are currently being conducted to compare the epidemiologic characteristics of women with breast cancer whose tumors do and do not have estrogen (and progesterone) receptors. An assessment of the value of hormone receptors for studying etiology will have to await the results of these investigations.

EXOGENOUS FEMALE HORMONES

Because endogenous hormones apparently play a role in the genesis of mammary carcinomas, it is reasonable to ask whether risk of breast cancer is altered by use of exogenous hormones. Oral contraceptives and estrogens, used for replacement therapy at menopause, are of particular concern because of their widespread use in some parts of the world. The epidemiologic evidence for a relationship between both benign and malignant breast tumors and these preparations have recently been reviewed (186).

There is strong evidence that oral contraceptives reduce the risk of benign breast diseases. At least six case-control studies (187–192) and three prospective studies (193–195), have shown the risk of benign breast diseases to be lower in pill users than nonusers. The apparent protective effect of oral contraceptives appears to be particularly strong for cystic diseases of the breast (188,190–193), although most studies in which specific histologic types of lesions were considered also showed oral contraceptives to reduce the risk of fibroadenoma (188,190,192,193). Risks of both cystic disease (188,190,191) and fibroadenoma (188,190), as well as all types of benign lesions combined (188–192), have been shown to diminish with increasing duration of use.

Recent data from a prospective study of the Royal College of General Practitioners (196) showed the incidence rates of benign breast disease to be inversely related to the amount of progestogen in the preparations used; and four case-control studies (190,191,197,198), have failed to show menopausal estrogens (which have no progestogen) to be protective against benign breast disease. These observations suggest that it is the progestational component of oral contraceptives that is responsible for their protective influence.

Although one of these four case-control studies (198) showed the relative risk of benign breast lesions to be significantly increased in users of menopausal estrogens, as discussed elsewhere (186), this is probably a spurious finding. There is no other evidence that non-contraceptive estrogens increase the risk of benign breast conditions.

As discussed in a subsequent section, women with fibrocystic breast lesions tend to be at increased risk of breast cancer. A number of histologic characteristics of these benign lesions have been shown to distinguish women at particularly high risk. One of these characteristics is the degree of atypia in the mammary epithelium. One case-control study (199) has shown the risk of benign lesions in oral contraceptive users relative to nonusers to be less than one for lesions with no or mild atypia, but greater than one for lesions with severe atypia. Although the 95% confidence limits of all of the relative risks included unity, these findings, if confirmed by others, imply that oral contraceptives do not protect against, and may even increase the risk of, benign lesions most likely to be precursors of breast cancer.

Available results from eight case-control studies of breast cancer and oral contraceptives are summarized in Table 14 (74,187–191,200). None shows a significant overall increase or decrease in risk of breast cancer in oral contraceptive users. This consistency of results is striking, considering the varied settings in which the different studies were conducted and the numerous methodologic differences between studies. However, in the two studies that

TABLE 14. Case-Control Studies of the Relationship of Oral Contraceptives to the Risk of Breast Cancer

(1) First author (reference)	(2) Type of control	(3) No. of cases	(4) Age of cases	(5) Years cases were diagnosed	(6) Relative risk in ever users	(7) Relative risk on long-term users	(8) Minimum years of use by long-term users
Vessey (200)	Hospital	322	16–45	1968–74	0.89	0.94	2
BCDSP (187)	Hospital	23	20–75	1972	0.60	—	—
Paffenbarger (189)	Hospital	452	<50	1970–72	1.1	1.7	8
Henderson (74)	Office	308	40–64	1971–73	0.74	—	—
Sartwell (191)	Hospital	284	20–73	1969–72	0.86	0.97	5
Kelsey (188)	Hospital	99	20–44	1971–73	1.35	1.7	5
Lilienfeld[a]	Hospital	342	18–74	1973–75	0.80	—	—
	Neighborhood	254		1973–75	1.50	—	—
Ravnihar (190)	Hospital	190	20–49	1972–74	0.91	0.86	2

[a]Personal communication.

were restricted to relatively young women (188,189) and that provided information on fairly long-term use, users of more than 8 and more than 5 years duration had a relative risk of 1.7. Although this value does not differ significantly from unity in either study, and in neither was there evidence of a consistent increase in risk with duration of use, these findings indicate the need for additional information on long term users.

Only two studies (189,200) provide information on relative risk of breast cancer in relation to time since initial use of oral contraceptives. Neither shows a consistent change in risk with the passage of time. Analysis of data published by Vessey, et al. (200) yields a relative risk of 0.87 after 8 years; Paffenbarger (189) observed a relative risk of 1.1 after 6 years from first use. Information is needed on the risk of breast cancer after longer periods of time since initial exposure.

The Paffenbarger study (189) also showed that oral contraceptives were associated with an increased risk of breast cancer in parous women who first used them prior to the birth of their first child, and in 15- to 39-year-old nulliparous women. These findings suggest that early use of oral contraceptives does not afford the protection against breast cancer that an early first birth provides, and may increase the risk of breast cancer. However, at variance with this is the observation, in a case-control study by Stavraky et al. (88), that the relative risk of breast cancer tended to increase with age at first pill use, although the trend was not statistically significant. Additional information on the relationship of age of oral contraceptive use to breast cancer risk is obviously needed.

Women with a history of benign breast disease prior to use of oral contraceptives have been shown in one study (189) to be at increased risk of breast cancer.

Results from three prospective studies of oral contraceptives and breast cancer (193–195) are shown in Table 15. The Royal College of General Practitioners (RCGP) study shows no relationship between oral contraceptives and breast cancer. The other two studies show a negative association, but in neither study is the relationship statistically significant. In the Ory study (193), the rate was the same for women who had used oral contraceptives for less than 2 years and for women who had used them for 2 or more years.

Results from seven case-control studies of noncontraceptive estrogens and breast cancer are summarized in Table 16 (74,97,190,191,197,201,202). None

TABLE 15. Prospective Studies of the Relationship of Oral Contraceptives to the Risk of Breast Cancer

First author (reference)	Incidence per 1000 woman-years (number of cases) by use of oral contraceptives: Users	Nonusers	Relative risk
RCGP (194)	0.36 (11)	0.34 (16)	1.08
Vessey (195)	0.18 (5)	0.44 (11)	0.41
Ory (193)	0.6 (22)	1.0 (115)	0.60

TABLE 16. Studies of the Relationship of Noncontraceptive Estrogens to the Risk of Breast Cancer

Type of study	First author (reference)	Type of controls	No. of cases	Years of breast cancer diagnosis	Measure of estrogen use	Relative risk[a]
Hospital-based	Sartwell (191)	Hospital	284	1969–1972	Ever	0.82
Case-control	BCDSP (197)	Hospital	51	1972	Ever	1.0
	Ravnihar (190)	Clinic	374	1972–1974	Ever	0.78
Population-based	Henderson (74)	Office	100	1969–1972	Ever	0.75
Case-control	Casagrande (201)	Neighborhood	47	1972–1973	Ever	3.1
	Craig (97)	Population and neighborhood	134	1949–1967	Ever	1.0
	Mack (202)	Population	111	1971–1975	Ever	1.6
Practice-based	Burch (203)	None	19	1948–1973	≥5 yr.	1.2
Prospective	Hoover (204)	None	49	1939–1972	≥6 mo.	1.3

[a]Risk in women who used estrogens relative to risk in nonusers.

shows a significant association between these preparations and mammary carcinoma. The Casagrande study (201) is small and the relative risk of 3.1, though impressive, is not statistically significant. Mack et al. (202) conducted a study to examine the relationship of Reserpine to breast cancer. A small relative risk in excess of 1 was noted for four classes of drugs in addition to estrogens, suggesting that selection bias may have been operative in this study.

Two prospective studies of noncontraceptive estrogens and breast cancer have been conducted (203,204). Results of these studies are summarized in the last two lines of Table 16. Methodologic errors in the design and analysis of the Burch study (203) render the results questionable, and the relative risk of 1.2 is not statistically significant.

The study of Hoover (204) consisted of following up, through the end of 1972, a total of 1891 women who had been given between 1939 and 1960 conjugated estrogens for menopausal symptoms. Observed numbers of breast cancer in the study group were compared with expected numbers that were derived from incidence rates from the Second and Third National Cancer Surveys. Although the overall risk of breast cancer was slightly increased in the study group (relative risk = 1.3) and was of borderline statistical significance, the questionable appropriateness of the source of the expected numbers makes this a difficult finding to interpret. More importantly, the risk increased with duration of follow-up. Risk did not appreciably increase until 12 years after initial use; after that time it approximately doubled. This observation is consistent with the long latent period that follows exposure to known carcinogens. So far studies of oral contraceptives have not provided data on risk of breast cancer long after initial use. This finding emphasizes the need for such information, particularly for sequential oral contraceptives.

In Hoover's study (204) the increase in risk was greatest in women who took the preparations of highest strength, but also in those who took their medication less frequently than daily. Risk was not related to duration of use.

This study also showed that the risk of breast cancer in women who developed benign breast disease after starting on estrogens was increased sevenfold. The risk was approximately doubled in women who had a history of benign breast disease prior to taking estrogens. These findings are consistent with Paffenbarger's observation (189) that oral contraceptives predispose women with benign breast disease to breast cancer.

The case-control study by Henderson (74) showed somewhat different findings relating risk of breast cancer to time since initial use of estrogens. The relative risk was actually observed to be less than unity in users less than 10 years after initial use but was greater than 1 for users 10 or more years after first use. This is what one would observe if estrogens delayed the development of preexisting breast cancer.

Additional information regarding the possible relationship of exogenous estrogens to breast cancer is needed. Of particular interest is the effect of oral contraceptives on breast cancer risk after prolonged use, long after initial use, in women with various histologic types of benign breast diseases, and in young nulliparous women. The effects of sequential and combined preparations also must be assessed separately, as well as the influence of noncontraceptive estrogens.

Long-acting injectable progestational agents have been used for contraception in many parts of the world during the past decade. The influence of these preparations on the risk of breast cancer is unknown but is currently being investigated.

RAUWOLFIA DERIVATIVES

In 1973, an association between breast cancer and use of reserpine was observed in women studied by the Boston Collaborative Drug Surveillance Program (205). This program is designed to detect associations between use of all commonly used drugs and a large number of conditions that result in hospitalization. As a result, the investigators recognized that their observation could have been a chance phenomenon. Before reporting their findings, they stimulated two additional studies (206,207), the results of which tended to confirm the original observation. Findings from all three studies were published in 1974. Considerable debate followed, the three studies were criticized on methodological grounds, and the need for additional information from more rigorously designed investigations became apparent.

At least eight more studies have now been conducted (202,208–214). Results from these, plus the three original investigations, are summarized in Table 17. In general, subsequent findings do not support the original observations. None of the relative risks estimated from the eight additional studies is significantly greater than one.

Rauwolfia derivatives are known to stimulate prolactin production in humans, and it has been suggested that these drugs could alter the risk of breast cancer by stimulating growth of preexisting neoplastic foci (205). In support of this, some studies showed an association between breast cancer and current or recent use of rauwolfia derivatives (205,206,208,212). However, other investigations have failed to confirm this observation (211,214), and a number of studies have not shown an association between breast cancer and other drugs known to stimulate prolactin production (202,205–207,209–211). Thus, if rauwolfia derivatives were found to be related to breast cancer, a mechanism other than prolactin production would have to be operative.

Evidence against a more direct carcinogenic effect of rauwolfia derivatives on the human breast is also considerable. The eight more recent studies were conducted in different populations, and varied in methodologic details. Yet, the consistency of their negative findings is striking. Seven studies dealt with any use of rauwolfia compounds (202,207–210,212,214), not just recent use, so a relatively long-term carcinogenic effect would likely have been observed, if present. Also, various rauwolfia alkaloids were used with varying frequencies in the various study areas; thus, if one compound were particularly carcinogenic, this would likely have resulted in more inconsistent findings among the various investigations.

On balance, it thus seems that the findings of the original three studies were spurious, and that subsequent investigations have provided little evidence that rauwolfia alkaloids exert either a direct carcinogenic effect on the breast, or act to promote the growth of preexisting neoplastic foci. However,

TABLE 17. Case-Control Studies of the Relationship of Rauwolfia Derivatives to Breast Cancer

First author (reference)	Year of publication	Location of study	Source of study subjects		No. of cases	Relative risk	95% C.L.
			Cases	Controls			
1. BCDSP (205)	1974	Boston	Hospital	Medical and surgical patients	150	3.4	1.6–8.0
2. Armstrong (206)	1974	England	Cancer registry	Other cancer patients	708	2.04	0.74–5.53
3. Heinonen (207)	1974	Finland	Hospital	Surgical patients	438	2.0	1.2–3.4
4. Laska (208)	1975	New York	Psychiatric hospital	Psychiatric hospital	55	1.08[a]	Unavailable
5. O'Fallon (209)	1975	Olmstead Co.	County residents	Residents with gallbladder disease	167[b]	1.02[a]	Unavailable
6. Mack (202)	1975	Los Angeles	Retirement community	Residents of same community	99	1.2	0.7–2.2
7. Lilienfeld (210)	1976	Baltimore	Hospital	Hospital	164	1.57	0.85–2.94
				Neighborhood	139	0.88	0.44–1.70
8. Aromaa (211)	1976	Finland	Cancer registry	Hypertensive patients	109[b]	1.16	0.59–2.28
9. Armstrong (212)	1976	England and Wales	Death certificates	Other deaths	33[b]	2.1	0.94–4.9
				Other cancer deaths	35[b]	1.4	0.56–3.4
10. Kewitz (213)	1977	Berlin	Hospital	Benign breast disease	181	0.6	0.4–1.1
				Nonmalignant surgical	181	0.9	0.4–1.7
11. Kodlin (214)	1978	California	Prepaid health plan	Hypertensive patients	77[b]	1.3	Unavailable

[a]Calculated from data in published report.
[b]Study subjects with hypertension.

because of the long latent period between exposure to some human carcinogens and development of neoplasia, rauwolfia derivatives should continue to be monitored for potential long-term carcinogenic effects on the breast.

BENIGN BREAST LESIONS

A large number of studies of the relationship of benign breast lesions to breast cancer have been conducted. These were extensively reviewed by Davis et al. (215) in 1964. Early investigations were of two types: pathologic studies of the prevalence of concomitant benign lesions in breasts with cancer, and follow-up studies of the incidence of subsequent breast cancer in women with benign breast lesions.

The pathologic studies showed that a high proportion of breasts in which cancer had arisen also had evidence of various benign conditions. However, such observations do not indicate a causal relationship between benign and malignant breast lesions in the absence of comparable information on the prevalence of benign lesions in cancer-free breasts. The prevalence of benign lesions in some independent autopsy series was as high as the prevalence in some series of cancerous breasts. Although this suggests that the simultaneous occurrence of both malignant and benign lesions is not evidence of a cause and effect relationship, the observed prevalance of benign lesions can vary with the pathologic techniques used to detect them, making comparisons of prevalence rates among independent studies of little value.

Many of the early follow-up studies reviewed by Davis et al. (215) were small in size and provided only the percentage of women that developed breast cancer (not rates per women-years at risk). In addition, most provided no estimates of the number of cases that would be expected to occur if women with benign breast lesions were not at increased risk of breast cancer; and those that did used crude and often inappropriate methods. More recently, however, four more rigorous follow-up studies (216–219) have shown that rates of breast cancer are from 2.1 to 2.7 times greater in women with histologically confirmed benign breast diseases than in women in the general population. These studies are summarized in Table 18.

Two of these studies (218,219), and a study by Black, et al. (220), provide information on the relationship of breast cancer to specific histologic types or characteristics of benign lesions. Using a system of grading lesions for the degree of atypia in various sized ducts, Black et al. (220) compared prior benign breast lesions from women with breast cancer with benign lesions from cancer-free individuals. Lesions from women who had developed breast cancer more frequently had evidence of duct atypia. Using the same grading system, Kodlin et al. (218) also showed the risk of breast cancer to be directly related to the degree of ductal atypia in prior benign lesions.

The follow-up studies of both Kodlin (218) and Hutchinson (219) also showed risk of breast cancer to be related to one or more traditional classes of benign lesions, and Kodlin found those classes to be as effective as the Black grading system in distinguishing women at increased risk of breast cancer.

Kodlin et al. (218) categorized women with benign breast diseases into five

TABLE 18. Prospective Studies of Breast Cancer in Women with Benign Breast Diseases

First author (reference)	Study population	Type of benign lesions	No. of women	No. of breast cancers		Relative risk	Basis of expected numbers
				Observed	Expected		
Donnelly (216)	Residents of Rochester, Minn.	Any type	370	14	8.5	2.12	Incidence rates for Rochester, Minn.
Monson (217)	Hospital Admissions Boston, Mass.	Chronic mastitis	733	49	18.8	2.61	Mortality for Mass.
Kodlin (218)	Prepaid plan, Oakland, Calif.	Any type	2900	64	23.8	2.69	Third National Cancer Survey, San Francisco Area
Hutchinson (219)	Private practice	Any type	1356	64	29.8	2.15	Second and Third National Cancer Surveys and SEER data

mutually exclusive categories; they did not consider the simultaneous occurrence of multiple histologic features. In the Hutchinson study (219), benign lesions were classified according to the presence or absence of a number of histologic characteristics, and their simultaneous occurrence was taken into account in the data analysis. Both studies showed the risk of breast cancer to be increased in women with fibroadenoma, intraductal papilloma, and fibrocystic disease. The risk in women with the latter condition was particularly increased if their lesions were characterized by adenosis or sclerosing adenosis, or ductal hyperplasia (including metaplasia and papillomatosis). However, after taking into account the simultaneous occurrence of various histologic features, Hutchinson et al. found that only the relationship of subsequent breast cancer to fibrocystic disease that was characterized by ductal hyperplasia persisted. Women with such lesions were not at further increased risk if their lesions showed evidence of atypia, although the number of women with atypias was too small to confidently rule out atypia as a risk factor. It thus appears that fibrocystic disease characterized by proliferation of ductal epithelial cells best distinguished women with benign breast diseases who are at increased risk of breast cancer.

The Hutchinson study (219) also showed the risk of breast cancer to be directly related to the size of the initial benign mass, and greater for women with bilateral than unilateral benign lesions. Monson (217) observed that excess risk in women with benign lesions persisted up to 30 years after the diagnosis of the initial benign condition.

Women with benign lesions could be at increased risk of breast cancer for three reasons: (a) benign lesions may be early stages of the same pathologic process that eventuates in breast cancer, (b) breasts with benign lesions may be more vulnerable to carcinogenic insults, or (c) breast cancer and benign breast lesions are both caused by some of the same factors but are otherwise unrelated entities. Current epidemiologic studies to identify risk factors associated with various kinds of benign breast lesions, as well as with breast cancer, may provide data needed to determine which of these explanations is correct.

In 1976, Wolfe (221) described a scheme for classifying breasts according to the radiographic appearance of the breast parenchyma. He reported an increased incidence of breast cancer in women whose breasts were characterized by either of two mammographic patterns. The two high-risk mammographic patterns were designated P_2, characterized by a prominent ductal pattern occupying more than one-fourth of the volume of the breast, and DY, or "dysplasia," characterized by epithelial and connective tissue densities. A subsequent histopathological study (222) showed the prominent ductal pattern to be due to periductal and periolobular fibrosis such as seen in some forms of fibrocystic disease, focal "dysplasia" to be due to the presence of atypical and other lesions of lobular and terminal duct origin, and more extensive "dysplasia" to reflect generalized fibrosis.

Table 19 summarizes the results of four studies (221,223–225) providing ratios of incidence and prevalence rates of breast cancer in women with P_2 and DY mammographic patterns relative to women with other, more normal, patterns. The incidence rates are for women followed for from 6 months to an average of 3 years in the Wolfe study (221), and for from 6 months up to 3 years

TABLE 19. Ratios of Rates of Breast Cancer in Women with Mammographic Patterns Classified as P_1 and DY Relative to Rates in Women with More Normal Patterns[a]

First author (reference)	Rates in women with mammograms classified as P_2 or DY ÷ rates in women with mammograms classified N_1 P_1	
	Ratios of prevalence rates	Ratios of incidence rates
Wolf (221)		10.5[b]
Mendel (223)	1.23	
Wilkinson (224)	2.10[b]	
Krook (225)	1.33	3.5

[a]Classified according to the method of Wolfe (221).
[b]Calculated from published reports.

in the Krook study (225). In all four studies, the ratios are higher for women in the P_2 and DY categories. The studies of Wolfe (221), Wilkinson (224), and Krook (225) also showed rates to be higher in women with DY than P_2 patterns. Wilkinson et al. (224) found that the association between these patterns and the prevalence of breast cancer persisted after controlling for three risk factors for breast cancer: age at birth of first child, age at menopause, and family history of breast cancer.

There are at least two possible interpretations of these observations: either the abnormal mammographic patterns reflect benign changes that are precursors of breast cancer or in some other way are associated with an increased risk of developing mammary carcinoma, or they are manifestations of an existing cancer that is not yet detectable. If the first (etiologic) interpretation is correct, and these patterns precede the development of cancer, then, as Krook has noted (225), one would expect an increase in the relative risk of breast cancer in women with P_2 and DY patterns with time following the initial observation of these characteristics. If the second interpretation is correct, the relative risk would be expected to decrease with duration of follow-up. Data in Table 19 show the ratio of incidence rates to be greater than the ratio of prevalence rates. This suggests that the relative risk might increase with time, which supports the etiologic interpretation of these findings. Also in support of this interpretation is the observation by Wilkinson et al. (224) that the breast cancer risk factors, age at first birth, age at menopause, and family history of breast cancer all tend to distinguish currently cancer-free women with abnormal mammographic patterns.

Additional follow-up studies of women with these mammographic patterns who are followed for longer periods of time, and more adequately described with respect to other known risk factors for breast cancer, are currently being undertaken to provide better information regarding the etiologic significance of these radiologic patterns.

PREVIOUS CANCERS

Women who have had one cancer of the breast are at increase risk of developing a second primary carcinoma in the opposite breast. This risk has been reported to be about twice as great in American than Japanese women (226), a ratio considerably smaller than the ratio of incidence or mortality rates of breast cancer in the United States and Japan. The etiologic significance of this observation is unclear.

The risk of a second breast carcinoma has also been found to be inversely related to the age of the woman at the time of her initial cancer (227), a finding consistent with the observation that women with carcinomas occurring simultaneously in both breasts tend to be younger than women with unilateral lesions (228,229).

The risk of a second primary breast cancer is greater for women with than without a family history of breast cancer (230). In addition, second breast cancers in women under 55 years of age with two or more first-degree relatives with this disease have been found to occur either before the sixth or after the thirteenth post-operative year (231), a finding that suggests a different mechanism for the genesis of second breast cancers at different times following development of an initial mammary carcinoma.

Women with cancers of the colon (232), ovary (233,234), and endometrium (233,235,236) have also been reported to be at increased risk of breast cancer. The most likely explanation for this is that all of these neoplasms, including cancer of the colon (237,238) have some epidemiologic features in common with breast cancer. A high risk of breast cancer in women with salivary gland tumors has also been reported (239), the etiologic implications of which are unclear.

GENETIC FACTORS

As described in a previous section, incidence rates of breast cancer in migrants from low- to high-risk countries gradually increase to levels comparable to those in women within the high-risk country. This finding suggests that racial and international differences in rates are not due to genetic factors. On the other hand, some women with all of the known risk factors for breast cancer develop the disease, but others do not. Those spared are either not subjected to other, unknown environmental causes of breast cancer to which those who developed the disease were exposed, or those who develop the disease have a genetic predisposition to do so when the proper complex of risk factors is operating. If genetic factors do play a role, they must be distributed with nearly equal frequency in all populations from which migrants to high-risk countries have come, and with the same frequency in these populations as in the high-risk countries.

In a study conducted in the United States, less than 15% of all women with breast cancer reported a family history of this disease (240), a finding that suggests that most breast cancer is probably not explainable on the basis of hereditary factors. There is evidence, however, that genetic factors do contribute to the development of some cases of breast cancer.

Table 20 summarizes results from 12 case-control studies of breast cancer in which a history of this disease in first-degree relatives was ascertained (74,241–251). With very few exceptions (243,246,247), the risk of breast cancer was found to be increased in mothers, sisters, and daughters of women with breast cancer. On balance, it appears that the risk in these three types of

TABLE 20. Observed and Expected Numbers of Breast Cancer Cases in First-Degree Relatives of Women with Breast Cancer[a]

First author (reference)	Year of publication	No. of cases	Mothers			Sisters			Daughters		
			O	E	O/E	O	E	O/E	O	E	O/E
Jacobsen (241)	1946	200	21	7	3.0	13	5	2.6			
Penrose (242)	1948	300[b]	25	11	2.3	23	7	3.3			
Passay (243)	1952	585	23	20	1.1						
Smithers (244)	1952	556	29	13.9	2.1						
Woolf (245)	1955	200	4	2.1	1.9	8	3.2	2.5			
Anderson (246)	1958	544	9	7.7	1.2	28	12.4	2.3			
Murphy (247)	1959	200	7	3	2.3	2	6	0.3			
Macklin (248)	1959	295	11	5.6	2.0	14	5	2.8			
Tokuhata (249)	1969	551							10	2.1	4.8
Morgan (250)	1974	48							6	0.85	7.0
Henderson (74)	1974	308	22	5	4.4	26	10.3	2.5	2	0	∞
Albert (251)	1977	348				20	5.3	3.8	9	6.3	1.4

[a] Expected numbers based on rates of breast cancer in relatives of controls.
[b] Approximate number.

relatives is somewhat more than doubled. As shown in Table 21, risk is increased by a similar, or perhaps even greater, amount in both paternal and maternal grandmothers and aunts of cases (74,248,252).

Familial aggregation of a disease can result from either common environmental or genetic factors. The data in Tables 20 and 21 are generally compatible with either explanation (although the higher risk of breast cancer in second than first degree relatives of cases fits neither). If genetic factors are involved, they are unlikely to be x-linked, because of the comparable elevations of risk in paternal and maternal relatives. Studies of a large number of genetic markers in breast cancer cases, controls, and their relatives, have not shown any genetically determined biochemical or immunological factors to be associated with susceptibility to breast cancer (253,254). Studies of additional genetic markers are currently underway.

Some evidence for genetic factors playing a causative role comes from studies of twins, which show the degree of concordance for breast cancer to be roughly twice as great for monozygotic than dizygotic twins (255). However, even these findings could be a result of monozygotic twins having more common environments than dizygotic twins. Also, concordance for monozygotic twins was estimated to be only 0.28, which suggests that environmental factors also play a considerable role.

Perhaps the best evidence that genetic factors are operative in the genesis of some breast cancers comes from studies in the United States by Anderson (229,240,252). He has found the subsequent risk of breast cancer in sisters (252) and daughters (229) of cases to be lowest if the case had no other family member with breast cancer, somewhat higher if the case had an affected second degree relative, higher yet if the case had a sister with prior breast cancer, and highest if the case's mother had also had the disease. Also, the relatives of premenopausal cases were at higher risk of breast cancer than the relatives of postmenopausal cases, an observation also noted by others (74,97). Bilateral breast cancer tended to occur at an earlier age than unilateral disease, and to occur in women with a family history of breast cancer. The latter finding has also been reported in Japan (226). Unilateral cases with a family history of breast cancer also tended to be younger than unilateral cases without a family history of breast cancer.

TABLE 21. Observed and Expected Numbers of Breast Cancer Cases in Maternal and Paternal Second-Degree Relatives of Women with Breast Cancer[a]

First author (reference)	Year of publication	Relative	Maternal O	Maternal E	Maternal O/E	Paternal O	Paternal E	Paternal O/E
Macklin (248)	1959	Grandmother	10	2.53	3.95	7	1.96	3.57
		Aunt	21	7.7	2.72	22	6.8	3.24
Henderson (74)	1974	Aunt	23	15.6	1.48	21	7.77	2.70
Anderson (252)	1974	Aunts and Grandmother	15	3.8	3.95	8	1.4	5.71

[a]Expected numbers based on rates of breast cancer in relatives of controls.

In some groups of women, these various factors appeared to have synergetic effects. In 20- to 39-year-old sisters of premenopausal cases with bilateral disease whose mothers also had breast cancer, the risk was increased 40-fold. These findings, plus others from the same studies, led Anderson to hypothesize that there are two forms of inherited breast cancer: one that tends to be bilateral and occur premenopausally, and one that tends to occur unilaterally in the postmenopausal years. A predisposition to the first kind is vertically transmitted from mother to daughter, such that the probability of developing the disease in one's lifetime is 30–35%. Reported pedigrees that appear to represent each of these hypothesized hereditary types of breast cancer have been sited as additional evidence for their existence (240).

Knudson has developed a two-step mutation model to explain the occurrence of childhood tumors that tend to occur both unilaterally and bilaterally (and at an earlier age when bilateral). Based on the assumption that all bilateral breast cancer is hereditary, this model was used to estimate the proportion of all breast cancer cases that are hereditary (255). An estimate of 30% was derived. The validity of the model for breast cancer is conjectural, however, and this estimate should consequently be viewed with caution.

Other evidence for a genetic role in breast cancer development comes from reports of high-risk families in which cancer of the breast and various other organs have occurred with unusually high frequency (256–258). In some of these families, a simple dominant form of inheritance appears to explain the observed patterns if all cancers are treated as a single disease. This, however, may be a dubious analytic technique, and some of the reported familial occurrences of cancers could represent chance phenomena.

It thus seems likely that at least a small portion of all breast cancers have a genetic component to their etiology, but that the mode of inheritance is a complicated one, not conforming to currently understood laws of inheritance, and not the same for all cases with a genetic component.

The mechanism of action of any implicated gene may well be an indirect one. Compatible with this are the findings already described of Wang et al. (135), and of Pike et al. (150). The former group found lower levels of plasma and urinary androgen metabolites in sisters of breast cancer cases than controls, and the latter group found luteal phase plasma levels of prolactin, estradiol, and estrone to be higher in daughters of cases than controls. Also, Lemon (259) has suggested that the rate of conversion of estradiol and estrone to estriol could vary according to the degree of activity of the enzyme estradiol 16-alpha-hydroxylase, and that this activity could be genetically determined. These observations suggest that studies to more clearly elucidate the genetic determinants of various endocrinologic patterns of hormone production and metabolism might be fruitful.

VIRUSES

Evidence that viruses may play a role in the genesis of breast cancer in humans comes mainly from laboratory studies and has been reviewed a number of times in recent years (5,260–262). Attention was first seriously focused on viruses as a possible cause of breast cancer as a result of studies in mice in the

1930s by Bittner (263), which showed that a factor that induced breast cancer was transmitted through milk from mother to offspring.

It is now known that this factor is an RNA virus, and that in some strains of mice the viral genome (but not the whole virus) is transmitted via the gametes and is integrated into the chromosomes of all cells of the offspring (264). This Murine Mammary Tumor Virus (MMTV) has not been found to induce breast tumors in other species of animals, and even viruses from one strain of mice are less efficient inducers of breast tumors in mice of other strains than in mice of the same strain as the source mouse. Hormonal and dietary factors can also alter rates of tumor production in mice infected with the MMTV (261).

There is considerable evidence that human breast cancer may be caused by a virus similar to the MMTV. There are two types of RNA viruses that are oncogenic: C-type particles that can cause leukemia and sarcomas in some animals, and B-particles that include the MMTV. Particles morphologically identical to both B- and C-particles have been found in human milk. Early studies showed the presence of B-particles to be more frequent in milk from women with a family history of breast cancer than in women without such a family history (265,266), but this was not confirmed by additional observations (267). Virtually all known B- and C-type RNA oncogenic viruses contain an enzyme, RNA-directed DNA polymerase (RDDP). This enzyme has been demonstrated in human milk and its presence has been correlated with the presence of B-particles, but also more strongly with the presence of C-particles (267). There is additional evidence, however, that the enzyme in humans is B-particle associated. The human enzyme, like that of the MMTV, is activated by magnesium, whereas this enzyme in animal C-particles is activated by manganese (261).

Cross hybridization studies have shown, in human breast cancers, the presence of RNA molecules with portions identical to the RNA of the MMTV (261). Such RNA molecules have not been found in other human neoplasms. Neutralization and immunofluorescent studies have demonstrated that some human sera have antibodies against MMTV, the presence of which suggests prior infection with an agent closely related to the MMTV. Additionally, although the differences were small, serum from breast cancer patients was shown to more effectively reduce the infectivity of the MMTV than serum from normal women (268). Also, by leukocyte inhibition techniques, cross-sensitization of leukocytes to MMTV has been demonstrated in leukocytes from breast cancer patients, but not from healthy women or women with other cancers (261).

Although these observations are highly suggestive of a virus similar to the MMTV being involved in the genesis of mammary cancer in humans, epidemiologic studies have not shown a mode for its transmission. No clustering of cases in time or space have been reported that would suggest person-to-person spread or exposure of unrelated persons to a common source.

Numerous epidemiologic observations also tend to rule out transmission via breast feeding. The incidence of breast cancer in the United States increased slightly during a time when the popularity of breast feeding declined; and there are many examples of high breast cancer rates in countries with relatively little breast feeding, and low rates in countries where most babies are breast fed. Case-control studies have shown that women with breast cancer and controls do not differ in their history of having been breast fed (25,73,74). Prospective studies have also shown the incidence of breast cancer to be the same in women who were and were not breast fed. This was true for the daughters of predominantly normal women (250), as well as for the daughters of women with benign and malignant breast disease (249). The data in Tables 21 and 22 showing comparable rates of breast cancer in maternal and paternal second-degree relatives of women with breast cancer also are unsupportive of transmission by nursing, or by the transplacental route.

One possible explanation consistent with both the virologic and epidemiologic observations is the presence of a viral genome similar to the MMTV that is distributed with uniform frequency in human populations, and whose carcinogenic potential is expressed only under certain conditions. Such conditions might be achieved in some women in the presence of the known risk factors for breast cancer, and this would explain the epidemiologic characteristics of the disease. Those with the same risk factors but not the viral genome would not get the disease. The presence of such a genome would be a situation similar to that observed in some strains of mice in which the virus is transmitted as a viral genome to all progeny, and in which the rate of tumor production can be altered by nutritional, reproductive, and hormonal manipulation. Although B-particles, which might represent the complete virus, are not found in all women with breast cancer, and other tests for evidence of prior or current infection by an agent related to the MMTV are negative in many breast cancer patients, such results could well be due to limitations in current laboratory techniques, and therefore are not firm evidence against the concept of a viral genome for human breast cancer. As advances are made in the laboratory, they will provide the tools needed for additional epidemiologic studies, such as those suggested by Shah et al. (269), to test the hypothesis of a viral causation of human mammary carcinomas.

CONCLUSIONS

Although we know much more about breast cancer today than we did 30 years ago, there are also more unanswered questions now than then. We have learned that its etiology is complex and multifactorial. Attempts to develop unifying etiologic hypotheses that explain all of the observed characteristics of the disease have failed. These failures have stemmed not from lack of imagination on the part of responsible investigators, but from lack of information. In my opinion, there are at the present time insufficient facts to be synthesized into a single unifying explanation for the cause of breast cancer. Many of today's unanswered questions, some of which have been mentioned in this review, are the subject of current investigations. When these and subsequent generations of studies are completed, our perception of breast cancer etiology will change, just as it has changed during the past three decades. Eventually our perceptions will coincide with the truth, and the means to prevent this disease will become known. However, the process will undoubtedly be a gradual one in which investigators from many disciplines will participate during the next several decades.

REFERENCES

1. Logan, W. P. D. (1975) Cancer of the female breast international mortality trends. Bull. World Hlth. Org. 28, 232–251.
2. Zdeb, M. S. (1977) The probability of developing cancer. Am. J. Epidemiol. 106, 6–16.
3. Campbell, H. (1972) A review of studies of breast cancer in human populations excluding endocrine studies. Proc. Royal Soc. Med. 65, 641–648.
4. Seidman, H. (1972) Cancer of the Breast: Statistical and Epidemiological Data, New York: American Cancer Society, pp. 1–63.
5. MacMahon, B., Cole, P., Brown, J. (1973) Etiology of human breast cancer: a review. J. Natl. Cancer Inst. 50, 21–42.
6. Vakil, D. V., Morgan, R. W. (1973) Etiology of breast cancer. I. Genetic aspects. Can. Med. Assoc. 109, 29–32.
7. Vakil, D. V. and Morgan, R. W. (1973) Etiology of breast cancer. II. Epidemiologic aspects. Can. Med. Assoc. 109, 201–206.
8. Cole, P. (1974) Epidemiology of human breast cancer. J. Invest. Dermatol. 63, 133–137.
9. Papaioannou, A. N. (1974) Etiologic factors in cancer of the breast in humans. Surgery 138, 257–287.
10. Schottenfeld, D. (1975) Epidemiology of breast cancer. Clin. Bull. 5, 135–143.
11. Doll, R. (1975) The epidemiology of cancers of the breast and reproductive system. Scott. Med. J. 20, 305–315.
12. Thomas, D. B., Lilienfeld, A. M. (1976) Geographic, reproductive and sociobiological factors. *In:* Risk Factors in Breast Cancer. Stoll (ed.). London: Heinemann, Vol. II, pp. 25–53.
13. Vorherr, H., Messer, R. H. (1978) Breast cancer: potentially predisposing and protecting factors. Am. J. Obstet. Gynecol. 130, 335–358.
14. Segi, M. (1977) Graphic Presentation of Cancer Incidence by Site and by Area and Population. Segi Institute of Cancer Epidemiology, Nagoya, Japan.
15. Blot, W. J., Fraumeni, J. F., Stone, B. J. (1977) Geographic patterns of breast cancer in the United States. J. Natl. Cancer Inst. 59, 1407–1411.
16. Moolgavkar, S. H., Lee, J. A. H., Hade, R. D. (1978) Comparison of age-specific mortality from breast cancer in males in the United States and Japan. Cancer 60, 1223–1226.
17. Hems, G., Stuart, A. (1975) Breast cancer rates in populations of single women. Br. J. Cancer 31, 118–123.
18. Third National Cancer Survey: Incidence Data (1975) Cutler, S. J., Young, J. L. (eds.). Washington, D.C.: U.S. Government Printing Office, National Cancer Institute Monograph No. 41.
19. Enstrom, J. E. (1975) Cancer mortality among Mormons. Cancer 36, 825–841.
20. Phillips, R. L., Kuzma, J. W. (1977) Rationale and methods for an epidemiologic study of cancer among Seventh-Day Adventists. Natl. Cancer Inst. Monogr. 47, 107–112.
21. Lilienfeld, A. M., Levin, M. L., Kessler, I. I. (1972) Cancer in the United States. Cambridge: Harvard University Press.
22. Zippin, C., Petrakis, N. L. (1971) Identification of high risk groups in Breast Cancer. Cancer 28, 1385.
23. Paymaster, J. C., Gangadharan, P. (1972) Some observations on the epidemiology of cancer of the breast in women of Western India. Int. J. Cancer 10, 443.
24. Shapiro, S., Strax, P., Venet, L., et al. (1968) The search for risk factors in breast cancer. Am. J. Publ. Hlth. 58, 820.
25. Wynder, E. L., Bross, I. J., Hirayama, T. (1960) A study of the epidemiology of cancer of the breast. Cancer 13, 559.

26. Ramazzini, B. (1713) Diseases of Workers. (The Latin text of 1713.) W. C. Wright (translator). New York: Hafner, 1964, p. 191.
27. Wagoner, J. K., Chiazze, L., Lloyd, J. W. (1967) Cancer of the breast at menopausal ages. Cancer 20, 354.
28. Fraumeni, J. F., Lloyd, J. W., Smity, E. M., et al. (1969) Cancer mortality among nuns: role of marital status in etiology of neoplastic disease in women. J. Natl. Cancer Inst. 42, 455.
29. Lancaster, H. O. (1971) The mortality in Australia from cancers peculiar to the female. Med. J. Australia July 7, pp. 1–7.
30. Stewart, H. L., Dunham, L. J., Casper, J., et al. (1966) Epidemiology of cancers of uterine cervix and corpus, breast and ovary in Israel and New York City. J. Natl. Cancer Inst. 37, 1.
31. Lilienfeld, A. M. (1956) The relationship of cancer of the female breast to artificial menopause and marital status. Cancer 9, 927.
32. MacMahon, B., Lin, T. M., Lowe, C. R., et al. (1970) Lactation and cancer of the breast. A summary of an international study. Bull. World. Hlth. Org. 42, 185.
33. Lilienfeld, A. M., Coombs, J., Bross, I. D. J., Chamberlain, A. (1975) Marital and reproductive experience in a community-wide epidemiological study of breast cancer. Johns Hopkins Med. J. 136, 157–162.
34. Bjarnason, O., Day, N., Snaedal, G., Tulinius, H. (1974) The effect of year of birth on the breast cancer age-incidence curve in Iceland. Int. J. Cancer 13, 689–696.
35. DeWaard, F., Baanders-van Halewijn, E. A., Huizinga, J. (1964) The bimodal age distribution of patients with mammary carcinoma. Cancer 17, 141–151.
36. DeWaard, F. (1966) Adrenal Oestrogens and the Geographical Distribution of Breast Cancer. Utrecht: Instituut Voor Sociale Geneeskunde, pp. 191–201.
37. DeLisi, C. (1977) The age incidence of female breast cancer—simple models and analysis of epidemiological patterns. Math. Biosci. 37, 245–266.
38. Lee, J. A. H., Chin, P. G., Kukull, W. A., Tompkins, R. S., Weatherall, A. L. (1976) Relationship of age to incidence of breast cancer in young women. J. Natl. Cancer Inst. 57, 753–756.
39. Tulinius, H., Day, N. E., Johannesson, G. et al. (1978) Reproductive factors and risk for breast cancer in Iceland. Int. J. Cancer 21, 555–561.
40. DeWaard, F. (1978) Recent time trends in breast cancer incidence. Prev. Med. 7, 160–167.
41. Hirayama T. (1978) Epidemiology of breast cancer with special reference to the role of diet. Prev. Med. 7, 173–195.
42. Arellano, M. G., Linden, G., Dunn, J. E. (1972) Cancer patterns in Alameda County, California. Br. J. Cancer 26, 473–482.
43. Armstrong, B. (1976) Recent trends in breast cancer incidence and mortality in relation to changes in possible risk factors. Int. J. Cancer 17, 204–211.
44. Fabia, J., Bernard, P. M., Hill, G. (1977) Recent time trends of age-specific death rates for breast cancer: Quebec and other provinces, 1965 through 1974. Can. Med. Assoc. 116, 1135–1138.
45. Wigbe, D. T. (1977) Breast cancer and fertility trends in Canada. Am. J. Epidemiol. 105, 428–438.
46. Devesa, S. S., Silverman, D. T. (1978) Cancer incidence and mortality trends in the United States: 1935–74. J. Natl. Cancer Inst. 60, 545–571.
47. Thomas, D. B. (1979) Epidemiologic Studies of Cancer in Minority Groups in the Western United States. Natl. Cancer Inst. Monogr. 53, 103–113.
48. King, H., Haenszel, W. (1973) Cancer mortality among foreign and native born Chinese in the United States. J. Chron. Dis. 26, 623–646.
49. Buell, P. (1973) Changing incidence of breast cancer in Japanese-American women. J. Natl. Cancer Inst. 51, 1479.

50. International Agency for Research on Cancer (1976) Cancer Incidence in Five Continents. Lyon: I.A.R.C. Scientific Publications, Vol. III, No. 15.
51. Staszewski, J., Haenszel, W. (1965) Cancer mortality among the Polish-born in the United States. J. Natl. Cancer Inst. 35, 291.
52. Buell, P., Dunn, J. E., Jr. (1965) Cancer mortality among Japanese Issei and Nisei of California. Cancer 18, 656.
53. Mackenzie, I. (1965) Breast cancer following multiple fluoroscopies. Br. J. Cancer 19, 1–8.
54. Myrden, J. A., Hiltz, J. E. (1969) Breast cancer following multiple fluoroscopies during artificial pneumothorax treatment of pulmonary tuberculosis. Can. Med. Assoc. J. 100, 1032–1034.
55. Cook, D. C., Dent, O., Hewitt, D. (1974) Breast cancer following multiple chest fluoroscopy: the Ontario experience. Can. Med. Assoc. J. 111, 406–410.
56. Delarue, N. C., Gale, G., Ronald, A. (1975) Multiple fluoroscopy of the chest: carcinogenicity for the female breast and implications for breast cancer screening programs. Can. Med. Assoc. J. 112, 1405–1411.
57. Boice, J. D., Monson, R. R. (1977) Breast cancer in women after repeated fluoroscopic examinations of the chest. J. Natl. Cancer Inst. 59, 823–832.
58. Mettler, F. A., Hempelmann, L. H., Dutton, A. M., et al. (1969) Breast neoplasms in women treated with x-rays for acute postpartum mastitis. A pilot study. J. Natl. Cancer Inst. 43, 803–811.
59. Shore, R. E., Hempelmann, L. H., Kowaluk, E., et al. (1977) Breast neoplasms in women treated with x-rays for acute postpartum mastitis. J. Natl. Cancer Inst. 59, 813–822.
60. Baral, E., Larsson, L-E., Mattsson, B. (1977) Breast cancer following irradiation of the breast. Cancer 40, 2905–2910.
61. Simon, N., (1977) Breast cancer induced by radiation: relation to mammography and treatment of acne. J.A.M.A. 237, 789–790.
62. Wanebo, C. K., Johnson, K. G., Sato, K., Thorslund, T. W. (1968) Breast cancer after exposure to the atomic bombings of Hiroshima and Nagasaki. N. Engl. J. Med. 279, 667–671.
63. McGregor, D. H., Land, C. E., Choi, K., et al. (1977) Breast cancer incidence among atomic bomb survivors, Hiroshima and Nagasaki, 1950–1969. J. Natl. Cancer Inst. 59, 799–811.
64. Bross, I. D. J. (1978) Letter to the Editor. J. Natl. Cancer Inst. 60, 727–728.
65. Shore, R. E. (1978) Letter to the Editor. J. Natl. Cancer Inst. 60, 728.
66. Land, C. E., McGregor, D. H. (1978) Letter to the Editor. J. Natl. Cancer Inst. 60, 728–729.
67. Boice, J. D. (1978) Letter to the Editor. J. Natl. Cancer Inst. 60, 729–730.
68. Swartz, H. M., Reichling, B. A. (1977) The risks of mammograms. J.A.M.A. 237, 965–966.
69. Bross, I. D. J. (1977) Possible hazards of radiologic surveillance of high risk groups. N. Engl. J. Med. 296, 232.
70. Gur, D., Sashin, D. (1977) Evaluation of benefits and risks of breast cancer screening. Radiology 124, 261–262.
71. Thier, S. O. (1977) Breast cancer screening: a view from outside the controversy. N. Engl. J. Med. 297, 1063–1065.
72. Shapiro, S. (1976) Statistical evidence for mass screening for breast cancer and some remaining issues. Cancer Detect. Prev. 1, 347–363.
73. Bucalossi, P. and Veronesi, U. (1959) Researches on the etiological factors in human breast cancer. Acta Union Internationale Contre le Cancer 15, 1056.
74. Henderson, B. E., Powell, D., Rosario, I., et al. (1974) An epidemiologic study of breast cancer. J. Natl. Cancer Inst. 53, 609.

75. Kaplan, S. D., Acheson, R. M. (1966) A single etiological hypothesis for breast cancer? J. Chron. Dis. 19, 1221.

76. Herity, B. A., O'Halloran, M. J., Bourke, G. J., Wilson-Davis, K. (1975) A study of breast cancer in Irish women. Br. J. Prev. Soc. Med. 29, 178–181.

77. Sartwell, P. E., Arthes, F. G., Tonascia, J. A. (1977) Exogenous hormones, reproductive history, and breast cancer. J. Natl. Cancer Inst. 59, 1589–1592.

78. Choi, N. W., Howe, G. R., Miller, A. B., et al. (1978) An epidemiologic study of breast cancer. Am. J. Epidemiol. 107, 510–521.

79. Levin, M. L., Sheehe, P. R., Graham, S., et al. (1964) Lactation and menstrual function as related to cancer of the breast. Am. J. Publ. Hlth. 54, 580.

80. Paymaster, J. C., Gangadharan, P. (1972) Epidemiology of breast cancer in India. J. Natl. Cancer Inst. 48, 1021.

81. Soini, I. (1977) Risk factors of breast cancer in Finland. Int. J. Epidemiol. 6, 365–373.

82. Adami, H. O. (1977) Epidemiology and Endocrinology in Breast Cancer. Abstracts of Uppsala Dissertations from the Faculty of Medicine, No. 286.

83. MacMahon, B., Cole, P. (1972) The ovarian etiology of human breast cancer. *In:* Recent Results in Cancer Research: Current Problems in the Epidemiology of Cancer and Lymphomas. Grundman, E. and Tulinius, H. (eds.). New York: Springer-Verlag.

84. Shapiro, S., Goldberg, J., Venet, L., Strax, P. (1973) Risk factors in breast cancer—a prospective study. *In:* Host Environment Interactions in the Etiology of Cancer in Man. Proceedings of Meeting at Primosten. Doll, R., Vodopija, I. (eds.). Lyon: I.A.R.C., pp. 189–192.

85. Farewell, V. T. (1977) The combined effect of breast cancer risk factors. Cancer 40, 931–936.

86. Farewell, V. T., Bulbrook, R. D., Hayward, J. L. (1978) Risk factors in breast cancer: a prospective study in the Island of Guernsey. Cancer Campaign 1, 43–51.

87. Staszewski, J. (1971) Age at menarche and breast cancer. J. Natl. Cancer Inst. 47, 935.

88. Stavraky, K., Emmons, S. (1974) Breast cancer in premenopausal and postmenopausal women. J. Natl. Cancer Inst. 53, 647–654.

89. Wynder, E. L., MacCormack, F. A., Stellman, S. D. (1978) The epidemiology of breast cancer in 785 United States Caucasian Women. Cancer 41, 2341–2354.

90. Trichopoulas, D., MacMahon, B., Cole, P. (1972) Menopause and breast cancer. J. Natl. Cancer Inst. 48, 605.

91. Hirayama, T., Wynder, E. L. (1962) A study of the epidemiology of cancer of the breast. II. The influence of hysterectomy. Cancer 15, 28.

92. Feinleib, M. (1968) Breast cancer and artificial menopause: a cohort study. J. Natl. Cancer Inst. 41, 315.

93. Schneider, R., Dorn, C. R., Taylor, D. O. N. (1969) Factors influencing canine mammary cancer development and postsurgical survival. J. Natl. Cancer, Inst. 43, 1249.

94. Swerdlow, M., Humphrey, L. J. (1964) The relationship of breast disease to gynecologic disease. Cancer 17, 1165.

95. MacMahon, B., Cole, P., Lin, T. M., et al. (1970) Age at first birth and breast cancer risk. Bull. World. Hlth. Org. 43, 209–221.

96. Chew, L. C. (1977) The Relationship Between Breast Cancer and Rauwolfia Derivatives. Master of Science Thesis, Johns Hopkins University School of Hygiene and Public Health.

97. Craig, T. J., Comstock, G. W., Geiser, P. B. (1974) Epidemiologic comparison of breast cancer patients with early and late onset of malignancy and general population controls. J. Natl. Cancer Inst. 53, 1577–1581.

98. Mirra, A. P., Cole, P., MacMahon, B. (1971) Breast cancer in an area of high parity: Sao Paulo, Brazil. Cancer Res. 31, 77–83.
99. Grattarola, R. (1964) The premenstrual endometrial pattern of women with breast cancer. Cancer 17, 1119.
100. Swain, M. C., Bulbrook, R. D., Hayward, J. L. (1974) Ovulatory failure in a normal population and in patients with breast cancer. J. Obst. Gynaecol. Brit. Commonwealth 81, 640.
101. Sherman, B. M., Korenman, S. G. (1974) A pathophysiological interpretation of human breast cancer epidemiology. Cancer 33, 1306.
102. Anderson, J. D. (1975) Breast feeding and breast cancer. S.A. Med. J. 49, 479–482.
103. MacMahon, B., Feinleib, M. (1960) Breast cancer in relation to nursing and menopausal history. J. Natl. Cancer Inst. 24, 733–753.
104. Kamoi, M. (1960) Statistical study on relation between breast cancer and lactation period. Tohoku J. Exp. Med. 72, 59–65.
105. Abrahmson, J. L. (1966) Breastfeeding and breast cancer. Israel J. Med. Sci. 2, 457–464.
106. Meyer, M. F. (1968) Breast feeding in the United States. Report of a 1966 National Survey with comparable 1946 and 1956 data. Clin. Pediat. 7, 708.
107. Segi, M., Fukushima, I., Fujisaku, S., et al. (1957) An epidemiological study on cancer in Japan. Gann. 48 (supplement), 1–63.
108. Ing, R., Ho, J. H. C., Petrakis, N. L. (1977) Unilateral breast-feeding and breast cancer. Lancet 2, 124–127.
109. DeWaard, F., Baanders-van Halewijn, E. A., Huizinga, J. (1964) The bimodal age distribution of patients with mammary carcinoma. Evidence for the existence of 2 types of human breast cancer. Cancer 17, 141.
110. Adami, H. O., Rimsten, A., Stenkvist, B., Vegelius, J. (1977) Influence of height, weight, and obesity on risk of breast cancer in an unselected Swedish population. Br. J. Cancer 36, 787–792.
111. Valaoras, U. G., MacMahon, B., Trichopoulos, D., et al. (1969) Lactation and reproductive histories of breast cancer patients in greater Athens, 1965–67. Int. J. Cancer 4, 350–363.
112. DeWaard, F. (1975) Breast cancer incidence and nutritional status with particular reference to body weight and height. Cancer Res. 35, 3351–3356, 1975.
113. DeWaard, F., Cornelis, J. P., Aoki, K., Yoshida, M. (1977) Breast cancer incidence according to weight and height in two cities of the Netherlands and in Aichi Prefecture, Japan. Cancer 40, 1269–1275.
114. Ravnihar, B., MacMahon, B., Lindtner, J. (1971) Epidemiologic features of breast cancer in Slovenia, 1965–1967. Eur. J. Cancer 7, 295–306.
115. Lin, T. M., Chen, K. P., MacMahon, B. (1971) Epidemiologic characteristics of cancer of the breast in Taiwan. Cancer 2, 1497–1504.
116. DeWaard, F., Baanders-van Halewijn, E. A. (1974) A prospective study in general practice on breast-cancer risk in postmenopausal women. Int. J. Cancer 14, 153.
117. Kagawa, Y. (1978) Impact of Westernization on the nutrition of Japanese: changes in physique, cancer, longevity and centarians. Prev. Med. 7, 205–217.
118. Frisch, R. E., McArthur, J. W. (1974) Menstrual cycles: fatness as a determinant of minimum weight for height necessary for their maintenance or onset. Science 185, 949–951.
119. Rikiya, A., Kumagai, N., Kimura, M., et al. (1976) Biological characteristics of breast cancer in obesity. Tohuku J. Exp. Med. 120, 351–359.
120. Donegan, W. L., Hartz, A. J., Rimm, A. A. (1978) The association of body weight with recurrent cancer of the breast. Cancer 41, 1590–1594.
121. Hems, G. (1970) Epidemiological characteristics of breast cancer in middle and late age. Br. J. Cancer 24, 226.

122. Draser, B. S., Irving, D. (1973) Environmental factors and cancer of the colon and breast. Br. J. Cancer 27, 167.

123. Armstrong, B., Doll, R. (1975) Environmental factors and cancer incidence and mortality in different countries with special reference to dietary practices. Int. J. Cancer 15, 617–631.

124. Phillips, R. L. (1975) Role of life-style and dietary habits in risk of cancer among Seventh-Day Adventists. Cancer Res. 35, 3513–3522.

125. Miller, A. B., Kelly, H., Choi, N. W., et al. (1978) A study of diet and breast cancer. Am. J. Epidemiol. 107, 499–509.

126. Nomura, A., Hirohata, T., Kolonel, L., et al. (1977) Diet and Exogenous Estrogens in Three Populations at Different Levels of Risk for Breast Cancer. National Cancer Institute Monograph 47, 165–167.

127. International Agency for Research on Cancer. Directory of On-Going Research in Cancer Epidemiology (1977) Muir, C. S., Wagner, G. (eds.). Lyon: I.A.R.C., Publication No. 17.

128. Carroll, K. K., Gammal, E. B., Plunkett, E. R. (1968) Dietary fat and mammary cancer. Can. Med. Assoc. J. 98, 590.

129. Chan, P., Cohen, L. A. (1974) Effect of dietary fat, antiestrogen, and antiprolactin on the development of mammary tumor in rats. J. Natl. Cancer Inst. 52, 25.

130. Hill, M. J., Goddard, P., Williams, R. E. O. (1971) Gut bacteria and aetiology of cancer of the breast. Lancet 2, 472.

131. Lipsett, M. B. (1973) Consideration of steroid metabolism in breast cancer. *In:* Host Environment Interactions in the Etiology of Cancer in Man. Doll, R., Vodopija, I. (eds.). Lyon: I.A.R.C., pp. 105–113.

132. Bulbrook, R. D., Greenwood, F. C., Hayward, J. L. (1960) Selection of breast cancer patients for adrenalectomy or hypophysectomy by determination of urinary 17-hydroxycorticosteroids and aetiocholanolone. Lancet 2, 1154–1157.

133. Bulbrook, R. D., Hayward, J. L., Spicer, C. C. (1971) Relation between urinary androgen and corticoid excretion and subsequent breast cancer. Lancet 2, 395–398.

134. Bulbrook, R. D., Thomas, B. S., Utsunomiya, J. (1964) Urinary 11-deoxy-17-oxosteroids in British and Japanese women with reference to the incidence of breast cancer. Nature 201, 189–190.

135. Wang, D. Y., Bulbrook, R. D., Hayward, J. L. (1975) Urinary and plasma androgens and their relation to familial risk of breast cancer. Eur. J. Cancer 11, 873–877.

136. Brennan, M. J., Bulbrook, R. D., Deshpande, N., et al. (1973) Urinary and plasma androgens in benign breast disease. Lancet 1, 1076–1079.

137. Miller, W. R., Hamilton, T., Champion, H. R., et al. (1975) Urinary aetiocholanolone in patients with early breast cancer from South East Scotland and South Wales. Br. J. Cancer 32, 619–627.

138. Lemon, H. M. (1969) Endocrine influences on human mammary cancer formation. Cancer 23, 781–790.

139. Cole, P., MacMahon, B. (1969) Oestrogen fractions during early reproductive life in the aetiology of breast cancer. Lancet 1, 604–606.

140. MacMahon, B., Cole, P., Brown, J. B., et al. (1971) Oestrogen profiles of Asian and North American Women. Lancet 2, 900–902.

141. Briggs, M. (1972) Ethnic differences in urinary oestrogens. Lancet 1, 324.

142. MacMahon, B., Cole, P., Brown, J. B., et al. (1974) Urine oestrogen profiles of Asian and North American women. Int. J. Cancer 14, 161–167.

143. Dickinson, L. E., MacMahon, B., Cole, P., Brown, J. B. (1974) Estrogen profiles of Oriental and Caucasian women in Hawaii. N. Engl. J. Med. 291, 1211–1213.

144. Bulbrook, R. D., Swain, M. C., Wang, D. Y., et al. (1976) Breast cancer in Britain and Japan: plasma oestradiol-17B, oestrone and progesterone, and their urinary metabolites in normal British and Japanese women. Eur. J. Cancer 12, 725–735.

145. Gross, J., Modan, B., Bertini, B., et al. (1977) Relationship between steroid excretion patterns and breast cancer incidence in Israeli women of various origins. J. Natl. Cancer Inst. 59, 7–11.
146. Cole, P., Brown, J. B., MacMahon, B. (1976) Oestrogen profiles of parous and nulliparous women. Lancet 2, 596–599.
147. Rudali, G., Apiou, F., Muel, B. (1975) Mammary cancer produced in mice with estriol. Eur. J. Cancer 11, 39–41.
148. Flood, C., Pratt, J. H., Longcope, C. (1976) The metabolic clearance and blood production rates of estriol in normal non-pregnant women. J. Cancer Epidemiol. Med. 42, 1–8.
149. Longcope, C., Pratt, J. H. (1977) Blood production rates of estrogens in women with differing ratios of urinary estrogen conjugates. Steroids 29, 483–492.
150. Pike, M. C., Casagrande, J. T., Brown, J. B., et al. (1977) Comparison of urinary and plasma hormone levels in daughters of breast cancer patients and controls. J. Natl. Cancer Inst. 59, 1351–1355.
151. Morgan, R. W., Vakil, D. V., Brown, J. B., et al. (1978) Estrogen profiles in young women: effect of maternal history of breast cancer. J. Natl. Cancer Inst. 60, 965–967.
152. Longcope, C. (1971) Metabolic clearance and blood production rates of estrogens in post-menopausal women. Am. J. Obstet. Gynecol. 111, 778–781.
153. MacDonald, P. C., Grodin, J. M., Siiteri, P. K. (1969) The utilization of plasma androstenedione for estrone production in women. *In:* Progress in Endocrinology. Gual, C. (ed.). Amsterdam: Excerpta Medica, Internatl. Congress Series No. 184, pp. 770–776.
154. Edman, C. D., MacDonald, P. C. (1978) Effect of obesity on conversion of plasma androstenedione to estrone in ovulatory and anovulatory young women. Am. J. Obstet. Gynecol. 130, 456–461.
155. MacDonald, P. C., Edman, C. D., Hemsell, D. L., et al. (1978) Effect of obesity on conversion of plasma androstenedione to estrone in postmenopausal women with and without endometrial cancer. Am. J. Obstet. Gynecol. 130, 448–455.
156. Fishman, J., Bradlow, H. L. (1977) Effect of malnutrition on the metabolism of sex hormones in man. Clin. Pharmacol. Ther. 22, 721–728.
157. Poortman, J., Prenen, J.A.C., Schwarz, F., et al. (1975) Interaction of Δ^5-andiostene-3B, 17B-diol with estradiol and dihydrotestosterone receptors in human myometrial and mammary cancer tissue. Metabolism 40, 373–379.
158. Sherman, B. M., Korenman, S. G. (1974) Inadequate corpus luteum function: a pathophysiological interpretation of human breast cancer epidemiology. Cancer 33, 1306–1312.
159. Swain, M. C., Bulbrook, R. D., Hayward, J. L. (1974) Ovulatory failure in a normal population and in patients with breast cancer. J. Obstet. Gynaecol. Br. Commonwealth 81, 640–643.
160. Sassin, J. F., Frantz, A. G., Weitzman, E. D., Kapen, S. (1972) Human prolactin: 24-hour pattern with increased release during sleep. Science 177, 1205–1207.
161. Sheth, N. A., Ranadive, K. J., Suraiya, J. N., Sheth, A. R. (1975) Circulating levels of prolactin in human breast cancer. Br. J. Cancer 32, 160–167.
162. Wilson, R. G., Buchan, R., Roberts, M. M., et al. (1974) Plasman prolactin and breast cancer. Cancer 33, 1325–1327.
163. Boyns, A. R., Cole, E. N., Griffiths, K., et al. (1973) Plasma prolactin in breast cancer. Eur. J. Cancer 9, 99–102.
164. Mittra, I., Hayward, J. L., McNeilly, A. S. (1974) Hypothalamic-pituitary-prolactin axis in breast cancer. Lancet 1, 889–891.
165. Kwa, H. G., Engelman, E., Bakker, M. D., Cleton, F. J. (1974) Plasma-prolactin in human breast cancer. Lancet 1, 433–435.
166. Hill, P., Wynder, E. L., Kumar, H., et al. (1976) Prolactin levels in populations at risk for breast cancer. Cancer Res. 36, 4102–4106.

167. Kwa, H. G., Wang, D. Y. (1977) An abnormal luteal phase evening peak of plasma prolactin in women with a family history of breast cancer. Int. J. Cancer 20, 12–14.

168. Hellman, L., Bradlow, H. L., Zumoff, B., et al. (1959) Thyroid-androgen interrelationships and the hypercholesteremic effect of androsterone. J. Clin. Endocrinae. Metabol. 19, 936–948.

169. Fishman, J., Hellman, L., Zumoff, B., et al. (1965) Effect of thyroid on hydroxylation of estrogen in man. J. Clin. Endocrinol. Metabol. 25, 365–368.

170. Myhill, J., Reeve, T. S., Heald, I. B. (1966) Thyroid function in breast cancer. Acta Endocrinol. 51, 290–300.

171. Sider, K., Waterhouse, J. A. H. (1961) Thyroid function in relation to mammary cancer. Br. J. Cancer 15, 45–49.

172. Mittra, I., Hayward, J. L. (1974) Hypothalamic-pituitary-thyroid axis in breast cancer. Lancet 1, 885–889.

173. Wanebo, H. J., Benua, R. S., Rawson, R. W. (1966) Neoplastic diseases and thyrotoxicosis. Cancer 19, 1523–1526.

174. Chalstrey, L. J., Benjamin, B. (1966) High incidence of breast cancer in thyroid cancer patients. Br. J. Cancer 20, 670–675.

175. Itoh, K., Maruchi, N. (1975) Breast cancer in patients with Hashimoto's thyroiditis. Lancet 2, 1119–1126.

176. Backwinkel, K., Jackson, A. S. (1964) Some features of breast cancer and thyroid deficiency. Cancer 17, 1174–1176.

177. Bogardus, G. M., Finley, J. W. (1961) Breast cancer and thyroid disease. Surgery 49, 461–468.

178. Schottenfeld, D. (1968) The relationship of breast cancer to thyroid disease. J. Chron. Dis. 21, 303–313.

179. Maruchi, N., Annegers, J. F., Kurland, L. T. (1976) Hashimoto's thyroiditis and breast cancer. Mayo Clin. Proc. 51, 263–265.

180. Mittra, J., Perrin, J., Kumaoka, S. (1976) Thyroid and other auto-antibodies in British and Japanese women: An epidemiological study of breast cancer. Br. Med. J. 1, 257–259.

181. Kapdi, C. C., Wolfe, J. N. (1976) Breast cancer: relationship to thyroid supplements for hypothyroidism. J.A.M.A. 236, 1124–1127.

182. Mustacchi, P., Greenspan, F. (1977) Thyroid supplementation for hypothyroidism: an iatrogenic cause of breast cancer? J.A.M.A. 237, 1446–1447.

183. Wallace, R. B., Sherman, B. M., Bean, J. A., Leeper, J. (1978) Thyroid hormone use in patients with breast cancer. J.A.M.A. 239, 958.

184. McGuire, W. L. (1975) Current status of estrogen receptors in human breast cancer. Cancer 36, 638–644.

185. Trams, G., Maass, H. (1977) Specific binding of estradiol and dihydrotestosterone in human mammary cancers. Cancer Res. 37, 258–261.

186. Thomas, D. B. (1978) Role of exogenous female hormones in altering the risk of benign and malignant neoplasms in humans. Cancer Res. 38, 3991–4000.

187. Boston Collaborative Drug Surveillance Program (1973) Oral contraceptives and venous thromboembolic disease, surgically confirmed gall bladder disease and breast tumors. Lancet 1, 1399–1404.

188. Kelsey, J. L., Holford, T. R., White, C., et al. (1978) Oral contraceptives and breast disease: an epidemiological study. Am. J. Epidemial. 107, 236–244.

189. Paffenbarger, R. S., Fasal, E., Simmons, M. E., Kampert, J. B. (1977) Cancer risk as related to use of oral contraceptives during fertile years. Cancer 39, 1887–1891.

190. Ravnihar, B., Seigel, D. G., Lindtner, J. (1979) An epidemiologic study of breast cancer and benign breast neoplasias in relation to the oral contraceptive and estrogen use. Eur. J. Cancer, 15, 395–405.

191. Sartwell, P. E., Arthes, F. G., Tonascia, J. A. (1977) Exogenous hormones, reproductive history, and breast cancer. J. Natl. Cancer Inst. 59, 1589–1592.

192. Vessey, M. P., Doll, R., Sutton, P. M. (1972) Oral contraceptives and breast neoplasia: a retrospective study. Br. Med. J. 3, 719–724.

193. Ory, H., Cole, P., MacMahon, B., Hoover, R. (1976) Oral contraceptives and reduced risk of benign breast diseases. N. Engl. J. Med. 294, 419–422.

194. Royal College of General Practitioners (1974) Oral Contraceptives and Health. London: Pitman Medical Publishing, Ltd.

195. Vessey, M., Doll, R., Peto, R., Johnson, B., Wiggins, P. (1976) A long-term follow-up study of women using different methods of contraception—an interim report. J. Biosocial Sci. 8, 373–427.

196. Royal College of General Practitioners' Oral Contraception Study (1977) Effect on hypertension and benign breast disease of progestogen component in combined oral contraceptives. Lancet 1, 624.

197. Boston Collaborative Drug Surveillance Program (1974) Surgically confirmed gall bladder disease, venous thromboembolism, and breast tumors in relation to postmenopausal estrogen therapy. N. Engl. J. Med. 290, 15–19.

198. Nomura, A., Comstock, G. W. (1976) Benign breast tumor and estrogenic hormones: a population-based retrospective study. Am. J. Epidemiol. 103, 439–444.

199. LiVols, V. A., Stadel, B. V., Kelsey, J. L., et al. (1978) Fibrocystic breast disease in oral-contraceptive users. A histopathological evaluation of epithelial atypia. N. Engl. J. Med. 299, 381–385.

200. Vessey, M. P., Doll, R., Jones, K. (1975) Oral Contraceptives and Breast Cancer. Progress Report of an Epidemiological Study. Lancet 1, 941–944.

201. Casagrande, J., Gerkins, J., Henderson, B. E., et al. (1976) Exogenous estrogens and breast cancer in women with natural menopause. J. Natl. Cancer Inst. 56, 839–841.

202. Mack, T. M., Henderson, B. E., Gerkins, V. R., et al. (1975) Reserpine and breast cancer in a retirement community. N. Engl. J. Med. 292, 1366–1371.

203. Burch, J. C., Byrd, B. F., Vaughn, W. K. (1974) The effects of long-term estrogen on hysterectomized women. Am. J. Obstet. Gynecol. 118, 778–782.

204. Hoover, R., Gray, L. A., Cole, P., MacMahon, B. (1976) Menopausal estrogens and breast cancer. N. Engl. J. Med. 295, 401–405.

205. Boston Collaborative Drug Surveillance Program (1974) Reserpine and breast cancer. Lancet 2, 669.

206. Armstrong, B., Stevens, N., Doll, R. (1974) Retrospective study of the association between use of Rauwolfia derivatives and breast cancer in English women. Lancet 2, 672–674.

207. Heinonen, O. P., Shapiro, S., Tuominen, L., Turunen, M. I. (1974) Reserpine use in relation to breast cancer. Lancet 2, 675–677.

208. Laska, E. M., Siegel, C., Meisner, M., et al. (1975) Matched pairs study of reserpine use and breast cancer. Lancet 2, 296.

209. O'Fallon, W. M., Labarthe, D. R., Kurland, L. T. (1975) Rauwolfia derivatives and breast cancer. Lancet 2, 292–297.

210. Lilienfeld, A. M., Chang, L., Thomas, D. B., Levin, M. L. (1975) Rauwolfia derivatives and breast cancer. Johns Hopkins Med. J. 139, 41–50.

211. Aromaa, A., Hakama, M., et al. (1976) Breast cancer and use of Rauwolfia and other antihypertensive agents in hypertensive patients: a nationwide case control study in Finland. Int. J. Cancer 18, 727–738.

212. Armstrong, B., Skegg, D., White, G., Doll, R. (1976) Rauwolfia derivatives and breast cancer in hypertensive women. Lancet 2, 8–12.

213. Kewitz, H., Jesdinsky, H. J., Schrofer, P. M., Lindtner, E. (1977) Reserpine and breast cancer in women in Germany. Eur. J. Clin. Pharmacol. 11, 79–83.

214. Kodlin, D., McCarthy, N. (1978) Reserpine and breast cancer. Cancer 41, 761–768.

215. Davis, H. M., Simons, M., Davis, J. B. (1964) Cystic disease of the breast: relationship to carcinoma. Cancer 17, 957–978.

216. Donnelly, P. K., Baker, K. W., Carney, J. A., O'Fallon, W. M. (1975) Benign breast lesions and subsequent breast carcinoma in Rochester, Minnesota. Mayo Clin. Proc. 50, 650–656.
217. Monson, R. R., Yen, S., MacMahon, B., Warren, S. (1976) Chronic mastitis and carcinoma of the breast. Lancet 2, 224–226.
218. Kodlin, D., Winger, E. E., Morgenstern, N. L., Chen, U. (1977) Chronic mastopathy and breast cancer. A follow-up study. Cancer 39, 2603–2607.
219. Hutchinson, W. B., Thomas, D. B., Hamlin, W. B. et al. (1980) Risk of breast cancer in women with benign breast diseases. J. Natl. Cancer Inst. 64 (in press).
220. Black, M. M., Barclay, T. H. C., Cutler, S. J., et al. (1972) Association of atypical characteristics of benign breast lesions with subsequent risk of breast cancer. Cancer 29, 338–343.
221. Wolfe, J. N. (1976) Breast patterns as an index of risk for developing breast cancer. Am. J. Roentgenol. 126, 1130–1139.
222. Wellings, S. R., Wolfe, J. M. (1978) Pathology of xeroradiographic images (Meeting Abstract). Proc. Am. Assoc. Cancer Res. 19, 32.
223. Mendell, L., Rosenbloom, M., Naimark, A. (1977) Are breast patterns a risk index for breast cancer? A reappraisal. Am. J. Roentgenol. 128, 547.
224. Wilkinson, E., Clopton, C., Gordonson, J., et al. (1977) Mammographic parenchymal pattern and the risk of breast cancer, J Natl. Cancer Inst. 59, 1397–1400.
225. Krook, P. M., Carlile, T., Bush, W., Hall, M. H. (1978) Mammographic parenchymal patterns as a risk indicator for prevalent and incident cancer. Cancer 41, 1093–1097.
226. Sakamoto, G., Sugano, H., Kasumi, F. (1978) Bilateral breast cancer and familial aggregations. Prev. Med. 7, 225–229.
227. Prior, P., Waterhouse, J. A. H. (1978) Incidence of bilateral tumors in a population-based series of breast cancer patients. I. Two approaches to an epidemiological analysis. Br. J. Cancer 37, 620–634.
228. Finney, G. G. Jr., Finney, G. G., Montague, A. C. W., et al. (1972) Bilateral breast cancer, clinical and pathological review. Ann. Surg. 175, 635–645.
229. Anderson, D. E. (1977) Breast cancer in families. Cancer 40, 1855–1860.
230. Anderson, D. E. (1970) Genetic considerations in breast cancer. *In* Breast Cancer: Early and Late. Chicago: Year Book Medical Publishers, Inc.
231. Harris, R. E., Lynch, H. T., Guirgis, H. A. (1978) Familial breast cancer: risk to the contralateral breast. J. Natl. Cancer Inst. 60, 955–960.
232. Schottenfeld, D., Berg, J., Vitsky, B. (1969) Incidence of multiple primary cancers. II. Index cancers arising in the stomach and lower digestive system. J. Natl. Cancer Inst. 43, 77–86.
233. Schottenfeld, D., Berg, J. (1971) Incidence of multiple primary cancers. IV. Cancer of the female breast and genital organs. J. Natl. Cancer Inst. 46, 161–170.
234. Schoenberg, B. S., Greenberg, R. A., Eisenberg, H. (1969) Occurrence of certain multiple primary cancers in females. J. Natl. Cancer Inst. 43, 15–32.
235. MacMahon, B., Austin, J. H. (1969) Association of carcinomas of the breast and corpus uteri. Cancer 23, 275–280.
236. Vongtama, V., Kurohara, S. S., Badib, A. O., Webster, J. H. Second primary cancers of endometrial carcinoma. Cancer 26, 842–846.
237. Jansson, B., Seibert, G. B., Speer, J. F. (1975) Gastrointestinal cancer—its geographic distribution and correlation to breast cancer. Cancer 36, 2373–2384.
238. Howell, M. A. (1976) The association between colorectal cancer and breast cancer. J. Chron. Dis. 29, 243–261.
239. Dunn, J. E., Bragg, K. U., Sautter, C., et al. (1972) Breast cancer risk following a major salivary gland carcinoma. Cancer 29, 1343–1346.
240. Anderson, D. E. (1976) Genetic predisposition to breast cancer. *In:* Recent Results in Cancer Research. St. Arneault, G., Band, P., Israel, L. (eds). Berlin: Springer-

Verlag, Vol. 57, pp. 10–20.

241. Jacobsen, O. (1946) Heredity in Breast Cancer: A Genetic and Clinical Study of Two Hundred Probands, London: H. K. Lewis.

242. Penrose, L. S., MacKenzie, H. J., Karn, M. N. (1948) A genetical study of human mammary cancer. Ann. Eugenics 14, 234–266.

243. Passay, R. D., Waiman, M., Armstrong, E. C., Rhodes, J. (1952) Heredity in human breast cancer. Acta Unio. Internat. contra Cancrum 8, 184–186.

244. Smithers, D. W. (1948) Family histories of 459 patients with cancer of the breast. Br. J. Cancer 2, 163–167.

245. Woolf, C. M. (1955) Investigations on Genetic Aspects of Carcinoma of the Stomach and Breast. University of California Publications in Public Health 2, 265.

246. Anderson, V. E., Goodman, H. O., Reed, S. C. (1950) Variables Related to Human Breast Cancer. Minneapolis: University of Minnesota Press.

247. Murphy, D. P., Abbey, H. (1959) Cancer in Families (A Study of the Relatives of 200 Breast Cancer Probands). Cambridge: Harvard University Press.

248. Macklin, M. T. (1959) Comparison of the number of breast-cancer patients and the number expected on the basis of mortality rates. J. Natl. Cancer Inst. 22, 927–951.

249. Tokuhata, G. K. (1969) Morbidity and mortality among offspring of breast cancer mothers. Am. J. Epidemiol. 89, 139–153.

250. Morgan, R. W., Vakil, D. V., Chipman, M. L. (1974) Breast feeding, family history, and breast disease. Am. J. Epidemiol. 99, 117–122.

251. Albert, S., Child, M. (1977) Familial cancer in the general population. Cancer 40, 1674–1679.

252. Anderson, D. E. (1974) Genetic study of breast cancer: identification of a high risk group. Cancer 34, 1090–1097.

253. Petrakis, N. L. (1977) Genetic factors in the etiology of breast cancer. Cancer 39, 2709–2715.

254. Petrakis, N. L., King, M. C. (1977) Genetic markers and cancer epidemiology. Cancer 39, 1861–1866.

255. Knudson, A. G. Jr., Strong, L. C., Anderson, D. E. (1973) Heredity and cancer in man. Prog. Med. Genet. 9, 113–158.

256. Li, F. P., Fraumeni, J. F. Jr. (1969) Soft tissue sarcomas, breast cancer and other neoplasms. A familial syndrome? Ann. Intern. Med. 71, 747–752.

257. Lynch, H. T., Krush, A. J. (1971) Carcinoma of the breast and ovary in three families. Surg. Gynecol. Obstet. 131, 644–648.

258. Lynch, H. T., Krush, A. J., Gurgis, H. (1973) Genetic factors in families with combined gastrointestinal and breast cancer. Am. J. Gastoenterol. 1, 31–40.

259. Lemon, H. M., Reilly, D. (1974) Genotypic variations in Caucasian leukocyte estradiol 16 hydroxylase activity: a measurable deterrent of breast cancer risk? Nebr. Med. J. 59, 151–155.

260. Schlom, J., Spielman, S. (1974) Breast cancer. Molecular basis for a viral etiology. N.Y. State J. Med. 74, 1373–1383.

261. Moore, D. H., Charney, J. (1975) Breast cancer: etiology and possible prevention. Am. Scientist 63, 160–168.

262. Rapp, F., Reed, C. (1977) The viral etiology of cancer. Cancer 40, 419–429.

263. Bittner, J. J. (1936) Some possible effects of nursing on the mammary gland tumor incidence in Mice. Science 84, 162.

264. Bentvelzen, P., Daams, J. H., Hageman, P., Calafat, J. (1970) Genetic transmission of viruses that incite mammary tumor in mice. Proc. Nat. Acad. Sci. U.S.A. 67, 377–384.

265. Moore, D. H., Sarkar, N. H., Kelly, C. E., et al. (1969) Type B particles in human milk. Tex. Rep. Biol. Med. 27, 1027–1039.

266. Moore, D. H., Charney, J., Kramarsky, B., et al. (1971) Search for a human breast cancer virus. Nature (London) 229, 611–614.

267. Sarkar, N. H. and Moore, D. H. (1972) On the possibility of a human breast cancer virus. Nature (London) 236, 103–106.

268. Charney, J., Morre, D. H. (1971) Neutralization of murine mammary tumor virus by sera of women with breast cancer. Nature (London) 229, 627–628.

269. Shah, K. V., Bang, F. B., Abbey, H. (1972) Considerations for epidemiologic studies to test the hypothesis of viral causation of human breast cancer. J. Nat. Cancer Inst. 48, 1035–1038.

APLASTIC ANEMIA

MOYSES SZKLO, M.D., Dr.P.H.

CONTENTS

INTRODUCTION

Aplastic anemia is characterized by cytopenia in the peripheral blood and in the bone marrow. It is apparently the result of a wide variety of pathogenetic mechanisms which give rise to defects within the hematopoietic system, resulting in pancytopenia. As a totally aplastic marrow is unlikely, perhaps a better designation for the disorder would be hypoplastic anemia. However, for practical reasons the universally accepted term, aplastic anemia, will be used in this review.

In general, the term aplastic anemia has been used to describe pancytopenia of varying degrees of severity with hypocellular, hypercellular, or truly aplastic bone marrows. The diagnosis is strongly suspected when a pancytopenia is associated with morphologic evidence of bone marrow aplasia. Marrow depression in which evidence of increased blood destruction or infiltrative disease of the marrow are present is usually not included among the true aplastic anemias (1).

Aplastic anemia may not be fully developed at the time of the initial examination and each of the three cellular elements may not decline at the same rate. Williams and colleagues (2) have analyzed the clinical characteristics of 110 patients with aplastic anemia and observed that neutropenia, thrombocytopenia and anemia were present in 83% of the patients when first seen. However, pancytopenia developed in all patients thereafter, and the authors could not pinpoint one specific cellular element as being the first or last to be depressed. It was also noted by these authors that in all patients the bone marrow biopsy was hypocellular when first obtained, although this is not always true (3).

The pathogenesis of aplastic anemia is somewhat obscure, and the primary problem could be a result of a defect either in the microenvironment or "soil," or in the pluripotential stem cell. Thus, aplasia could result from a failure of the microenvironment to sustain growth of granulocyte, platelet and red cell precursors, or from a lesion located at the level of the stem cell. The fact that there is damage to all three major marrow cell lines, and the presence of endogenous erythropoietin in the absence of morphologic evidence of erythropoiesis suggests that the basic defect is situated prior to the committed compartments (3). Boggs and Boggs (4) have suggested that in aplastic anemia a chronic state of stem-cell depletion arises because its rate of differentiation exceeds the required rate of self-renewal.

The occurrence of aplastic anemia either in association with or followed by paroxysmal nocturnal hemoglobinuria (PNH) has been considered symptomatic of stem cell injury (5). This disorder was present in about 15% of aplastic anemia patients studied by Lewis and Dacie (6), who postulated that a new clone of cells emerges as a result of somatic mutation of the stem cell, leading to PNH. A fair degree of success with marrow transplants from HLA-matched sibling donors is also taken as evidence that most cases of aplastic anemia are due to a persistent abnormality induced in the stem-cell population, since

From the Johns Hopkins University School of Hygiene and Public Health, Baltimore, Maryland 21205.

otherwise infusion of normal, syngeneic stem cells would not be expected to correct the abnormality (7,8). However, the opposite argument that isogeneic transplants can fail to repopulate the marrow of patients with aplastic anemia has been also used to advance the hypothesis that aplastic anemia may sometimes be caused by destruction of the sinusoidal microcirculation of the bonemarrow or "soil," rather than by stem-cell or "seed" failure (9). Probably the truth lies somewhere in between these theories and aplastic anemia may in fact be caused by several mechanisms (5,7,10,11).

Aplastic anemia may be a recessively determined hereditary disease. When accompanied by multiple congenital anomalies, it is called Fanconi anemia (12,13). A congenital form of "pure" red cell aplasia, the Blackfan-Diamond syndrome, has also been described (14).

Presumably the acquired types are sometimes caused by an identifiable chemical or other toxic agent which depresses the bone marrow through either an idiosyncratic or a dose-related action (2,3,15–20). In other instances, aplastic anemia follows bacterial or viral infections, mostly hepatitis (1,3,20–25). However, although some risk factors—such as chloramphenicol (26) or ionizing radiation (27)—have been identified or are strongly suspected in connection with aplastic anemia, "idiopathic" cases in whom no prior exposure to environmental agents can be demonstrated seem to comprise at least 50% of all non-congenital aplastic anemia cases (1,3,20,28–30).

Given this high proportion of "idiopathic" cases, and since most of the evidence that many drugs and other environmental factors are related to aplastic anemia come from case-history reports, it is surprising that to date only a few epidemiologic studies have been carried out to examine factors which could explain the "idiopathic" cases, or to distinguish coincidental from truly causal associations with specific exposures.

Aside from reviewing the available information on the descriptive epidemiology of aplastic anemia and the few epidemiologic studies carried out to examine the relationship of chloramphenicol and ionizing radiation to aplastic anemia, the present report will limit itself to presenting data gathered from case-history reports and speculating on etiologic hypotheses based on these reports. In addition, since the hereditary forms of aplastic anemia seem to comprise only about 5% of all cases (31), studies cited in this review by necessity had to deal mostly with the acquired forms of aplastic anemia.

MORTALITY

Official mortality statistics for the United States concerning aplastic anemia have been available since 1949, and an analysis of crude death rates from 1947 to 1960 fails to show appreciable changes (Table 1). Although mortality data for other countries are generally not available, examination of data from Canada over a similar time period shows that mortality rates from aplastic anemia in that country were very similar to those in the United States (32). The time trend shown in Table 1 persisted in more recent years, with rates remaining stable within a range of about 4 to 5 per million population (Table 2).

When age-adjusted death rates from aplastic anemia are examined accord-

TABLE 1. Death Rates From Aplastic Anemia (I.C.D. 7th Revision 292.4) Per 1 Million Population, United States, 1949–1961

Year	Number of deaths	Rate
1949	638	4.3
1950	610	4.0
1951	671	4.4
1952	828	5.3
1953	774	4.9
1954	681	4.2
1955	633	3.9
1956	656	3.9
1957	669	3.9
1958	843	4.9
1959	921	5.2
1960	971	5.4

Source: California State Department of Public Health, "Particularly Chloromycetin. A Study of Antibiotic Drugs," Report of Senate Fact Finding Committee on Public Health and Safety, California State Department of Public Health, Senate of the State of California, p. 167.

TABLE 2. Age-Adjusted Death Rates From Aplastic Anemia Per 1 Million Population, According To Race, Sex, and Time Period, United States[a]

		Whites		Nonwhites		
ICD Code	Year	Males	Females	Males	Females	Total
292.4[b]	1964	5.2	4.4	3.8	3.0	4.6
284[c]	1968	6.3	5.0	5.2	5.5	5.6
284[c]	1972	6.0	4.3	4.6	4.9	5.1
284[c]	1976	5.3	3.9	4.5	3.2	4.4

Source: Population Estimates and Projections, Bureau of the Census, Vital Statistics of the United States. . . . Washington: Department of Health, Education and Welfare.

[a]Rates adjusted using the direct method, with the 1960 population as standard.

[b]7th Revision.

[c]8th Revision.

ing to race and sex in four recent time periods (Tables 2–4), it can be shown that both male : female and white : non-white ratios are not very marked. Males have slightly higher age-adjusted rates than females, mainly among whites. Rates among whites, especially in males, appear to be greater than those of nonwhites.

Annual average age-specific death rates for the 3-year period around the census year 1970 are shown for whites and nonwhites in Tables 5 and 6. Since death rates in nonwhites are based on extremely small numbers of deaths, Figure 1 shows the age distribution for whites only, according to sex. In addition, because of the relatively small death rates in ages below 50 years,

TABLE 3. Male To Female Ratios Of Age-Adjusted Death Rates From Aplastic Anemia, According To Race And Time Period, United States[a]

Year	Whites	Nonwhites
1964	1.2	1.3
1968	1.3	0.9
1972	1.4	0.9
1976	1.4	1.4

[a]Rates on which ratios are based were adjusted using the direct method, with the 1960 population as standard.

TABLE 4. White To Nonwhite Ratios Of Age-Adjusted Death Rates From Aplastic Anemia, According To Sex And Time Period, United States[a]

Year	Males	Females
1964	1.4	1.5
1968	1.2	0.9
1972	1.3	0.9
1976	1.2	1.2

[a]Rates on which ratios are based were adjusted using the direct method, with the 1960 population as standard.

the death rates in Figure 1 are plotted in a semilogarithmic scale, so that the pattern for the younger ages can be observed more clearly.

For both white males and females, the mortality curve seems to have two components. Relatively low rates characterize the younger ages, with the antimode seen at approximately ages 35–39 in both sexes. Subsequently, rates seem to increase in a log-linear pattern and after around age 50 years, there is an almost constant rate of increase with a ratio of one 5-year age group rate to the previous one of about 1.5 to 2.0.

It can be also seen in Figure 1 that death rates in males are consistently greater than those of females after ages 50–54 years. Furthermore, there is a suggestion that in males a peak in adolescence may occur. In females, death rates gradually decrease from the very young ages to reach a minimum at ages 35–39. Thus, for both sexes, there is a suggestion of a bimodal curve, which may indicate that aplastic anemia in younger subjects may be of a different nature from that in older individuals. In the series reported by Hagler and colleagues (20) of 174 predominantly male patients developing aplastic anemia after an acute episode of viral hepatitis, the mean age of cases was 19.9 years, which is similar to the modal age for the mortality rates from aplastic anemia among young male subjects. Thus, the distribution of mortality rates by age suggests that viral infections may be important in the etiology of aplastic anemia, at least among young subjects.

TABLE 5. Average Annual Age-Specific Death Rates From Aplastic Anemia (I.C.D. 8th Revision 284) Per 1 Million Population, According To Sex, 1969–1971, U.S. Whites

	Male		Female		Both sexes	
Age	Number of deaths[a]	Rate	Number of deaths[a]	Rate	Number of deaths[a]	Rate
0–4	37	1.7	39	1.8	76	1.7
5–9	47	1.8	40	1.6	87	1.7
10–14	31	1.1	41	1.6	72	1.3
15–19	63	2.5	40	1.6	103	2.1
20–24	48	2.3	30	1.3	78	1.8
25–29	24	1.3	23	1.3	47	1.3
30–34	21	1.4	18	1.2	39	1.3
35–39	11	0.8	12	0.8	23	0.8
40–44	16	1.0	25	1.5	41	1.3
45–49	39	2.5	39	2.3	78	2.4
50–54	57	3.9	46	2.9	103	3.4
55–59	95	7.3	87	6.1	182	6.7
60–64	114	10.4	103	8.2	217	9.2
65–69	159	18.7	137	13.0	296	15.6
70–74	192	30.3	188	21.7	380	25.3
75–79	216	49.8	218	34.1	434	40.5
80–84	187	76.8	203	50.8	390	60.7
85+	137	101.5	194	74.8	331	84.0

Source: Population Estimates and Projections, Bureau of the Census Vital Statistics of the United States. Washington: Department of Health, Education and Welfare.

[a]Although rates are annual averages, number of deaths are given for the total 3–year period.

INCIDENCE

Very little data exist on incidence rates for aplastic anemia. Modan and colleagues (30), in a nationwide study of aplastic anemia in Israel, found the overall mean annual incidence rates to be 7.1 per million in males and 8.7 in females for the period 1961–65. For males, mean annual incidence rates in this study were 4.6 per million for ages 0–14, 6.2 for ages 15–49, and 13.1 for ages 50 and over. Among females, corresponding incidence rates were 5.4, 6.6, and 17.2. Thus, female predominance seemed to occur, mainly in the older ages, where the incidence rate of females was about 30% greater than that of males. The authors did not find any differences in incidence rates among different migrant groups, which suggests that aplastic anemia may have been caused by an environmental agent after migration. However, no further subclassification was provided for these rather broad age groups which could allow confirmation of the peak in adolescence seen for mortality data in the U.S. males.

The overall incidence rate for aplastic anemia was also determined in a study done in Upsala, Sweden, which has a population corresponding to about 15% of the entire population of the country (33,34). The authors collected information on all patients discharged with a diagnosis of aplastic ane-

TABLE 6. Average Annual Age-Specific Death Rates From Aplastic Anemia (I.C.D. 8th Revision 284) Per 1 Million Population, According To Sex, 1969–1971, U.S. Nonwhites

	Male		Female		Both sexes	
Age	Number of deaths[a]	Rate	Number of deaths[a]	Rate	Number of deaths[a]	Rate
0–4	8	2.0	11	2.7	19	2.3
5–9	7	1.5	6	1.3	13	1.4
10–14	10	2.1	7	1.5	17	1.8
15–19	4	1.0	9	2.2	13	1.6
20–24	8	2.7	6	1.8	14	2.2
25–29	5	2.2	2	0.7	7	1.4
30–34	2	1.0	3	1.3	5	1.1
35–39	4	2.2	8	3.6	12	2.9
40–44	6	3.2	8	3.6	14	3.4
45–49	5	2.8	5	2.5	10	2.6
50–54	10	6.5	8	4.5	18	5.5
55–59	7	5.2	8	5.3	15	5.2
60–64	11	9.7	11	8.4	22	9.1
65–69	15	16.1	14	12.4	29	14.1
70–74	12	19.2	10	13.0	22	15.8
75–79	10	27.1	6	12.5	16	18.8
80–84	5	23.8	7	24.3	12	24.2
85+	5	35.5	8	37.5	13	36.7

Source: Population Estimates and Projections, Bureau of the Census Vital Statistics of the United States. Washington: Department of Health, Education and Welfare.

[a]Although rates are annual averages, numbers of deaths are given for the total 3–year period.

mia during the 5-year period 1964–68, and were thus able to compute a crude annual incidence rate of 13.2 per million population, which is about 1.7 times greater than the total crude incidence of 7.8 per million found by Modan et al. in Israel over a similar time period.

No incidence data are available for the United States, although Wallerstein and colleagues, who conducted a death certificate study in California between 1957 and 1967 (26), used an overall 50% case-fatality rate to estimate the annual incidence of aplastic anemia as being 4.8 per million population.

SURVIVAL

Aplastic anemia is a serious disease with a poor survivorship, as can be seen in Table 7, which summarizes data from several studies examining prognosis. In spite of differences in characteristics of the patients studied and in the time periods covered, the survival pattern of patients with aplastic anemia does not seem to vary much from study to study. The initial year after the onset of symptoms or diagnosis is characterized by an extremely high case-fatality rate of about 30–50%. With the possible exception of patients undergoing bone marrow transplantation, survival rates continue to decline after the first year,

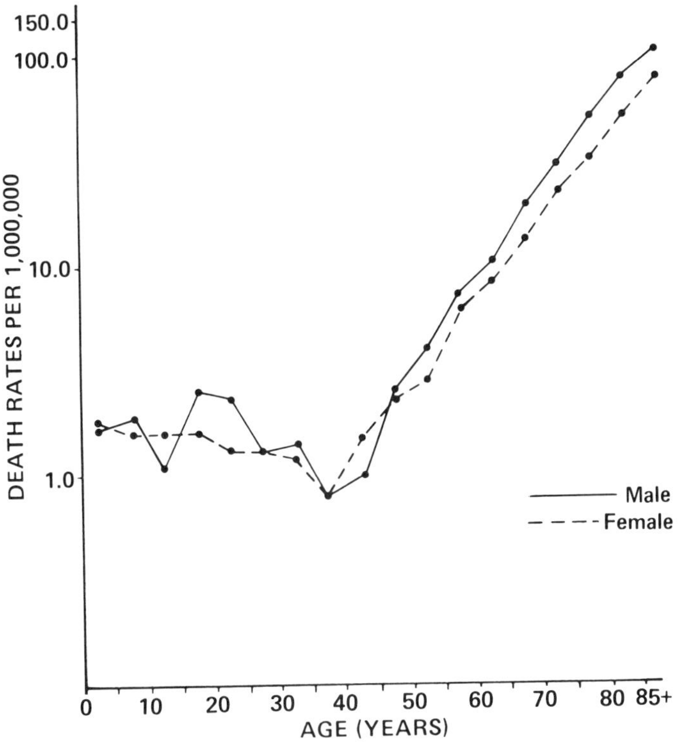

FIGURE 1. Average annual age-specific death rates from aplastic anemia (I.C.D. 8th Revision 284) per 1,000,000 population, according to sex, 1969–1971, United States, whites only.

although at a slower pace. Complete recovery seems to be a rare phenomenon and in the large series reported by Williams et al. (2) of patients not receiving a bone marrow transplant, it was attained for only 7.3% of the 110 cases. These findings certainly suggest that primary prevention of aplastic anemia, when it becomes possible, will be the ideal approach to prevent deaths and disability from this disease.

Factors identified with poor survival have included male sex, a hemorrhagic onset, a short mean interval from onset to first visit, a high proportion of nonmyeloid elements in the bone marrow indicative of severe reduction in erythroid and granulocytic cells, low reticulocyte count, lowest total neutrophil count during the clinical course, and a low mean platelet count (2,29,37,38). On the other hand, survival seems to be unrelated to age (30). In the study by Modan et al. cases in which there was a history of chloramphenicol use seemed to have a worse survivorship than those without such history (30), although this finding was not confirmed in other studies (39).

TABLE 7. Selected Studies of Survivorship in Cases of Aplastic Anemia at Specified Time Intervals

Author	Years covered by report	Country	Number of cases	Point of entry	Survival rates: 3 mo	5 mo	6 mo	12 mo	24 mo	36 mo	48 mo	60 mo
Scott et al. (1)[a]	1945–1957	United States	39	Onset of symptoms			75%	65–70%	55%	40%	40%	
Williams et al. (2)	1947–1971	United States	101	Onset of symptoms		75%		50%	45%		35%	29%
Modan et al. (30)[a,d]	1961–1965	Israel	Males= 42	Diagnosis			55–60%	45–50%				
			Females=51				70–75%	55–60%				
Bottiger (33)[c]	1964–1968	Sweden	80	Onset of symptoms	70%			55%	39%			
Haak et al. (35)[a]	1964–1976	Switzerland	40	First examination			60%	50–55%	40–45%	35–40%	30%	
Storb et al. (36)[a,b]	1970–1977	United States	110	Transplantation			50–55%			45–50%		45–50%

[a]A range is sometimes presented because rates were extrapolated from survival curves in which scales were not sufficiently detailed.

[b]Only study shown in summary table dealing with transplant patients.

[c]Population-based study including the Upsala region population, comprising about 15% of the entire Swedish population.

[d]Population-based study including the entire population of Israel.

Males =42
Females=51

ENVIRONMENTAL FACTORS

Industrial and Therapeutic Chemicals

A few industrial chemicals have been sporadically reported to be associated with aplastic anemia, including benzene and trinitrotoluene (40). On the other hand, many therapeutic drugs have been reported to have caused aplastic anemia (Table 8), of which the most commonly cited is chloramphenicol (1–3,16–19,26,30,42–44).

Chloramphenicol. Chloramphenicol is a broad spectrum antibiotic which has been available commercially in the United States since 1949, which is also the year when mortality data concerning aplastic anemia became available. Chloramphenicol has been an extremely popular antibiotic. It is estimated that in 1959 it accounted for almost half of hospital purchases and almost 15% of the new prescription market of leading antibiotics, other than penicillin and streptomycin (32).

Reports of cases of aplastic anemia with a history of exposure to chloramphenicol began to appear in the medical literature shortly after it entered the antibiotic market (45). Nationwide surveys conducted by the Food and Drug Administration and data from the Blood Dyscrasia Registry of the American Medical Association indicated a high frequency of chloramphenicol usage among the aplastic anemia cases studied (46–48).

At the request of the California State Senate, two studies were conducted by the State Department of Public Health to examine the relationship of chloramphenicol to fatal aplastic anemia (26,32,49). In the first study (32), the authors examined the relationship between chloramphenicol sales data and death rates from aplastic anemia in the years between 1950 and 1960. They were able to show that when the number of grams sold per million population was correlated with mortality for the United States 1 year later, a strikingly high correlation coefficient of +.92 ($P<0.01$) was found (Figure 2). According to the authors, the time lag of 1 year consisted of the period from company sales to consumption of drugs, from drug consumption to clinical onset of aplastic anemia, and from onset of aplastic anemia to death. However, no significant correlation was found for Canada, whereas in the State of California, a significant correlation was found only when a 2-, rather than a 1-year time lag between chloramphenicol sales and death rates from aplastic anemia was assumed.

In this study, a random sample of California death certificates listing aplastic anemia as an underlying cause was also examined from January 1957 through June 1961. Of 138 deaths identified in the sample, 86 met the study criteria for aplastic anemia upon review of data obtained from medical charts. Thus, 52 deaths that had been mistakenly coded as aplastic anemia were available for comparison with the 86 true aplastic anemia deaths. In Table 9, selected exposures noted on the medical charts are compared between the two groups. As seen, marked differences seem to exist with regard to certain drugs, including chloramphenicol and tetracyclines. Some of the chemicals studied may be also responsible for blood dyscrasias other than aplastic anemia, thus leading to an underestimation of differences. On the other hand, the

TABLE 8. Drugs Reported To Have Caused Aplastic Anemia

Acetazolamide	Methylphenylhydantoin
Allopurinol	Methylthiouracil
Aminopyrine	Naphtalene
Amitriptyline	Oxyphenbutazone
Amodiaquine	Para-aminosalicylic acid (PAS)
Amphotericin B	Paracetamol
Ampicillin	Penicillin
Antihistamines	Pentachlorophenol
Arsenicals	Pharathion
Aspirin	Phenacemide
Benzene	Phenacetin
Carbamazepine	Phenelzine
Carbimazole	Pheneturide
Carbon tetrachloride	Phenylenediamine
Carbutamide	Phenindione
Chloramphenicol	Phenylbutazone
Chlordane	Phenytoin
Chlordiazepoxide	Potassium perchlorate
Chloraquine	Primidone
Chlorothiazide	Prochlorperazine
Chlorphenothane (DDT)	Promazine
Chlorpromazine	Promethazine
Chlorpropamide	Propylthiouracil
Colchicine	Pyrimethamine
Co-trimoxazole	Quinacrine
Diazepam	Quick drying glues and cements
Dicophane	Quinidine
Diphenylhydantoin sodium	Ristocetin
Ethosuximide	Salicylamide
Flufenamic acid	Sodium aurothiomalate
Frusemide	Stoddard solvent
Gamma benzene hexachloride	Streptomycin
Gold Compounds	Sulphadimethoxine
Hydroflumethiazide	Sulphadimidine
Hydroxychloraquine	Sulphamethoxypyridazine
Indomethacin	Sulphasalazine
Isoniazid	Sulfisoxazole
Lithium	Sulfathiazole
Malathion	Tetrachlorethylene
Mepacrine	Tetracycline
Mepazine	Thiacetazone
Mephenytoin	Thiocyanate
Meprobamate	Thiouracils
Methaqualone with diphenhydramine	Tolbutamide
Methicillin	Trifluoperazine
Methimazole	Trimethadione
Methoin	Trinitrotoluene
Methyldopa	Troxidone

Source: Data from references 2, 3, 19, 41.

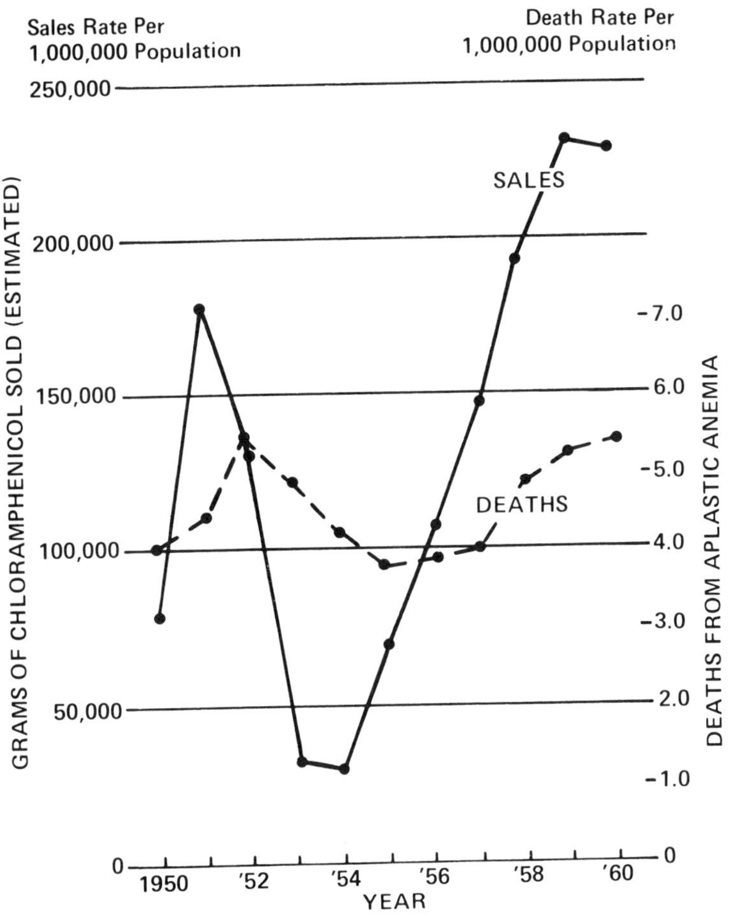

FIGURE 2. Death rates for aplastic anemia and sales rates for chloramphenicol.

Source: California State Department of Public Health, "Particularly Chloromycetin. A Study of Antibiotic Drugs." Report of Senate Fact Finding Committee on Public Health and Safety. California State Department of Public Health, Senate of the State of California, p. 167 (1963).

physicians' belief that the comparison cases may have also had aplastic anemia provided an opportunity to compare exposures noted on medical records probably free of reporting biases.

The second study conducted by the State Department of Public Health at the request of the California State Senate reviewed all fatal cases of aplastic anemia that had occurred during an 18-month period, January 1, 1963, through June 30, 1964 (26,49). Sixty fatal aplastic anemia cases were found in which the diagnosis was confirmed by means of review of clinical charts and interviews with physicians. Of these, no prior history of potentially myelotoxic exposure could be found in the clinical charts of 40 patients

TABLE 9. Percent Distribution of Fatal Confirmed Cases of Aplastic Anemia (AA) and of Fatal Cases Incorrectly Coded as Aplastic Anemia, According to Past Exposure to Selected Chemicals Within 6 Months Prior to Clinical Onset, California, 1957–1961[a]

Drug	Deaths from: Aplastic anemia (N=86)	Deaths from: Other blood dyscrasias and "undiagnosed"[b] (N=52)
Cloramphenicol	29.1%	9.6%
Penicillin	9.3%	5.8%
Tetracyclines	10.5%	1.9%
Aspirin	5.8%	5.8%
Meprobamate	7.0%	—
Barbiturates	9.4%	13.5%
All insecticides	13.9%	—
Paints, shellacs, lacquers, varnishes	9.4%	—
Paint thinners, cleaning fluids, solvents for automotive parts	9.3%	—
Miscellaneous[c]	8.1%	1.9%

Source: California State Department of Public Health. "Particularly Chloromycetin. A Study of Antibiotic Drugs," Report of Senate Fact Finding Committee on Public Health and Safety, California State Department of Public Health, Senate of the State of California, p. 167 (1963).

[a]Data were obtained from review of clinical charts. Table includes only exposures mentioned for a total of 5 or more cases.

[b]These 2 categories were coded as aplastic anemia in the death certificates, but did not meet the study criteria upon review of clinical charts. "Other Blood Dyscrasias" mostly included other types of anemia (7 cases), myeloproliferative disorders (6 cases) and myelofibrosis (4 cases). "Undiagnosed" includes cases in which data from clinical charts were insufficient to arrive at a diagnosis.

[c]Airplane glue and dope; bioychloheptadienedibromide; Christmas decorative spray; hair dye; hair spray; paint remover; unidentified "toxic chemical".

(67%). In 10 of the 60 deaths (17%), prior exposure to chloramphenicol was noted, but 7 of these had also received another potentially toxic agent.

In this study, two surveys were carried out involving a sample of physicians and pharmacies in the state in order to estimate the human consumption of nontopical chloramphenicol. On the basis of findings of these surveys and those of the review of fatal cases, the authors estimated the risk of death from aplastic anemia within one year of use of an average dose of 4.5 grams of chloramphenicol to be 24.6 per million. In the population not exposed, the yearly death rate was estimated to be 1.9 per million, thus indicating that the risk of dying from aplastic anemia after chloramphenicol use was 12.9 times the risk for the general population, i.e., the mortality ratio was 12.9.

Because the prevalence rate of chloramphenicol usage had been estimated in order to arrive at these mortality data, Levin's formula (50) could be applied to estimate the percent population attributable risk for fatal aplastic anemia cases. With an estimated prevalence rate of 2% for an average chloramphenicol use of 4.5 grams and a mortality ratio of 12.9, the percent of the total population death rate explainable on the basis of chloramphenicol use in California in 1964 was around 19%. These estimates of relative and attributable risks do not take into account the possibility of confounding exposures; thus it is possible that both these measures are overestimated.

In addition to these population-based studies, other studies have supported an etiologic role for chloramphenicol. For example, of 823 cases of aplastic anemia reported to the American Medical Association Registry, 44% had taken chloramphenicol prior to the onset of the disease, which is likely to be in great excess of the expected percent population usage (2). Armenian and Lilienfeld (51) analyzed a large series of cases of aplastic anemia occurring after the use of chloramphenicol and found that the distribution of intervals from use of the drug to the time of onset of aplastic anemia had a log-normal distribution similar to that found for epidemic curves of infectious diseases following a common exposure. In this study, the estimated median incubation period for all cases of pancytopenia following the use of chloramphenicol was 3.2 months.

In the aplastic anemia that results from chloramphenicol use, two main forms can be distinguished. In the first, prolonged administration of high doses of chloramphenicol will initially depress erythropoiesis and then other cellular elements of the marrow (3). At least in children, it has been postulated that bone marrow depression caused by chloramphenicol is the result of the daily, rather than the total, dose (52). This dose-related type of aplastic anemia is generally, but not always, reversible upon withdrawal of the drug (3,53).

The second, or "idiosyncratic," form of chloramphenicol-induced aplastic anemia is not dose-related and usually occurs weeks or months after the use of the drug has been terminated (53). Apparently, even chloramphenicol eye drops can cause aplastic anemia (15), although there is some indication that it may not occur when the drug is administered parenterally (44). While the first form seems to result from a direct toxic effect of chloramphenicol, which is known to inhibit mitochondria isolated from bone marrow cells (19,54), the second form is probably related to a prior genetic defect in the bone marrow stem cell (54). Because the second form often involves all three major cellular elements, it is presumed to be a defect of the pluripotential stem cell (3).

Although little doubt remains about the etiologic role of chloramphenicol in aplastic anemia, certain intriguing findings are still in need of explanation. For example, the lack of correlation between sales data and death rates both in Canada (32) and Japan (55), and the fact that death rates from aplastic anemia in the United States have not changed recently, in spite of a probable reduction in use of chloramphenicol are still unexplained. Thus, there is a need for further epidemiologic studies to obtain a more precise quantification of the risk associated with this drug.

Other Drugs and Chemicals. Of the other drugs suspected of being related to aplastic anemia, a good case seems to exist for phenylbutazone, which had been taken by 6.3% of the aplastic anemia cases reported to the American Medical Association Registry (2). In the California study by Wallerstein et al.

(26), although no case of aplastic anemia developed after use of phenylbutazone, the risk of developing fatal aplastic anemia after exposure to oxyphenbutazone was estimated to be 4 times greater than that of the general population. A population mortality ratio could also be obtained for use of quinacrine hydrochloride (Atabrine) among armed forces personnel stationed in the South and Southwest Pacific areas during the second world war (56). In this study, a death rate of 20 per million was found in areas where quinacrine was routinely used for the prevention of malaria, whereas a rate of only 2 per million was found in military installations not using quinacrine.

In prospective studies involving a follow-up of workers exposed to benzol and other organic solvents, there was either no excess risk for aplastic anemia (55) or the number of deaths from aplastic anemia was so small that the results were regarded to be inconclusive (57). In addition, a large prospective study involving 5 million workers employed by about 12,000 large and middle-size industries throughout Japan in 1970–1974 has not revealed any excess deaths from aplastic anemia (55).

Generally speaking, it is impossible to determine whether the association of most of the drugs listed in Table 8 with aplastic anemia is coincidental or causal, due to lack of control data. It is, therefore, important that aplastic anemia cases be compared with control subjects in well-designed retrospective studies, so that the independent contribution of each exposure can be properly estimated.

Ionizing Radiation

A few reports have suggested that ionizing radiation can play an etiologic role in aplastic anemia (Table 10). In general, studies examining the relationship of radiation to aplastic anemia have not been able to quantify the degree of exposure. Nevertheless, there is a strong suggestion that an association indeed exists, with relative risks varying from a minimum of 1.8 in the study of atomic bomb survivors (61) to a maximum of 43.0 in the Matanoski et al. follow-up of American radiologists and internists (58). In this latter study, an excess risk was only seen for the cohort of radiologists joining their specialty society in 1920–29. Because no excess risk was seen in subsequent cohorts, the inference can perhaps be made that lower level radiation exposure of radiologists associated with better protection devices does not play a role in the etiology of aplastic anemia.

Difficulties in diagnosing aplastic anemia from death certificates are illustrated by the study of Court-Brown and Doll (59), who examined the risk of fatal aplastic anemia among patients given x-ray therapy for ankylosing spondylitis at 81 British centers. In this study, of the 16 deaths initially identified as aplastic anemia, only 4 met the study criteria upon review of clinical and pathological data. Of the 12 nonconfirmed cases, a diagnosis of definite or probable leukemia was made in eight, whereas for 4, the information was not sufficient to arrive at any diagnosis.

According to Cronkite, radiation-induced aplasia is almost solely due to direct killing of stem cells (62).

Viruses

In recent years, a growing number of cases of aplastic anemia with a grave prognosis have been reported following hepatitis (2,20–22,25). Hagler and colleagues (20) reviewed case-reports published through the early 1970's of patients developing aplastic anemia after an episode of hepatitis. In general, there was no history of antecedent chronic liver disease; pancytopenia usually began within one year after the onset of hepatitis and all fatalities occurred within 16 months after onset of aplastic anemia. The case-fatality rate during this period was 85.1%, which is substantially higher than that for the largely nonhepatitis-associated total aplastic anemia cases (see Table 7).

Hagler et al. (20) presented detailed clinical information for 153 patients, of whom 137 (90.2%) developed aplastic anemia within one year after the episode of hepatitis. The time interval from the onset of hepatitis to that of aplastic anemia was available for 127 of these 137 patients who developed aplastic anemia within one year. Thus, it was possible to examine the distribution of cases according to this interval (Figure 3). Notwithstanding the possibility of reporting bias, there seems to be a similarity between the distribution of aplastic anemia cases by time interval from the hepatitis episode, and the log-normal configuration of the epidemic curve of infectious diseases. This suggests that the observed curve may result from a latent period between the exposure to infectious hepatitis and the development of disease. This distribution may resemble a logarithmic normal distribution, that is further illustrated by the fact that when cumulative percentages are plotted on a logarithmic probability graph paper, the resulting distribution seems to approximate a straight line (Figure 4).

Further examination of the data provided in the paper by Hagler et al. revealed that of the 137 cases in which aplastic anemia started within one year after hepatitis, 36 (26%) had been exposed to another potentially myelotoxic agent prior to the onset of hepatitis. In about 15% of these cases, chloramphenicol had been used. The authors suggest that these latter patients could have suffered idiosyncratic damage of the liver and the bone marrow, both resulting from exposure to chloramphenicol, or they might have developed marrow toxicity as a consequence of drug administration during unrecognized hepatitis.

The median incubation period for the chloramphenicol-associated aplastic anemia estimated by Armenian and Lilienfeld (3.2 months) (51) was shorter than that estimated from the data by Hagler et al. for cases occurring within one year after hepatitis (5.8 months). It is nevertheless possible that at least some of the cases following hepatitis can be due to the use of chloramphenicol or other drugs, rather than to the hepatitis virus. Other reports of the so-called chloramphenicol–hepatitis–aplastic anemia syndrome have been published (63), pointing to the need of conducting epidemiologic studies in order to assess the independent effect of one exposure while controlling for the effects of confounding variables, with regard to the risk of developing aplastic anemia.

Additional evidence that hepatitis may cause aplastic anemia comes from a population-based study by Böttiger and Westerholm (34) of 80 cases of aplas-

TABLE 10. Selected Studies Examining the Relationship of Ionizing Radiation to Aplastic Anemia

Author	Populations compared	Period of study	End-point measured	Results		Relative risk	P Value
Matanoski et al. (58)	U.S. radiologists vs. internists joining respective specialty societies in 1920–1929	1920–1969	Deaths	Rate per 1,000,000	Radiologists = 172.0[a] Internists = 4.0[a]	43.0	Not stated
Court-Brown and Doll (59)	Patients treated for ankylosing spondilitis at 81 radiotherapy centers in Britain vs. population of England and Wales.	1935–1955	Deaths	Number of deaths	Observed =4[b] Maximum expected =0.3[a,c]	16.0	Not stated

Lewis (27)	Male radiologists certified by the American Board of Radiology vs. U.S. white male population.	1948–1961	Deaths	Number of deaths { Observed = 4; Expected = .23[a]	17.4 (4.7–44.5)[d]	0.0001
Kitabatake (60)	Japanese radiological technicians vs. Japanese population.	1930–1960	Incident cases	Observed incidence/74,400 person–years = 3; Expected incidence = 0.5	6.0	"Statistically significant"
Ichimaru et al. (61)	Atomic bomb survivors exposed to 1 rad or more vs. those exposed to <1 rad.	1950–1967	Incident cases	Rate per 1,000,000 { 1 + rad = 10.7[e]; <1 rad = 6.0[e]	1.8	>0.05

[a] Age-adjusted.

[b] In only one of the four cases x-ray exposure alone was implicated.

[c] "Maximum expected" on the assumption that all patients who were lost to follow-up survived to the end of follow-up period.

[d] 95% confidence limits.

[e] Age and sex-adjusted.

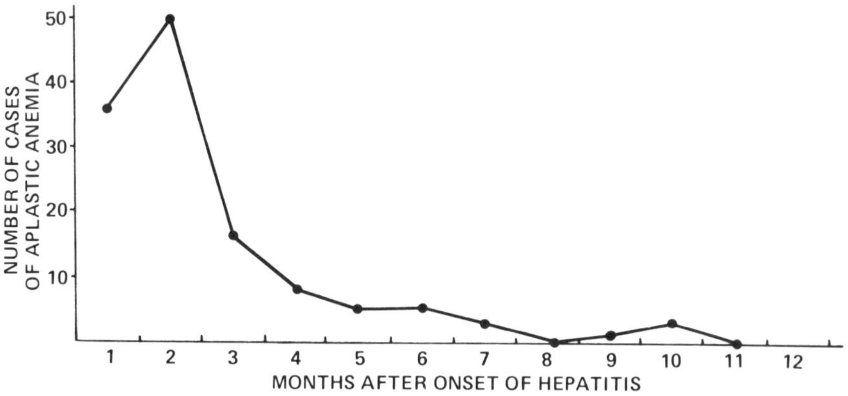

FIGURE 3. Number of cases of aplastic anemia following an episode of acute hepatitis within 1 year, according to time interval between onset of hepatitis and onset of aplastic anemia.

Source: Hagler, L. Pastore, R. A., Bergin, J. J., Aplastic anemia following viral hepatitis: report of two fatal cases and literature review. Medicine 54, 139–164 (1975). © 1975, The Williams and Wilkins Co., Baltimore.

tic anemia occurring between 1964 and 1968 in Upsala, Sweden. Eight hundred and ninety-five cases of infectious hepatitis were reported during this period, of whom 2 subsequently developed aplastic anemia. The average annual incidence rate of aplastic anemia following an episode of hepatitis was thus found to be 44.7 per 100,000 or 34.4 times greater than the estimated incidence of 1.3 per 100,000 for the non-exposed population.

The pathogenesis of aplastic anemia following hepatitis remains largely unexplained. When pancytopenia ensues, direct destruction of bone-marrow stem cells seems likely, but when only pure red-cell aplasia occurs, an autoimmune mechanism may be involved (64,65). If stem-cell failure is the chief mechanism, it could result from chromosomal damage, which has been noted to occur in viral hepatitis and other viral infections (66–68). On the other hand, if a virus is responsible, it could also act by destroying the microcirculation (22).

A hematodepressive potential of the hepatitis viral genome is indicated by the fact that experimental infection in animals with murine hepatitis virus (MHV-3) is able to produce changes in the peripheral blood and bone marrow (20). There is also the possibility that hepatocellular failure in viral hepatitis impairs the liver's ability to provide hematopoietic nutrients, or to detoxify intermediate metabolites or drugs which might become myelotoxic, as could well be the case in the chloramphenicol–hepatitis–aplastic anemia syndrome (20–22).

Aside from the hepatitis virus, other viruses may be involved in the etiology of aplastic anemia. For example, Mir and Delamore (24) have recently described a case of aplastic anemia following infectious mononucleosis. In addition, pancytopenia is known to sometimes occur during the course of severe infections, particularly chronic ones, such as tuberculosis and brucellosis (1).

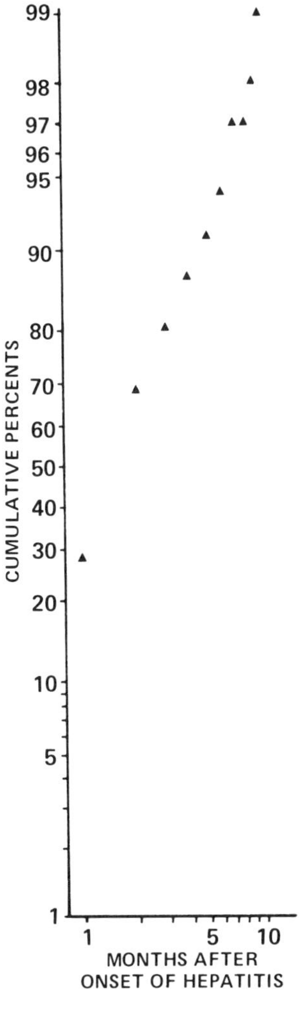

FIGURE 4. Cumulative percent of cases of aplastic anemia following an episode of acute hepatitis within 1 year, according to time interval between onset of hepatitis and onset of aplastic anemia.

Source: Hagler, L., Pastore, R. A., Bergin, J. J., Aplastic anemia following viral hepatitis: report of two fatal cases and literature review. Medicine 54, 139–164 (1975). © 1975, The Williams and Wilkins Co., Baltimore.

Because it has been suggested that subclinical hepatitis or other infections may be responsible for a significant percentage of cases of the so-called "idiopathic" aplastic anemia (20,22), there is a need for a detailed epidemiologic study of prior exposure to infections in patients with aplastic anemia.

APLASTIC ANEMIA AS AN IMMUNOLOGICAL DISORDER

There is evidence to suggest that aplastic anemia may have an immunological basis. Both the "pure" red cell aplasia and the fully developed pancytopenia forms of aplastic anemia have been found to be associated with autoimmune diseases (64,65,69), with the occasional presence of autoantibodies against hemopoietic cells (3). Knospe and Crosby (9) have postulated that the unique marrow sinusoidal structures, with an incomplete or absent basement membrane, may permit immune mechanisms to mount antigen–antibody or cellular immune reactions restricted to these structures. More recently, additional support for the role of immune processes in the pathogenesis of aplastic anemia has come from the observation that immunosuppressive agents, such as cyclophosphamide, can lead to successful recovery from aplastic anemia (70). These findings suggest that it is important to carry out studies to investigate personal and familial occurrence of autoimmune disorders as possible predictors of aplastic anemia.

APLASTIC ANEMIA AND ACUTE NONLYMPHOCYTIC LEUKEMIA

An important feature of aplastic anemia refers to its association with acute nonlymphocytic leukemia (ANLL). Although aplastic anemia is generally not regarded as a malignant disorder, it is significant that both hereditary and acquired cases are known to occasionally progress to ANLL (3,12,30,53,71). In the study by Modan et al. (30) involving the entire Israeli population, 22% of the 23 cases of aplastic anemia with a history of exposure to chloramphenicol and 6% of the 51 "idiopathic" cases developed ANLL. Overall, 11% of the 93 cases detected between 1961 and 1965 subsequently developed ANLL.

Aplastic anemia and ANLL may also share a number of etiologic agents such as benzene (72,73) and ionizing radiation (27,58,59,61). In addition, infection with feline leukemia virus has been shown to result in aplastic anemia in cats (74,75). Furthermore, analysis of mortality (and also incidence) rates from ANLL reveals a peak in adolescence (76) and a subsequent increase of rates with age (77), a trend which coincides with that for males with regard to aplastic anemia.

Common risk factors would, of course, be sufficient to explain the simultaneous occurrence in susceptible individuals of two disorders with similar latent periods. Court-Brown and Doll (59) have, for example, noted that the risk of aplastic anemia following x-ray therapy for ankylosing spondylitis is increased until 3–5 years after therapy, after which there is a decline. This trend is very similar to that of radiation-induced leukemia, although the decline in risk of aplastic anemia after 5 years is more marked (61).

Brauer and Dameshek (53) have postulated that leukemia may be a secondary, perhaps reparative, response to aplastic anemia. In support for this hypothesis, they have emphasized the tendency to neoplasia of hypoplastic tissue, such as atrophic gastritis and leukoplakia. These same authors have also suggested that both disorders may be thought of as growth disturbances of the bone marrow and thus may occur either together or sequentially as phases of the same pathogenetic mechanism.

These observations indicate that a comparison of the epidemiologic characteristics of aplastic anemia patients with those of ANLL patients may provide clues with regard to the pathogenesis of aplastic anemia with possible preventive or even curative implications.

CONCLUSIONS

Aplastic anemia is a disease of very poor prognosis in which at least 50% of all cases are considered of idiopathic origin (1,3,20,28–30). Although over the last few years much attention has been given to bone marrow transplantation as a potentially ideal therapy for severe aplastic anemia (8,78–80), serious problems remain: Graft rejection of HLA-matched siblings occurs in about one-third of the cases (79,80), and graft-versus-host disease seems to occur in as many as 70% of successful engraftments (8). These two conditions lead to a high case-fatality rate caused by infections (79); as a result, the survival rates for patients undergoing transplantation are far from ideal even in the most experienced centers (Table 7). Thus, identification of risk factors with adoption of preventive measures seems to be both less expensive and more productive than curative approaches to avoid disability and death from aplastic anemia.

From the many case-history reports and the few epidemiologic studies covered in the present review, three general categories of factors seem to emerge as likely etiologic factors in aplastic anemia: chemicals, ionizing radiation, and viruses. With regard to chemicals, a strong case can be made for an etiologic role of chloramphenicol, based on both clinical reports and population-based mortality studies. However, for most of the other drugs and chemicals, the evidence mostly comes from individual case reports in which comparisons with expected exposures in subjects without aplastic anemia have usually not been made. Thus, it is possible that in many instances, the association of aplastic anemia with these agents was coincidental rather than causal, which suggests that the presumed proportion of 50% for idiopathic cases may be even greater.

Evidence supporting a role for ionizing radiation has been chiefly epidemiologic in nature, derived from large scale prospective studies yielding relative risks or mortality ratios of between 1.8 and 43. However, information on the effect of dose is generally missing, making it difficult to determine whether or not the risk of aplastic anemia is dependent on a radiation exposure threshold.

Substantial additional clarification is also required for the role that viruses, particularly the hepatitis virus, may play in the etiology of aplastic anemia. In one population-based study in which the incidence of aplastic anemia following hepatitis was found to be more than 30 times greater than the incidence in the general population, the rate among hepatitis patients was based on only two cases of the disease (34). In addition, a distribution of times of onset of aplastic anemia after the hepatitis episode resembling a log-normal distribution (20) may be due to a latent period following the time of exposure to the hepatitis virus or to a myelosuppressive chemical taken by the patient during the prodromal phase of hepatitis.

Thus, even in studies that permitted the calculation of relative risks, the associations found could have been due to either the factor under study or to a confounding exposure. Consequently, there is a need both to identify additional risk factors related to the "idiopathic" cases and to estimate more precisely relative and attributable risks associated with suspected etiologic factors, such as chloramphenicol and ionizing radiation.

Given the rarity of the disorder, the choice of an appropriate study design to examine risk factors for aplastic anemia is a complex matter. Case-control studies would seem to represent a logical first step, in spite of the limitations in ascertainment of exposures. Prospective studies, on the other hand, would have to rely on collaborative efforts capable of yielding large samples that would have to be followed up for relatively long periods of time. Another possibility would be to take advantage of studies which have already collected baseline data on specific exposures for a defined population for which the risk of aplastic anemia could be ascertained. Thus, if prospective studies have already been or are being carried out on, for example, viral hepatitis, a more than welcome addition would be the examination of risk of aplastic anemia among the study cohort subjects, either concurrently or noncurrently.

Another problem in studying aplastic anemia prospectively is that of the estimation of the expected risk in non-exposed individuals. Since the risk in the non-exposed group can be much smaller than that of exposed subjects, large sample sizes may be involved to obtain a risk estimate in the former. Population estimates of incidence rates of aplastic anemia according to demographic variables such as sex, age and race, are not available in the United States. Perhaps one of the ways to resolve this problem would be to add aplastic anemia to the diseases to be reported to cancer registries around the country.

The reporting of aplastic anemia cases to cancer registries raises the question as to whether aplastic anemia should be regarded as a malignant disorder. Its association with acute leukemia has suggested that both disorders are different stages of the natural history of the same basic disease (53,71). Thus, it would also be useful to analyze the epidemiologic characteristics of acute nonlymphocytic leukemia in studies designed to examine aplastic anemia. Similarities in the epidemiologic patterns of aplastic anemia and acute nonlymphocytic leukemia may suggest that aplastic anemia should be placed in the general category of malignant disorders, with possible important implications regarding both primary and secondary prevention.

REFERENCES

1. Scott, J. L., Cartwright, G. E., Wintrobe, M. M. (1959) Acquired aplastic anemia: an analysis of thirty-nine cases and review of the pertinent literature. Medicine (Baltimore) 39, 119–172.
2. Willaims, D. M., Lynch, R. E., Cartwright, G. E. (1973) Drug-induced aplastic anemia. Semin. Hematol. 10, 195–223.
3. Jepson, J. H. (1973) Hypoplastic anemia. Pathophysiology and therapy. Med. Clin. North Am. 57, 1079–1094.
4. Boggs, D. R., Boggs, S. S. (1976) The pathogenesis of aplastic anemia: A defective pluripotent hematopoietic stem cell with inappropriate balance of differentiation and self-replication. Blood 48, 71–76.
5. Stohlman, F., Jr. (1972) Aplastic anemia (Editorial). Blood 40, 282–286.
6. Lewis, S. M., Dacie, J. V. (1967) The aplastic anemia-paroxysmal nocturnal hemoglobinuria syndrome. Br. J. Haematol. 13, 236–251.
7. Gavosto, F., Aglietta, M., Foe, R., Gabutti, V., Pagliardi, G. L. (1978) Stem cell kinetics in aplastic anemia. *In:* Aplastic Anemia. Hibino, S., Takaku, F., Shahidi, N. T. (eds.). Baltimore, London, Tokyo: University Park Press, pp. 19–28.

8. Thomas, E. D., Storb, R., Clift, R. A., Fefer, A., Johnson, L., Neiman, P. E., Lerner, K. G., Glucksberg, H., Buckner, C. D. (1975) Bone marrow transplantation. N. Engl. J. Med. 292, 832–843.
9. Knospe, W. H., Crosby, W. H. (1971) Aplastic Anaemia: a disorder of the bone-marrow sinusoidal microcirculation rather than stem-cell failure? Lancet i, 20–22.
10. Knospe, W. H. (1978) Hematopoietic microenvironment: role of sinusoidal microcirculation and other stromal elements. *In:* Aplastic Anemia. Hibino, S., Takaku, F., Shahidi, N. T. (eds.). Baltimore, London, Tokyo: University Park Press, pp. 95–105.
11. Speck, B. (1978) Present results of bone marrow grafts in primary aplastic anemia. *In:* Aplastic Anemia. Hibino, S., Takaku, F., Shahidi, N. T. (eds.). Baltimore, London, Tokyo: University Park Press, pp. 425–428.
12. Bloom, G. E., Warner, S., Gerald, P. S., Diamond, L. K. (1966) Chromosome abnormalities in constitutional aplastic anemia. N. Engl. J. Med. 274, 8–14.
13. Swift, M. R., Hirschhorn, K. (1966) Fanconi's anemia. Inherited susceptibility to chromosome breakage in various tissues. Ann. Intern. Med. 65, 496–503.
14. Tartaglia, A. P., Propp, S., Amarose, A. P., Propp, R., Hall, C. H. (1966) Chromosome abnormality and hypocalcemia in congenital erythroid hypoplasia (Blackfan-Diamond Syndrome). Am. J. Med. 41, 990–999.
15. Carpenter, G. (1975) Chloramphenicol eye-drops and marrow aplasia. Lancet ii, 326–327.
16. Dameshek, W., (1960) Chloramphenicol—a new warning. J.A.M.A. 174, 161–162.
17. Donski, S. T., Bucher, U. (1967/1968) Increase of the number of pancytopenias between 1954 and 1964. Helv. Med. Acta 34, 337–350.
18. Erslev, A. J. (1964) Drug-induced blood dyscrasias. I. Aplastic anemia. J.A.M.A. 188, 159–160.
19. Girdwood, R. H. (1976) Drug-induced anaemias. Drugs 11: 394–404.
20. Hagler, L., Pastore, R. A., Bergin, J. J. (1975) Aplastic anemia following viral hepatitis: report of two fatal cases and literature review. Medicine 54, 139–164.
21. Deller, J. J., Cirksena, W. J., Marcarelli, J. (1962) Fatal pancytopenia associated with viral hepatitis. N. Engl. J. Med. 266, 297–299.
22. Editorial (1971) Infectious hepatitis and aplastic anemia. Lancet i, 844–845.
23. Editorial (1973) The hepatitis–aplastic anemia syndrome. Med. J. Aust. 1, 918–919.
24. Mir, M. A., Delamore, I. W. (1973) Aplastic anaemia complicating infectious mononucleosis. Scand. J. Haematol. 11, 314–318.
25. Rosner, F. (1970) Aplastic anemia and viral hepatitis. Lancet ii, 1080.
26. Wallerstein, R. O., Condit, P. K., Kasper, C. K., Brown, J. W., Morrison, F. R. (1969) Statewide study of chloramphenicol therapy and fatal aplastic anemia. J.A.M.A. 208, 2045–2050.
27. Lewis, E. B. (1963) Leukemia, multiple myeloma and aplastic anemia in American radiologists. Science 142, 1492–1494.
28. Editorial (1976) Mechanisms in aplastic anemia. Lancet ii, 1179–1181.
29. Li, F. P., Alter, B. P., Nathan, D. G. (1972) The mortality of acquired aplastic anemia in children. Blood 40, 153–162.
30. Modan, B., Segal, S., Shani, M., Sheba, C. (1975) Aplastic anemia in Israel: evaluation of the etiological role of chloramphenicol on a community-wide basis. Am. J. Med. Sci. 270, 441–445.
31. Nakayama, K., Nakagawa, T. (1978) Prevalence and clinical states of aplastic anemia among children in Japan. *In:* Aplastic Anemia. Hibino, S., Takaku, F., Shahidi, N. T. (eds.). Baltimore, London, Tokyo: University Park Press, pp. 207–223.
32. California State Department of Public Health (1963) "Particularly Chloromycetin." A Study of Antibiotic Drugs. Report of Senate Fact Finding Committee on Public Health and Safety. California State Department of Public Health, Senate of the State of California, p. 167.

33. Bottiger, L. E. (1978) Prevalence and etiology of aplastic anemia in Sweden. *In:* Aplastic Anemia. Hibino, S., Takaku, F., Shahidi, N. T. (eds.). Baltimore, London, Tokyo: University Park Press, pp. 171–180.
34. Bottiger, L. E., Westerholm, B. (1972) Aplastic anemia. III. Aplastic anemia and infectious hepatitis. Acta Med. Scand. 192, 323–326.
35. Haak, H. L., Hartgrink-Groeneveld, C. A., Eernisse, J. G., Speck, B., vanRood, J. J. (1977) Acquired aplastic anemia in adults. I. A retrospective analysis of 40 cases: Single factors influencing the prognosis. Acta Haematol. 58, 257–277.
36. Storb, R., Thomas, E. D., Weiden, P. L., Buckner, C. D., Clift, R. A., Fefer, A., Goodell, B. W., Johnson, F. L., Neiman, P. E., Sanders, J. E., Singer, J. (1978) One-hundred-ten patients with aplastic anemia (AA) treated by marrow transplantation in Seattle. Trans. Proc. 10, 135–140.
37. Editorial (1975) Prognosis in aplastic anemia. Br. Med. J. 2, 126–127.
38. Lynch, R. E., Williams, D. M., Reading, J. C., Cartwright, G. E. (1975) The prognosis in aplastic anemia. Blood 45, 517–528.
39. Najean, Y., Pecking, A., Dresch, C. (1978) A prospective analysis of 350 cases of aplastic anemia. *In:* Aplastic Anemia. Hibino, S., Takaku, F., Shahidi, N. T. (eds.). Baltimore, London, Tokyo: University Park Press, pp. 181–184.
40. Fleming, A. J. (1959) The etiology of aplastic anemia. Industrial chemicals versus therapeutic chemicals. J. Occup. Med. 1, 97–100.
41. Toghill, P. G., Wilcox, R. G. (1976) Aplastic anemia and hair dye. Br. Med. J. i, 502–503.
42. Editorial (1974) Drug-induced aplastic anemia. Lancet i, 251–252.
43. Hodgkinson, R. (1954) Blood dyscrasias associated with chloramphenicol. An investigation into the cases in the British Isles. Lancet i, 285–287.
44. Polin, H. B., Plaut, M. E. (1977) Chloramphenicol. N.Y. State. J. Med. 77, 378–381.
45. Lewis, C. N., Putnam, L. E., Henricks, F. D., Kerlan, I., Welch, H. (1952) Chloramphenicol (Chloromycetin) in relation to blood dyscrasias with observations on other drugs. Antibiot. Chemother. 2, 601–608.
46. Anonymous (1960) Blood dyscrasias associated with chloramphenicol (chloromycetin) therapy. J.A.M.A. 172, 2044–2045.
47. Erslev, A. J., Wintrobe, M. M. (1962) Detection and Prevention of drug-induced blood dyscrasias. J.A.M.A. 181, 114–119.
48. Anonymous (1962) Registry of blood dyscrasias: Report to Council. J.A.M.A. 179, 888–890.
49. California Medical Association and State Department of Public Health (1967) Fatal Aplastic Anemia and Chloramphenicol. Report to the California State Assembly and Senate by the California Medical Association and State Department of Public Health, with cooperation and assistance of the California Pharmaceutical Association (mimeograph).
50. Levin M. L. (1953) Symposium on endemiology of cancer of lung: Occurrence of lung cancer in man. Acta Univ. Int. Cancer 9, 531–540.
51. Armenian, H. K., Lilienfeld, A. M. (1973) The distribution of incubation periods of neoplastic diseases. Am. J. Epidemiol. 99, 92–100.
52. Yodfat, Y. (1969) Toxic effects of chloramphenicol. A survey of children treated in general practice. Isr. J. Med. Sci. 5, 1184–1187.
53. Brauer, M. J., Dameshek, W. (1967) Hypoplastic anemia and myeloblastic leukemia following chloramphenicol therapy. N. Engl. J. Med. 277, 1003–1005.
54. Yunis, A. A. (1978) Pathogenetic mechanisms in bone marrow suppression from chloramphenicol and thiamphenicol. *In:* Aplastic Anemia. Hibino, S., Takaku, F., Shahidi, N. T. (eds.). Baltimore, London, Tokyo: University Park Press, pp. 321–331.
55. Aoki, K., Ohtani, M. Shimizu, H. (1978) Epidemiologic approach to the etiology of

aplastic anemia. *In*: Aplastic Anemia Hibino. S., Takaku, F., Shahidi. N. T. (eds.). Baltimore, London, Tokyo: University Park Press, pp. 155–170.

56. Custer, R. P. (1946) Aplastic anemia in soldiers treated with Atabrine (Quinacrine). Am. J. Med. Sci. 212, 211–224.
57. Ott, M. G., Townsend, J. C., Fishbeck, W. A., Langner, R. A. (1978) Mortality among individuals occupationally exposed to benzene. Arch. Environ. Health. 33, 3–10.
58. Matanoski, G. M., Seltser, R., Sartwell, P. E., Diamond, E. L., Elliott, E. A. (1975) The current mortality rates of radiologists and other physician specialists: Specific causes of death. Am. J. Epidemiol. 101, 199–210.
59. Court-Brown, W. M., Doll, R. (1957) Leukemia and aplastic anaemia in patients irradiated for ankylosing spondylitis. Med. Res. Counc. Spec. Rep. Ser. No. 295, 1–135.
60. Kitakatake, T., Watanabe, T., Saito, A., Nakamura, M. (1976) Epidemiology of aplastic anemia in Japanese radiological technicians. Nippon. Acta Radiol. 36, 225. Cited by: Aoki, K., Ohtani, M., Shimizu, H., Epidemiological approach to the etiology of aplastic anemia. *In*: Aplastic Anemia (1978) Hibino, S., Takaku, F., Shahidi, N. T. (eds.). Baltimore, London, Tokyo: University Park Press, pp. 155–170.
61. Ichimaru, M., Ishimaru, T., Tsuchimoto, T., Kirshbaum, J. D. (1972) Incidence of aplastic anemia in A-bomb survivors, Hiroshima and Nagasaki, 1946–1967. Radiat. Res. 49, 461–472.
62. Cronkite, E. P. (1967) Radiation-induced aplastic anemia. Semin. Haematol. 4, 273–277.
63. Hodgkinson, R. (1973) The chloramphenicol–hepatitis–aplastic anemia syndrome. Med. J. Aust. 1: 939–940.
64. Dameshek, W., Brown, S. M., Rubin, A. D. (1967) "Pure" red cell anemia (erythroblastic hypoplasia) and thymoma." Semin. Haematol. 4, 222–232.
65. Skikne, B. S., Lynch, S. R., Bezwoda, W. R., Bothwell, T. H., Berstein, R., Katz, J. (1976) Pure red cell aplasia. S. Afr. Med. J. 50: 1353–1357.
66. Matsaniotis, N., Kiossoglou, K. A., Maounis, F., Anagnostakis, D. E. (1966) Chromosomes in infectious hepatitis. Lancet, ii, 421.
67. Mella, B. (1967) Leukocyte mitosis: Suppression in vitro associated with acute infectious hepatitis. Science 155, 80–81.
68. Nichols, W. W. (1970) Virus-induced chromosome abnormalities. Ann. Rev. Microbiol. 24, 479–500.
69. Carcassonne, Y., Gastaut, J. A. (1976) Pancytopenia and scleroderma. Br. Med. J. 1, 1446.
70. Baran, D. T., Griner, P. F., Klemperer, M. R. (1967) Recovery from aplastic anemia after treatment with cyclophosphamide. N. Engl. J. Med. 295, 1522–1523.
71. Cohen, T., Creger, W. P. (1967) Acute myeloid leukemia following seven years of aplastic anemia induced by chloramphenicol. Am. J. Med. 43, 762–770.
72. Aksoy, M., Dincol, K., Erdem, S., Dincol, G. (1972) Acute leukemia due to chronic exposure to benzene. Am. J. Med. 52, 160–166.
73. Aksoy, M., Erdem, S., Dincol, G. (1974) Leukemia in shoe-workers exposed chronically to benzene. Blood 44, 837–841.
74. Mackey, L., Jarrett, W., Jarrett, O., Laird, H. (1975) Anemia associated with feline leukemia virus infection in cats. J. Natl. Cancer Inst. 54, 209–217.
75. Cotter, S. M., Essex, M. (1977) Animal model of human disease. Am. J. Pathol. 87, 265–268.
76. Lee, J. A. H. (1961) Acute myeloid leukaemia in adolescents. Br. Med. J. 1, 988–992.
77. Third National Cancer Survey (1975) Incidence Data. DHEW Publication No. (NIH) 75–787, Monograph No. 41.
78. Camitta, B. M., Thomas, E. D., Nathan, D. G., Santos, G., Gordon-Smith, E. C., Gale, R. P., Rappeport, J. M., Storb, R. (1976) Severe aplastic anemia: a prospective

study of the effect of early marrow transplantation on acute mortality. Blood 48, 63–70.

79. Storb, R., Thomas, E. D., Weiden, P. L., Buckner, C. D., Clift, R. A., Fefer, A., Fernando, L. P., Giblett, E. R., Goodell, B. W., Johnson, F. L., Lerner, K. G., Neiman, P. E., Sanders, J. E. (1976) Aplastic anemia treated by allogeneic bone marrow transplantations: a report of 49 new cases from Seattle. Blood 48, 817–841.

80. U.C.L.A. Bone Marrow Transplant Team (1976) Bone marrow transplantation in severe aplastic anemia. Lancet ii, 921–923.

EPIDEMIOLOGY OF BRAIN TUMORS

ELLEN B. GOLD, PH.D.

CONTENTS

INTRODUCTION

Primary malignant brain tumors constitute only about 2% of all cancers in humans. However, they are an important cause of cancer morbidity and mortality, particularly in children (1). Among children, brain tumors account for 20% of all cancers and are the second most frequent type of cancer (with leukemia being the most frequent). Brain tumors also constitute an important cause of death from cancer in children, with leukemia accounting for about 45% and brain tumors about 20% of deaths from cancer in children (2). Five-year survival rates of brain tumors are only about 25% in adults over 35 years of age, and in children under 15 about 45% (3–5). In addition, treatment of brain tumors has not significantly improved survival in recent years. Many patients with brain tumors who do survive more than 5 years are left with permanent disabilities, and some die later from recurrences (6).

Despite the importance of the morbidity and mortality associated with brain tumors, particularly in children, relatively little is known about risk factors or possible causative agents associated with the development of these tumors, although both genetic and environmental factors have been implicated. This paper will first discuss some of the methodologic issues involved in epidemiologic investigation of brain tumors and then the epidemiologic patterns of brain tumors—including age, race, and sex distributions, time trends, and geographic variations. In addition, the literature will be reviewed to summarize what is known about the etiology of brain tumors, associated risk factors, and possible mechanisms of brain tumor induction.

METHODOLOGIC ISSUES

Several methodologic problems often arise in attempts to study the epidemiology of brain tumors. The first, is that about 10 to 20% of brain tumors are difficult to diagnose histologically (7). This problem is due both to the difficulty in establishing a single, clear predominant cell type as well as to the fact that some brain tumors are not even biopsied for histologic diagnosis due to the life-threatening location of some of these tumors.

Another issue that arises is the need to specify whether the tumors are primary or metastatic. This is a potential problem in some studies, since the brain is a frequent site of metastatic spread from other cancer sites whose etiologic factors and epidemiologic characteristics may differ from those of primary brain tumors. Thus, in this paper, unless otherwise specified, the term brain tumors will denote primary brain tumors.

A final important methodologic issue concerns distinguishing malignant and benign brain tumors. To quote Doll and his colleagues (8):

> Tumours of the central nervous system present the special difficulty that benign and malignant tumors may have a similar clinical course. Even grossly malignant tumours seldom metastasize and both may produce death by pressure on vital centres in the brain. Since surgery is not always carried out, a substantial proportion of

From the Department of Epidemiology, School of Hygiene and Public Health, The Johns Hopkins University, Baltimore, Maryland, 21205.

these tumors are not examined histologically and they are commonly diagnosed as cerebral tumours, without specification of their malignant or benign character. The proportion of cases diagnosed histologically—or clinically by a sufficiently descriptive diagnosis—varies greatly from place to place and, within one place, from time to time . . .

HISTOLOGIC TYPES AND SITES OF BRAIN TUMORS

Despite the difficulties involved in establishing the histopathology of brain tumors, an understanding of some of the characteristics of the different types of brain tumors in different locations in the brain is essential in order to appreciate their epidemiologic patterns and to try to elucidate their causes. To quote Harvey Cushing (1931), (9), one of the early investigators of brain tumors:

. . . with the growing conviction that the point of origin of different kinds is not purely accidental, it is no longer highly profitable to discuss the effects of brain tumors in general, to describe the symptomatology of tumors in a given region irrespective of their specific nature, or to deal with tumors of comparable histology irrespective of their location.

Histologic Types

Gliomas, including astrocytomas, medulloblastomas, ependymomas, oligodendrogliomas, and pinealomas constitute about 70–75% of all intracranial tumors of childhood in the United States and approximately 65% of intracranial tumors in adults (10–16). Meningiomas, neurinomas, and pituitary tumors constitute about one-third of all intracranial tumors in adults but are rarely seen in children (11). Thus, as shown in Table 1, the frequencies of different histologic types of brain tumors differ greatly by age (17).

Astrocytoma, the most cellularly differentiated and localized glial tumor, is often a slow growing type of brain tumor (18). Astrocytoma tumor cells exhibit attachments to blood vessels, characteristic of the glial astrocyte from which astrocytomas are derived (19). These tumors occur in various areas of the brain and nervous system, with symptoms and survival dependent on their location (20). In children, astrocytomas frequently occur in the cerebellum, where they are considered to follow a relatively benign course, with a 60% 5-year survival rate (15,21–25). In adults, the astrocytomas are often located in the cerebrum and follow a more rapid course (26). Like many other types of brain tumors, invasion of the brain stem by the astrocytoma, rather than metastasis of the tumor, is the main factor responsible for death (27).

Glioblastoma multiforme frequently occurs in patients who are beyond middle age but rarely in children (14). It is sometimes classified as a highly malignant, rapidly growing, and undifferentiated form of astrocytoma and is usually found in the cerebral hemispheres (15). These tumors often contain cells of varying degrees of differentiation as well as areas of necrosis. Five-year survival rates are generally less than 10% (28).

Medulloblastoma is a rapidly growing and highly invasive tumor, most frequently arising in the roof of the fourth ventricle or in the periphery of the

TABLE 1. Histologically Confirmed Primary Intracranial Neoplasms: Frequency Distribution (Connecticut, 1935–1964)

Children (0 through 14 yr)			Adult (≥15 yr)		
Type	No.	Percentage	Type	No.	Percentage
Medulloblastoma	74	24.2	Glioblastoma	1,105	52.1
Astrocytoma	63	20.6	Meningioma	389	18.4
Glioblastoma	62	20.3	Astrocytoma	214	10.1
Ependymoma	20	6.5	Chromophobe adenoma	96	4.5
Craniopharyngioma	17	5.6	Neurilemoma	46	2.2
Meningioma	14	4.6	Hemangioma	41	1.9
Hemangioma	9	2.9	Craniopharyngioma	30	1.4
Neuroblastoma	8	2.6	Medulloblastoma	27	1.3
Teratoma	6	2.0	Ependymoma	27	1.3
Pinealoma	6	2.0	Acidophilic adenoma	26	1.2
Chordoma	5	1.6	Oligodendroglioma	22	1.0
Sarcoma	5	1.6	Sarcoma	19	0.9
Oligodendroglioma	2	0.7	Pinealoma	6	0.3
Neurilemoma	2	0.7	Chordoma	5	0.2
Others, specified	6	2.0	Others, specified	21	1.0
Others, unspecified	7	2.3	Others, unspecified	45	2.1
Total	306	100	Total	2,119	100

Source: Schoenberg, Bruce S., et al., Mayo Clin. Proc. 51, 51–56. (January 1976).

cerebellum (29,30). It is a tumor predominantly seen in children and only rarely observed in adults (31). Developing from the cerebellar medulloblasts, it is the only brain tumor associated with both neuronal and glial features, each of which may predominate in the tumor (29). This phenomenon may be due to the fact that medulloblasts, which were described as early as 1897 by Schaper (32), are cells which occur early in the development of the brain and nervous system and later normally differentiate into neuronal as well as glial tissue (Figure 1) (33,34).

Medulloblastoma is generally about twice as frequent in males as in females; other gliomas show little differences in frequency between the sexes (15,20,35–39). In contrast to other histologic types of brain tumors, this brain tumor has a marked tendency to disseminate through the subarachnoid space of the brain and spinal cord (13,19,20,22,24,35,38,40–45). Although medulloblastoma is the most radiosensitive type of brain tumor (12,41,42,46) the 5-year survival rate is only about 30–40% (12,24,36,47–50), and operative mortality alone is about 20% (22,38,50). The risk of recurrence of medulloblastoma after surgical and/or radiation treatment seems to be a function of age at diagnosis (51), with teenaged patients having a better prognosis than younger patients (52). In addition, females tend to have a better prognosis than do males (12,38,44,53).

Ependymomas are derived from the ependymal cells covering the brain and spinal cord and lining the lateral, third and fourth ventricles and thus often have cells with long processes in contact with blood vessel walls (18). They are most frequently seen in the fourth ventricle as a slow-growing type

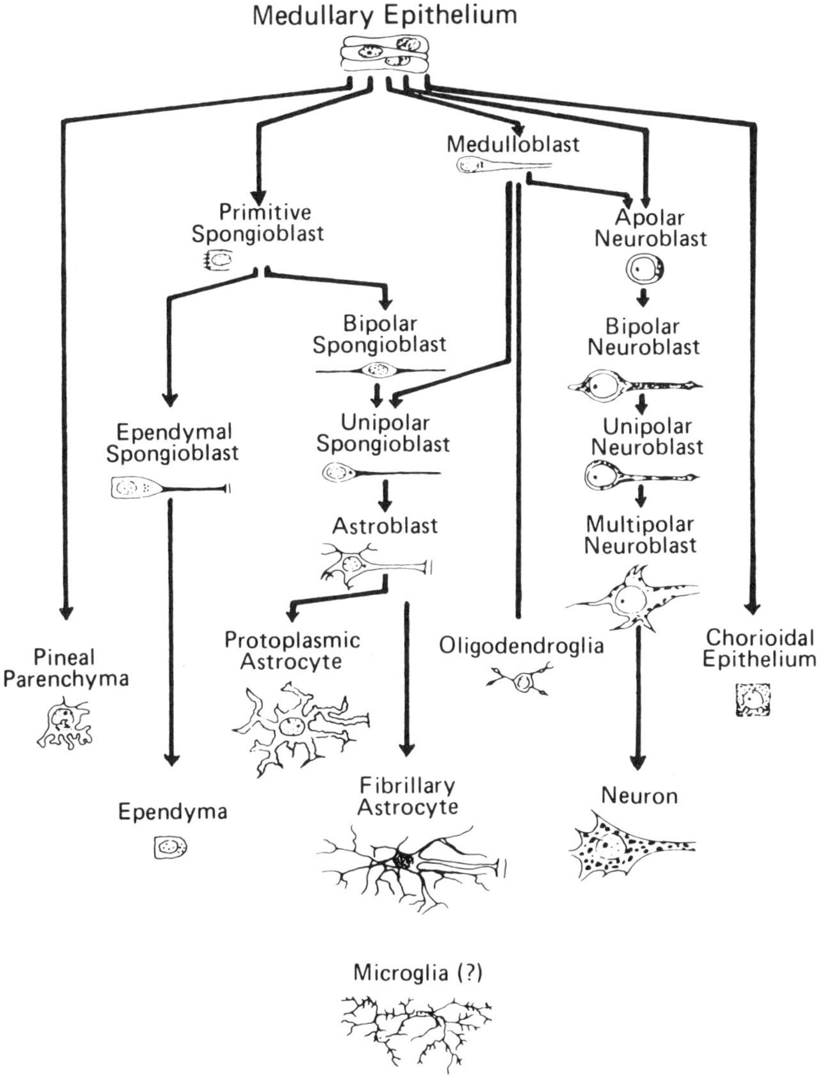

FIGURE 1. Cellular development of brain tissue.

Source: Bailey, P., Arch. Pathol. 4: 871–921, 1927. Copyright 1927, American Medical Association.

of tumor (24,29,51,54). However, unless located in the lateral ventricle, ependymomas may not be safely removed surgically and thus may cause death by their location through blockage of cerebrospinal fluid rather than by invasiveness (15,22). Operative mortality for ependymoma is about 30%, with median survival for more malignant types about two to three years. Five-year survival is about 30%, and aggressive treatment of less malignant ependymomas with surgery and radiotherapy may increase the 5-year survival to 80% (12,35,41,46,47,51,54,55). As with medulloblastoma, the period of greatest risk of recurrence of ependymomas, at least in children, is a function of age at the time of diagnosis, with younger children having a greater risk of recurrence (51).

Brain stem gliomas, including those in the pons and medulla, usually have an insidious onset and are fairly common in children, but not in adults (15,22,35,56,57). Because of their location in areas controlling vital functions, these tumors are generally surgically explored only when the neuroradiologic diagnosis is not clearcut (11,35,58). Few patients with brain stem gliomas survive longer than two years (12,57,59), and 5-year survivorship is only about 15% (23).

Oligodendrogliomas occur mainly in adults (15,35). They are slow growing tumors, generally arising in the cerebral hemispheres. They tend to infiltrate, reaching a large size before surgery and having a high rate of recurrence (13).

Sites of Brain Tumors

As early as 1889, Starr (60) observed that cerebellar tumors were much more frequent in children than adults. Many subsequent investigators have confirmed that about 65% of all brain tumors giving rise to symptoms before age 15 are found below the tentorium, a phenomenon in contrast with that seen at older ages, when infratentorial tumors are rare, and cerebral tumors are more common, as shown in Figure 2 (15,16,20,30,33,35,49,59,61–66).

SECULAR TRENDS IN INCIDENCE AND MORTALITY

Cancer is the second leading cause of death in the United States in children under the age of 14 years, as well as in adults (67–69). Cancer of the brain accounted for about 2% of all new cancer cases in all age groups in 1969–1971 (1). However, brain tumors comprised 20% of all new cancer in children under 15 years of age, second only to leukemia, which accounted for 32% (1,2,10,35,37,68,70–72).

Distributions by Age

In children, the incidence rate of brain tumors in the United States peaks in the 5–9 year age group and then decreases in adolescence; it then gradually increases, peaking again in the 65–70 year age group, after which it declines, as shown in Figure 3 (1,10,36,64). Other investigators have observed a peak in incidence rates in the 0–4 year age group in black children and a peak in about the 60–64 year age group in adults (8,73,74).

As shown in Table 2, mortality rates for malignant neoplasms of the brain and nervous system (most of which are brain tumors) increased in all age groups during the period 1930–1961 in the United States, with some leveling off in the rate of increase in 1959–1961, particularly in childhood (75,76). Overall mortality rates for all ages continued to increase from 1961 to 1974

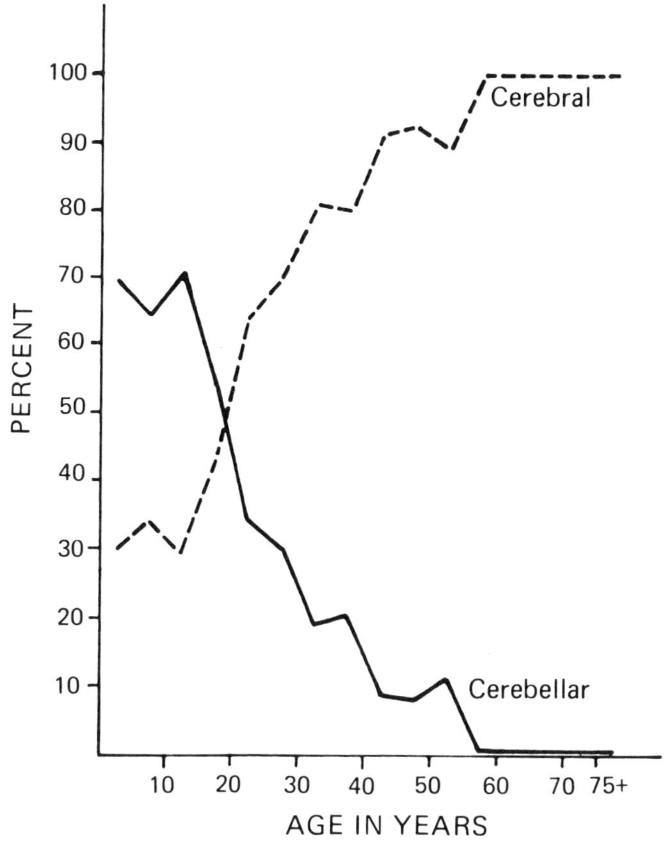

FIGURE 2. Percent distribution of cerebral and cerebellar brain tumors, by age.
Source: Cushing, H: Am. J. Dis. Child. 33: 551–584, 1927. Copyright 1927, American Medical Association.

(77). The incidence rates of brain tumors in the United States increased during the period 1937–1971, as shown in Figure 4, although in children incidence rates have declined in males and increased slightly in females (Figure 5 and 6) in recent years, i.e., 1960 to 1974 (1,73,78).

Data collected in the Mayo Clinic and Connecticut Tumor Registry from 1935 to 1964 showed that the peak annual incidence rate for astrocytoma in children occurred at three years of age (0.65/100,000), for medulloblastoma at 5 years (0.7/100,000), and for glioblastoma at seven years (0.55/100,000), while in adults peak annual incidence rates occurred in the age group 60–64 for glioblastoma (6.2/100,000), 80–84 for meningioma (2.6/100.000), and 50–54 for astrocytoma (0.8/100,000), as shown in Figure 7 (79). Medulloblastoma is almost exclusively seen in children (19,34,35,79), whereas incidence rates of ependymomas peak under age 10 (0.17/100,000) and again at about age 43

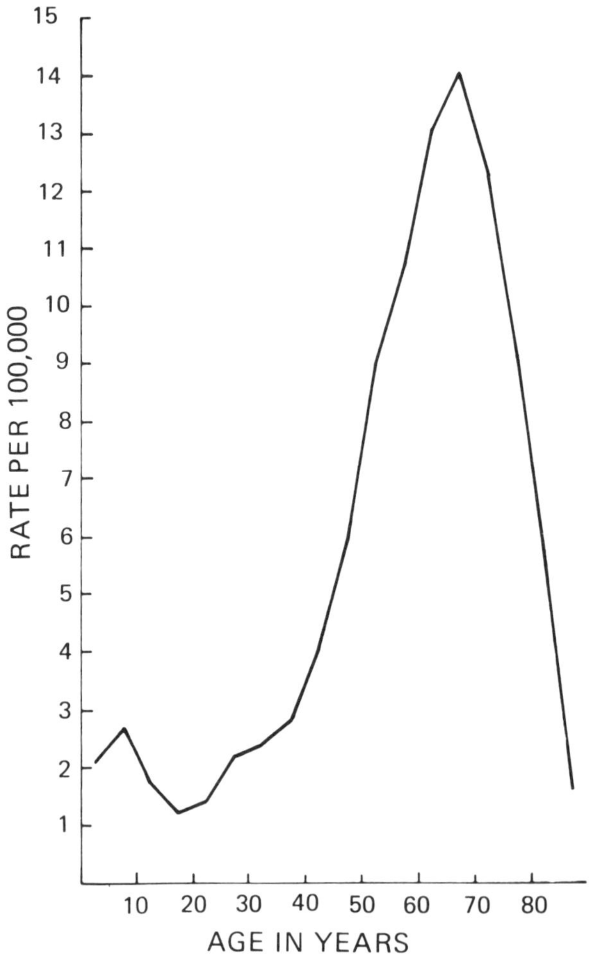

FIGURE 3. Average annual age-specific incidence rates for brain tumors, United States 1969–1971.

Source: Cutler and Young (1975).

(0.15/100,000) (Figure 8). In children, the peak age at which ependymoma was diagnosed in three hospitals in Seattle and Los Angeles varied by site of the tumor—2.3 years of age for tumors located in the fourth ventricle and 5.7 years for those in the lateral ventricles (51). The time between operation and signs or symptoms of recurrence also was related to the age at which the tumor was diagnosed, with younger age at diagnosis associated with a shorter symptom-free interval. Younger children, however, were not as likely to be given radiotherapy.

TABLE 2. Trends in Mortality Rates per 100,000 for Malignant Neoplasms of Brain and Nervous System by Age, Race, and Sex, United States, 1930–1961

Age and sex	White 1959–1961	White 1950	White 1940	White 1930	Nonwhite 1959–1961	Nonwhite 1950	Nonwhite 1940	Nonwhite 1930[a]
Male								
0–14	1.9	1.8	1.1	0.2	1.4	1.6	0.5	0.1
15–24	1.0	1.1	0.8	0.4	1.2	0.7	0.2	0.2
25–34	2.0	1.7	1.3	0.7	1.1	0.6	0.7	0.3
35–44	4.0	3.8	2.7	1.4	2.2	2.1	1.3	0.4
45–54	7.8	7.2	4.9	1.8	3.9	3.3	2.2	0.5
55–64	13.0	10.1	5.9	1.7	5.3	3.1	1.3	0.3
65–74	9.0	5.9	2.6	1.6	4.1	0.6	1.2	—
75–84	3.8	2.6	1.1	1.0	—	—	—	—
85+	1.7	1.4	0.7	—	—	—	—	—
Female								
0–14	1.5	1.6	1.1	0.3	1.4	1.2	0.4	0.1
15–24	0.9	0.9	0.7	0.2	0.9	0.4	0.4	0.2
25–34	1.4	1.3	1.0	0.5	0.9	0.8	0.3	0.2
35–44	2.7	2.4	1.9	0.9	2.7	1.9	0.1	0.4
45–54	5.0	4.1	3.5	1.4	2.5	1.0	1.1	0.4
55–64	7.0	6.0	3.5	1.3	2.8	1.7	2.0	0.4
65–74	5.6	3.4	1.8	0.9	1.8	0.6	0.9	—
75–84	2.2	1.6	1.3	1.3	0.9	1.0	—	—
85+	1.3	1.6	2.1	0.7	—	—	—	—

Source: Gordon, T., Crittenden, M., and Haenszel, W. (1961); Lilienfeld, A. M., Levin, L., and Kessler, I. I. (1972).

[a]1930 data for whites are for brain tumors only.

Distributions by Race and Sex

Brain tumors of all ages tend to be more frequent in males than females (male : female ratio = 1.4) and more frequent in whites than nonwhites (white : nonwhite ratio = 1.5) (1,67,80–82). Since the number of brain tumors in non–whites is often small, reported incidence and mortality rates vary greatly. Nevertheless, reported rates seem to be lower in non–whites for all intracranial tumors except meningiomas and pituitary adenomas (1,13,82–84).

In children, the sex ratio (male : female) for brain tumors in whites and non–whites is greater than one and in whites tends to increase with age until the age of 9 years (Table 3). At about the time of puberty, the sex ratio drops to about 1 or lower and then increases to over 1 in the post-pubertal period (1,67,73,78,85). In Baltimore, the sex ratio of incidence rates of brain tumors in children declined during the period 1960–1974 (73).

Spiers (85) postulated that the variation in the sex ratio with age may be

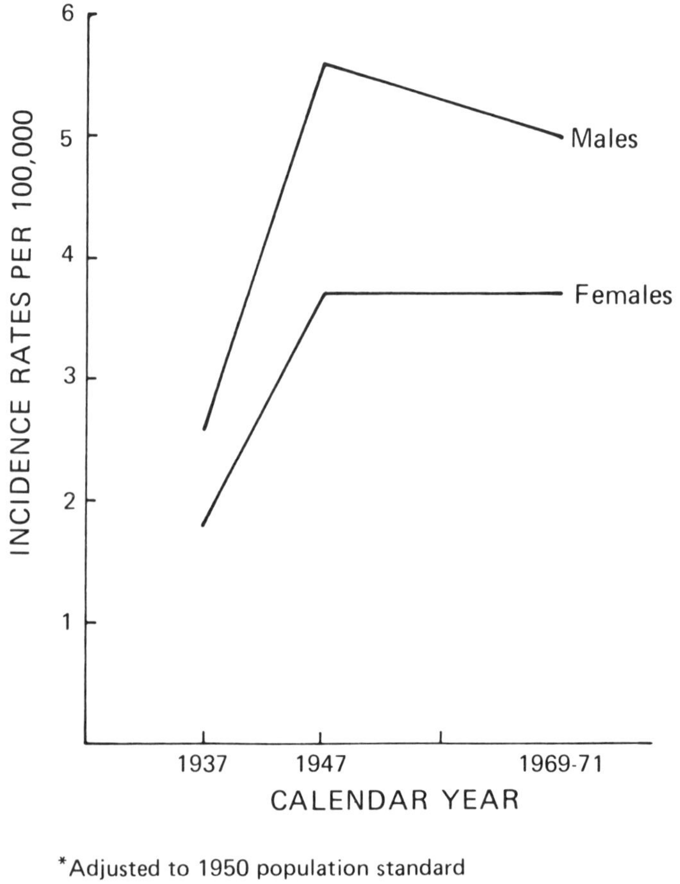

FIGURE 4. Average annual age-adjusted incidence rates for brain tumors, by sex and year (adjusted to 1950 population standard).

Source: Dorn and Cutler (1959); Cutler and Young (1975).

due to the differential effect of age and sex on the host's susceptibility to some carcinogenic agents. This argument is consistent with the fact that different histologic types of brain tumors have different sex ratios. Medulloblastoma is about twice as common in males as in females, whereas astrocytoma is about equally common in males and females (15,36,39,45,48,86–88). In addition, in Seattle and Los Angeles the sex ratio of ependymomas in three hospitals varied with the location of the tumor—1:1 in lateral ventricle and 2:1 in the fourth ventricle (51). According to Spiers (85): "The scarceness of the tumors at or around the ages of puberty and the predilection of certain types of tumors for one sex or the other as well as pronounced occurrences in certain age groups are suggestive of an hormonal effect or effects." These latter authors consider this possibility particularly important in light of animal experiments in this area, to be discussed later in this chapter.

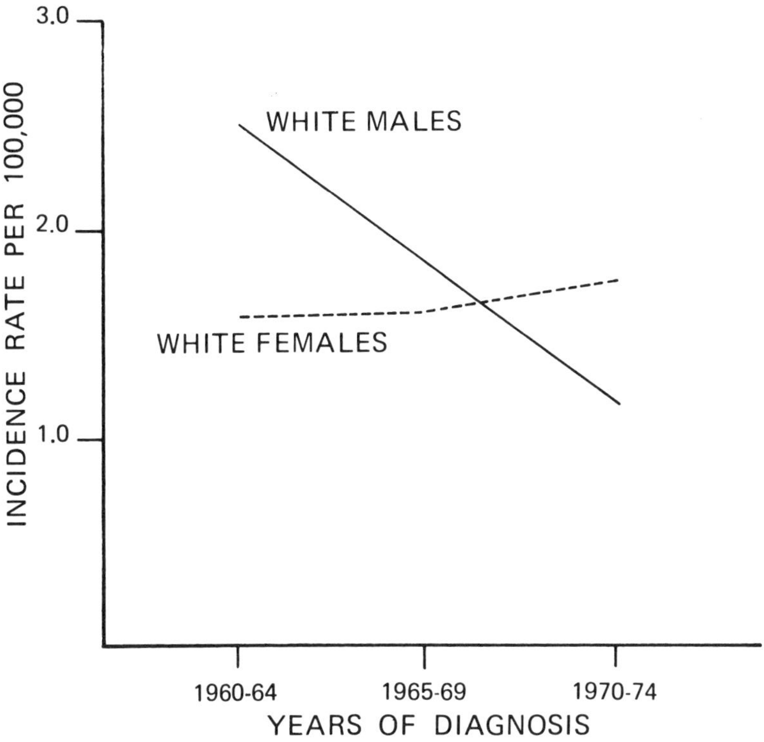

FIGURE 5. Average annual incidence rates per 100,000 for brain tumors in white children aged 0–19 years by year of diagnosis and sex, Baltimore SMSA.

Source: Gold and Gordis (1979).

In summary, the incidence of and mortality from brain tumors has increased in recent decades, particularly in adults. Peak incidence rates occur in the 5–9 year age group in children and the 65–70 year group in adults, and distributions of cell types differ by age, which may suggest different etiologic factors for adult and childhood brain tumors. Brain tumors also tend to occur more frequently in males than females and more frequently in whites than blacks, which may reflect a role for host or environmental factors.

GEOGRAPHIC VARIATIONS IN THE DISTRIBUTION OF BRAIN TUMORS

International Differences

As shown in Table 4, international differences in the frequency of brain tumors have been observed (8). However, some of these differences may have been due to difficulties associated with ascertainment of accurate diagnoses of

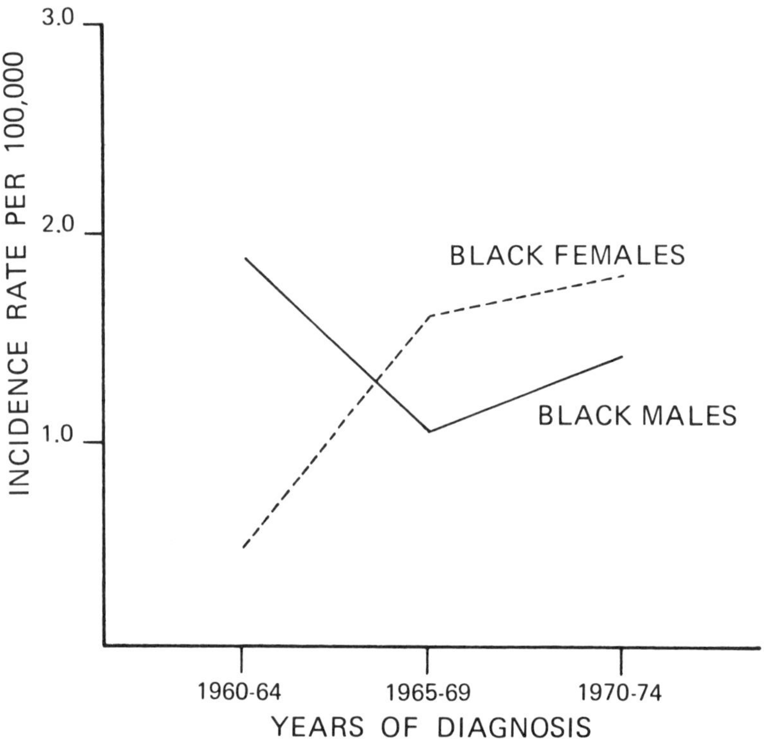

FIGURE 6. Average annual incidence rates per 100,000 for brain tumors in black children aged 0–19 years by year of diagnosis and sex, Baltimore SMSA.
Source: Gold and Gordis (1979).

brain tumors as well as problems in classification, under-ascertainment and under-reporting.

In one study, mortality rates for diseases of the nervous system, including benign and malignant neoplasms of the nervous system for cases of all ages were requested from 37 countries (89,90). For 5 additional countries, data from published reports were used. Data were received from all but 4 of the 37 countries, and mortality rates were age-adjusted to the 1950 U.S. population. The lowest mortality rates for brain and nervous system tumors were reported in Mexico, Chile, Poland, and Japan (0.7–2.3/100,000). In addition, Japanese migrants to the United States had mortality rates which approached those of U.S. whites (4.7/100,000 in males and 3.4/100,000 in females), suggesting that environmental factors may play an important role in the etiology of brain tumors. Mortality rates in all other countries except Israel varied between 3.4/100,000 (U.S. nonwhite) and 5.6/100,000 (Denmark).

Israel had the highest mortality rate for all brain and nervous system tumors (malignant, benign and unspecified) at 6.8/100,000. The authors state that this higher rate in Israel may have been due to differences in reporting prac-

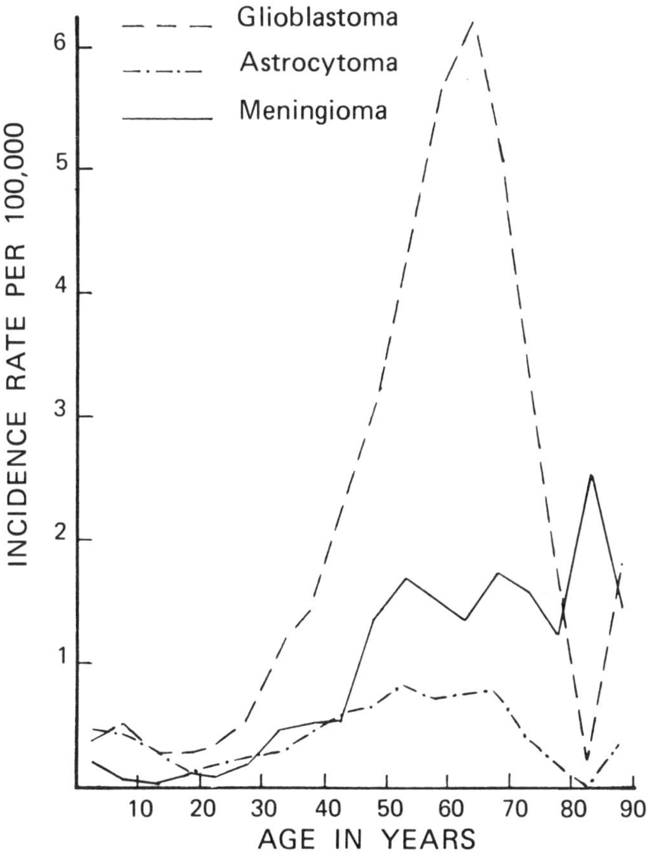

FIGURE 7. Average annual age-specific incidence rates for selected neoplasms of the brain and cranial meninges, Connecticut, 1935–1964.

Source: Schoenberg et al. (1976).

tices. Review of nervous system tumors reported to the Central Tumor Registry in Israel revealed that Israeli- and European-born residents in Israel had significantly higher age-adjusted incidence rates of malignant brain tumors than did Asian- or African-born Israelis (48,84,86). There were no significant differences in incidence rates of malignant or benign tumors between the residents who arrived in Israel before 1955 and those who came later, when rates were analyzed separately for the different ethnic and age groups. The investigators did not state, however, whether the differences in incidence rates between the various ethnic groups were found consistently in all age groups. A recent international study of age-standardized incidence rates for brain tumors showed rates to be highest in Israel and lowest in Japan, India, and Nigeria (74).

A more recent study also was conducted of the histopathologic distribution

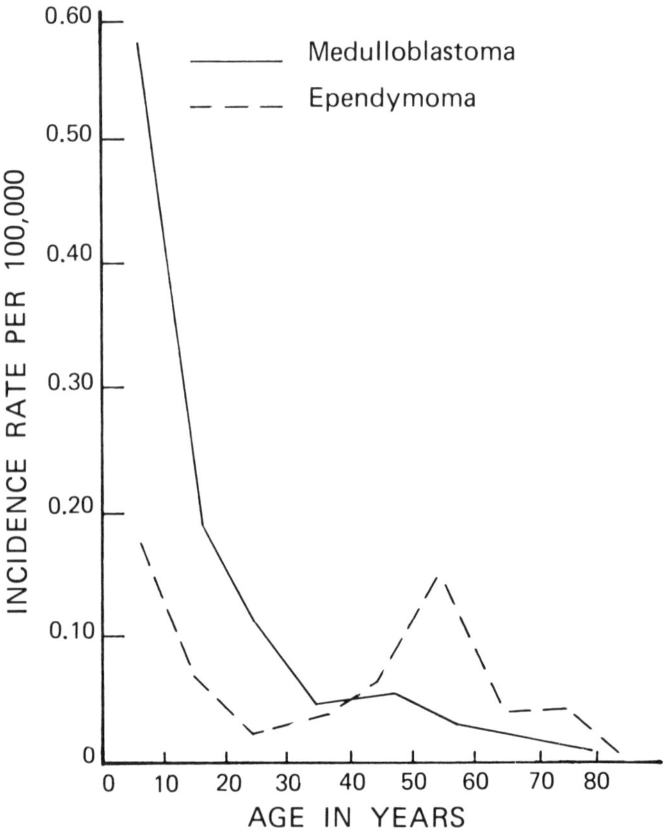

FIGURE 8. Average annual age-specific incidence rates for selected neoplasms of the brain, Connecticut, 1935–1964.

Source: Schoenberg et al. (1976).

TABLE 3. Sex Ratios of Male: Female Incidence Rates of Brain Tumors in Children by Age at Diagnosis and Race, Baltimore SMSA, 1960–1974

Age in years at diagnosis	Race	
	White	Black
0–4	1.14	0.98
5–9	1.32	1.14
10–14	0.61	0.61
15–19	1.12	3.24
0.19	1.10	1.06

Source: Gold, E., Gordis, L. (1978).

TABLE 4. Average Annual Incidence Rates per 100,000 for Cancer of the Brain and Nervous System by Age, Sex, and Country, 1956–1962

Location	Males	Females	Male:female ratio
Israel	9.8	9.1	1.08
Sweden	8.9	8.7	1.02
Norway	8.3	7.3	1.14
Iceland	7.7	6.2	1.24
Denmark	7.3	6.4	1.14
England and Wales	6.7	5.3	1.26
New York, United States	6.0	4.5	1.33
Connecticut, United States	5.9	4.3	1.37
New Zealand	5.9	3.8	1.55
Finland	5.5	4.8	1.15
Netherlands	5.5	4.5	1.22
Canada, five provinces	5.2	3.9	1.33
Slovenia, Yugoslavia	4.1	3.3	1.24
Hawaii	2.9	2.0	1.45
Cali, Colombia	2.9	1.4	2.07
Lourenco Marque, Mozambique	2.2	1.8	1.22
Jamaica, Kingston, St. Andrew	1.9	0.8	2.38
Puerto Rico	1.8	1.7	1.06
Johannesburg, Bantu, South Africa	1.8	1.6	1.12
Singapore, China	1.3	1.0	1.30
Chile	0.7	0.6	1.17
Ibadan, Nigeria	0.7	0.3	2.33
Miyagi, Japan	0.3	0.4	0.75
Kyadondo, Uganda	0.2	0.2	1.00

Source: Doll et al. (1966).

of intracranial neoplasms in children in four continents—North America, Europe, Africa, and Asia (91). The North American series was compiled from the Connecticut Tumor Registry and included all cases in children diagnosed in that state from 1935 through 1973. In the other areas, the cases were reported from one or more selected (though not necessarily representative) hospitals in each of the areas and were histologically verified. Astrocytoma was the most frequent tumor (26–38%) in children in all areas except Japan, where it comprised 15% of all tumors, with medulloblastoma being the second most frequent one in all areas. Craniopharyngiomas constituted 6–9% of tumors in children in all areas except Africa and Japan where they comprised 18% and 16%, respectively, of all brain tumors in childhood. Ependymomas accounted for 9-11% of all brain tumors in children in all areas except India where they constituted 19% of all tumors. Incidence rates were not available for the study areas, but differences in the distributions of cell types in the different areas were not thought to be due only to differences in histologic classification of intracranial tumors in the different regions.

Differences Within the United States

In a study of death certificates of all (39,235) deaths due to malignant neoplasms in children under the age of 15 years in the United States between 1950 and 1959, tumors of the brain and central nervous system, as well as leukemia, showed significantly higher standardized mortality ratios (SMRs) in children in the Pacific States (SMR = 113 for brain and central nervous system, 109 for leukemia) compared to children in the United States as a whole (80). In the Southern and Mountain areas, mortality rates from brain and central nervous system cancers in children were significantly lower than those in children in the rest of the United States, with SMRs ranging from 85 to 93.

This pattern is similar to that observed by Kurtzke (92) for deaths, at all ages, due to primary intracranial tumors in the United States in 1951–1953 and 1961–1963. It is also similar to the geographic pattern of mortality rates for all ages from brain and nervous system tumors reported by Lilienfeld et al. (75), who, in addition, observed high rates in the states along the Eastern seaboard. However, Kurtzke attributed this geographic variation to the geographic distribution of physicians in the United States, which was highly correlated with the distribution of mortality rates for brain tumors (92). This observation is similar to one made by MacMahon (93), in which the geographic distribution of leukemia mortality in the United States was found to be closely correlated with the physician : population ratio.

Urban-Rural Differences

In 1970, Choi and his associates (94) reported the results of a study of death certificates of all Minnesota residents of all ages who died with primary central nervous sytem neoplasms during the period 1958 through 1962, which is perhaps one of the only studies of urban-rural differences in mortality rates for brain tumors. A total of 760 such deaths were ascertained. Mortality rates for medulloblastoma and astrocytoma in males were higher in patients residing in rural than in those residing in urban areas (population greater than 2,500 people) in the first (1.4 times) and second (3 times) decades of life. In females mortality rates were higher for patients of urban residence for each tumor type and each age group, except that mortality rates for rural patients with medulloblastoma in the first two decades of life were approximately 2.3 times higher than the rates for patients residing in urban areas.

Temporal and Spatial Clustering

In 1972, Brooks (95) reported the findings of a study of clustering of brain tumors in Kentucky residents of all ages who were hospitalized from 1963 through 1969 in 29 hospitals in Kentucky and surrounding states. A total of 612 cases were ascertained. Only histologically confirmed tumors were included. Analysis by county of residence showed that only seven of 120 counties had five or more brain tumor patients per 100,000 population. Six of these seven counties were clustered in eastern Kentucky, a rural area isolated from the remainder of the state by rivers, mountains, and poor roads and containing 1.8% of the population of the state. The frequency of brain tumors in this area was 3.4 times that of the remainder of the state ($P < 4.5 \times 10^{-7}$), with gliomas occurring 4.4 times more frequently than the rest of the state, although no attempt was made to adjust the incidence rates of the counties for age. Availability of medical care was not thought to be a likely explanation for the cluster. Most of the cases in this eastern Kentucky area lived near two rivers. The author states that investigations are underway to investigate the possibility of the presence of carcinogens in the rivers in the area.

In a study of all deaths due to brain tumors at all ages in Denmark and the United States no evidence for clustering was found, although the reported mortality rates were neither age-specific nor age-adjusted (92,96). A further study of all cases of primary intracranial neoplasms in Newfoundland, an area relatively isolated from mainland Canada and providing most of the medical care for its own inhabitants, also found no evidence of clustering (97). Ninety-two cases were ascertained in this study from clinical and pathologic records as well as from the tumor registry for a 3-year period, yielding an average annual incidence rate of 6.04/100,000, which is slightly higher than that for the United States. The average annual incidence rate of intracranial neoplasms in children in Newfoundland also appeared to be slightly higher than for American children, though the age-groupings used for age-specific rates were not comparable for the two areas.

Nativity

In 1960, MacMahon (98) analyzed the death certificates of all residents of all ages in New York City dying in 1955 from neoplastic disease (15,594 deaths) to determine differences in cancer mortality between native- and foreign-born residents. For gliomas and other brain tumors, there were no major differences in mortality rates according to nativity. Newill (99) reported the same finding in a similar study in New York City whites dying during the period 1953–1958. However, Lilienfeld et al. (75) reported significantly lower mortality rates for the period 1959–1961 in American-born males than in males who were born in the Scandinavian countries of Sweden or Finland, or in Hungary, Yugoslavia, or the Soviet Union. In contrast, among females, mortality rates were higher in American-born women than in those born in Norway, Sweden, Finland, Czechoslovakia, or Lithuania.

In summary, the frequency of occurrence of brain tumors varies from one geographic region to another, regionally within the United States, as well as internationally. However, the magnitude of the differences are small, particularly when compared to those for other types of malignancies. In addition, migrants tend to reach the mortality rate of the country of adoption, which is suggestive of an environmental etiology for brain tumors.

HOST FACTORS

Birth Characteristics

In 1970, Choi and associates (94) reported a retrospective study of 157 patients of all ages with confirmed central nervous system neoplasms diagnosed during an 18-month period in four Minnesota hospitals. These cases were compared with hospital controls who did not have cancer or neurologic, lymphatic or ophthalmologic disorders and who were matched to cases by hospital, sex, age, race, and area of residence. There were no significant differences between cases and controls in history of epilepsy, alcohol consumption, or smoking. In the 30 patients who were children there also were no significant differences in birth order (although cases tended to have a lower mean birth order), maternal age at the time of pregnancy (also tending to be lower in cases), birth weight, delivery complications, x-rays during pregnancy, abortions or stillbirths subsequent to the birth of the case, malformations, or history of head trauma. However, more mothers of cases than of controls had a history of abortion prior to the birth of the child with the brain tumor ($P = 0.016$).

In Japan, a review of tumor registry data indicated that the frequency of brain tumors in childhood increased somewhat with advancing maternal age at birth of the index child (100). An increasing risk of brain tumors in children with increasing maternal age at birth of the child (as indicated on the birth certificate) also was reported in a study of all deaths due to neoplasms identified from death certificates in children (4,198) in New England during the period 1947–1958 (101). Controls were selected by taking the next birth certificate in the health department file of birth certificates after that of the index case. No significant differences were found between cases and controls with regard to number of live births in the family prior to the index child, number of previous stillbirths, mean birth weight of index child, or percent of index children weighing over 8.5 pounds or under 5.5 pounds at birth. However, there was a trend for mortality rates from cancer of the brain in children to increase with increasing maternal age at birth. The trend was more marked for cancer of the brain than for any other cancer, as shown in Table 5.

Unlike the findings of MacMahon and Newill (101) but in agreement with those of Choi et al. (94), the results of a recent study by Gold et al. (102), of brain tumors in children from 1965 to 1975 indicated that children with brain tumors had a greater but statistically insignificant tendency than nondiseased children to have been first births (odds ratio = 1.7, $P = 0.18$). In addition,

TABLE 5. Mortality Rates for Various Childhood Cancers per 100,000 Live Births by Age of Mother at Birth, Rates per 100,000

Maternal age	Whites: Leukemia	Whites: Cancer of brain	Whites: Cancer of kidney	Whites: Lymphoma	Whites: Other cancer	Whites: All cancer	Nonwhites: All cancer	Total
Under 20	27.2	10.0	5.4	3.5	7.5	53.8	34.6	50.4
20–24	30.5	13.5	5.6	4.2	6.4	60.2	38.0	58.4
25–29	31.4	13.7	5.4	3.7	7.6	61.7	38.9	60.4
30–34	33.7	13.9	5.6	4.0	6.0	63.3	37.7	62.0
35–39	33.4	16.0	4.2	4.7	6.5	64.7	57.6	64.3
40 or more	36.0	9.0	8.3	6.2	6.9	66.5	64.5	66.4
Total	31.6	13.6	5.4	4.0	6.8	61.5	39.3	59.9
χ^2	6.6	8.7	4.2	3.6	3.8	6.7	4.5	8.3

Source: MacMahon, B., Newill, V. A. (1962).

children with brain tumors were more likely to have had a birth weight of 8 pounds or more than were nondiseased children (odds ratio = 2.6, $P = 0.046$). This finding was of borderline statistical significance and can only be considered as being suggestive. The increased frequency of higher birth weights in cases in this study was noteworthy, since the cases tended to be of lower birth order. In general, however, first births tend to be of lower birth weight than subsequent births (103). Because the rate of growth of a child depends on the rate of cellular divisions and, therefore, on the number of cells (104), large babies would tend to have greater numbers of cells and increased rates of cellular division, which might make such babies more vulnerable to the effects of environmental carcinogens. Furthermore, as cell division and growth in the brain is largely completed by the sixth month of postnatal life, exposure to environmental carcinogens associated with brain tumors in children would have to occur prenatally or early in infancy.

Another study was conducted of all autopsies (9,223) performed at Kings County Hospital in Brooklyn, New York, from 1953 to 1963 that included the central nervous system and that had blood sugar levels available (105). In the entire series, including subjects of all ages, 3% of the diabetics and 10% of the nondiabetics had intracranial neoplasms, mainly glial tumors. Five hundred forty-four of the autopsies were of children 0–15 years old, only two of whom were diabetic, including one with an intracranial glioma. Seventeen percent of the nondiabetic children had brain tumors. Thus, it would appear that diabetes may not be an important risk factor for brain tumors in any age group.

Religion

Using the religious affiliation of the cemetery of burial as an indicator of religion of the deceased, MacMahon (98) analyzed differences in mortality for different cancer sites according to religion. Mortality from gliomas for both sexes was more than 1.5 times as frequent in Jews as in Catholics or Protestants. Newill (99) reported a similar finding for all types of brain tumors in adults over 45, whereas MacMahon found no major differences in mortality by religion for brain tumors other than gliomas. In a retrospective study of leukemia, Graham et al. (106) found no differences in religious or ethnic background of children with leukemia and controls, although in adults Jews had a higher risk of leukemia than other religious groups.

In 1970, Seidman (107) reported the findings of a study of cancer death rates by religious and socioeconomic status (SES) in 1949–1951 in New York City. Religious affiliation of the cemetery of burial was used as an indicator of religious preference. Mortality rates for brain and central nervous system tumors were significantly higher in low SES Catholics and in high SES Jews, and significantly lower in low SES and high SES Protestants than for New York City as a whole.

Gjerris (54) studied 316 children diagnosed with brain tumors in three neurologic, pediatric, and medical departments in Denmark between 1935 and 1939. He found that the social distribution of cases did not differ from that of the Danish population. In addition, he found no seasonal variation in onset of symptoms.

The data thus seem to indicate that Jewish adults have a higher risk of dying from brain tumors than do adults of other religions, but that in children no significant differences in risk exist between children of different religious or social backgrounds.

ENVIRONMENTAL FACTORS

Radiation

Several studies have demonstrated an increased risk of brain tumors following radiation exposure. In a retrospective study, Stewart and Kneale (108) interviewed the mothers of children with cancer diagnosed between 1952 and 1965, including 1,030 with "cerebral tumours," and the mothers of matched neighborhood controls. Radiation exposures reported by the mothers were not validated (109), but a greater percentage of mothers of children with brain tumors (15%) reported prenatal radiation exposure than did mothers of all controls (10.2%). The percentage of cases exposed relative to that of controls was of similar magnitude for leukemia, lymphosarcoma, neuroblastoma, and Wilm's tumor.

In an early study of x-ray exposure during pregnancy, children who were born and died of cancer in the Northeastern region of the United States from 1947 to 1959 were compared to a systematic sample of 7,242 single births in 37 large maternity hospitals in the nine states of the Northeastern region (110,111). Review of hospital pregnancy and delivery records for irradiation during pregnancy revealed a relative risk for intrauterine x-ray exposure and "cancer of the central nervous system" of 1.6, a very similar risk to that for leukemia and other cancers. The risk was highest for those who died of cancer between 5 and 7 years of age, with the observed number of deaths being about twice that expected. There were no significant differences with regard to abnormalities of pregnancy and delivery. Death rates from cancer of the nervous system also tended to be higher in first births, in males, in Jews, and in private as opposed to clinic patients. There were no major differences in mortality rates from cancer of the central nervous system between whites and non–whites or between children born in different time periods between 1947 and 1959. Mortality rates also tended to be higher for children whose mothers were under age 20 or over the age of 35.

A prospective study was also conducted of 11,000 children under 15 years of age in Israel who were identified from treatment records as having been irradiated for tinea capitis (112). Nonirradiated controls were selected and matched for sex, age, country of origin, and immigration period. In addition, nonirradiated siblings were also selected as controls, where possible. The Central Israeli Tumor Registry and death certificates were searched to identify the occurrence of tumors in exposed and non-exposed groups. The exposed group demonstrated a significantly increased risk of malignant (relative risk = 3) and benign (relative risk = 7) head and neck neoplasms. The increase was most striking for brain (absorbed dose estimated to be about 140 rads), parotid, and thyroid tumors, with most latent periods reported to be over 6 years. A similarly designed study conducted in New York found a relative risk of 1.6 for brain tumors induced by radiation administered for treatment of tinea capitis (113).

In an experiment with rhesus monkeys, 32 were given 200–1200 rads of whole body irradiation, and six were used as controls (114). Three of the 32 monkeys developed malignant ependymomas of the brain within five years after exposures of 600–800 rads. No long-term effects were seen in controls or in animals receiving less than 600 rads or more than 800 rads. Other, less well controlled studies have also reported the development of intracranial meningiomas in human adult patients and cerebral glioblastoma multiforme in monkeys following high doses of radiation to the head (115,116).

Thus, it seems that radiation exposure of moderate dose may induce brain tumors in humans as well as in animals, though the relative risks are not high. The role of low-dose radiation, however, remains unclear. Relative risks for brain tumors following high-dose radiation are high, but currently this type of radiation exposure is probably unusual. It is, therfore, unlikely that the attributable risk is very high for radiation-associated brain tumors. In fact, Berry (117) states that "the importance of radiation as a childhood carcinogen may have been overemphasized, and undoubtedly few tumours are induced in this way. However, even a very small risk of this type is worth preventing by changes in technique, and a valuable decrease in x-ray tumour induction has probably already taken place."

Infections

History of certain prior infections have been associated with an increased risk of brain tumors in brain cancer patients themselves or in children with brain tumors whose mothers had such infections during pregnancy. The principal infections which have been associated with brain tumors, include toxoplasmosis, tuberculosis, and chickenpox.

In 1967, Schuman and colleagues (118) analyzed sera for toxoplasma antibodies in 126 patients of all ages with central nervous system tumors and matched hospital controls. A significant excess of positive tests was found in the case group. Significantly more patients with gliomas had positive test results, with patients with astrocytomas accounting for most of the excess (nearly a twofold increase). The investigators stated that toxoplasma has a known affinity for nervous tissue and that gliomas have been observed in chickens experimentally exposed to toxoplasma. Toxoplasma is a protozoa that has been found in all tissues and organs except erythrocytes (119). It may remain dormant for a long time, though when active it causes various disorders, including encephalitis and eye lesions and may be found in the cerebrospinal fluid. In about 60% of those infected there are postencephalomyelitic calcium deposits in the cerebellum and cerebrum, hydrocephalus, and microcephalia.

In a study of 92 adult patients with gliomas and 100 hospital controls, Ward and associates (120) found a significant difference in history of past tuberculosis infection: 21.7% of cases and only 7% of controls ($P < 0.01$) gave a history of tuberculosis. Solitary tuberculomas in children are most often located in the cerebellum, pons, medulla, and brain stem—also the most common sites of brain tumors in children. The authors suggested that development of both tuberculosis and of gliomas may be due to an impaired immune system.

In a retrospective study of the relationship of malignancies in children to maternal history of infection during pregnancy, Bithell and associates (121) found an excess of mothers of children with medulloblastoma who had a history of having contracted chickenpox during the index pregnancy. Of 9,000 case-control pairs, seven mothers of cancer cases and no mothers of controls reported a history of chickenpox during pregnancy. Of the seven cases, three were leukemia, three were medulloblastoma, and one was Wilm's tumor. Only 0.3 case of medulloblastoma was expected.

In contrast, in a longitudinal study of influenza during pregnancy, influenza was not found to be associated with an increased risk of brain tumors (122). Women were questioned at the time of delivery about influenza during their pregnancy, and the children were then followed until age 11 years. A ninefold increase in risk for leukemia in children was reported for those exposed to influenza in utero compared to those not exposed. However, no brain tumors were reported in the exposed group compared to two medulloblastomas in the unexposed group. In still another study, no brain tumors developed in children exposed prenatally to maternal mumps, chickenpox, or rubella infections (123).

More recently, a retrospective study of tumors in children was conducted, based on the cancer registry of Finland (124,125). Information about illnesses, x-rays, drugs, and vaccinations during pregnancy, as well as other relevant maternal factors was obtained from Maternity Welfare Centers, where free antenatal care is provided. Cases were compared to children who were born after the cases and who were from the same Maternity Welfare Center. The study showed no significant differences between children with brain tumors and controls with regard to maternal illnesses during pregnancy.

Medications and Vaccinations

The study by Salonen and Saxen (124,125), cited above, also showed an apparent protective effect of maternal polio vaccination during pregnancy (relative risk = 0.29) associated with brain tumors in children (245 cases) and a slightly increased risk (relative risk = 1.4) of brain tumors in children associated with maternal intake of drugs of unspecified type during pregnancy.

In a follow-up study of epileptics treated with phenobarbitol, Clemmessen et al. (126) found no excess occurrence of cancer over that to be expected, except for tumors of the nervous system, which they stated would be "clinically expected" (127). However, results of a case-control study by Gold et al. (128) indicate a tendency for an increased risk of brain tumors in children exposed to barbiturates either prenatally or early in childhood. Such findings are consistent with the carcinogenic potential of barbiturates which has been suggested in animal experiments in which liver tumors have been induced (129–133). In addition, studies in humans have shown the teratogenic potential of barbiturates, particularly for malformations of the central nervous system (134–136). It has been suggested that substances which have been found to be teratogenic may also be carcinogenic when administered at a different phase of embryonic development during pregnancy (137).

Immunologic Factors

In recent years, research pertaining to the role of immunologic factors in the development of brain tumors has ranged from reports of brain tumor patients with immune system abnormalities (138) to reports of brain tumors in immunosuppressed patients (139), to differences in lymphocyte transformation in brain tumor patients (140) and studies of brain tumor-specific antigens (141).

To determine the role of cell-mediated immunity in brain tumor patients, Levy et al. (142) cultured biopsy specimens from different types of brain tumors from 14 patients, including one child, and normal brain and skin fibroblasts from patients and controls. Neoplastic cells grew to confluence in 7–21 days, normal glial cells in 20–40 days, and skin fibroblasts in 14–40 days. Lymphocytes from either the patients or normal controls were then added to the cultures. It was reported that, "In all cases, there was a significant inhibition of the neoplastic target cells by autogenous lymphocytes . . . however . . . the control lymphocytes effected equivalent reductions of both normal and neoplastic target cells, while the patient lymphocytes exerted a tumor-specific effect." Interestingly, one patient's lymphocytes worked against the same cell type of tumor cells in another patient, but not against the latter patient's normal glial cells. Mitts and Walker (143) also found that in explants of three intracranial tumors (including one from a child with an ependymoma), exposure to autogenous serum rendered the tumor cells nonviable, while unexposed cells remained viable. Levy et al. (142) stated that their studies demonstrated that different types of tumors of the central nervous system can generate a nonspecific cell-mediated immune response, regardless of the degree of malignancy of the host's tumor. In 1964, Scheinberg et al. (144) reported that chemically induced brain tumors in mice cured by subsequent irradiation rendered some immunity to subsequent tumor growth in the area with rejection of 37% of subsequently implanted intracerebral tumors.

ANIMAL EXPERIMENTS

The fact that most brain tumors are located in areas of the brain which may be vulnerable to blood-borne carcinogens (145) has suggested the need for investigating the development of brain tumors following exposure to environmental carcinogens. Many such investigations conducted in animals have provided etiologic clues to the development of brain tumors in humans. The study of brain tumors in animals has been focused primarily on two areas—induction of tumors with chemical carcinogens either by direct implantation or transplacentally and induction of tumors by known oncogenic viruses.

Chemical Carcinogenesis

Spontaneous gliomas in mice are relatively rare, but intracerebral implantation of small amounts of methylcholanthrene, benzpyrene, or dibenzanthracene have produced gliomas in mice (146,147). These chemically induced gliomas required 200–400 days to develop in mice. When a pellet of a chemical carcinogen is implanted in the brain, a tumor may grow on each side of it, each one being cytogenically distinct, suggesting that the development of gliomas may occur by simultaneous multiplication of different types of cells. Several early experiments succeeded in inducing gliomas and sarcomas in the brains of one-third to one-half of mice with intracerebral methylcholanthrene implantations (148–150). Similar results have been obtained with dimethylbenzanthracene (151) and ethylnitrosourea (152–154).

In studies of hydrocarbon-induced murine tumors, Kirsch and Schulz (155) report that Zimmerman has found that

> . . . if a carcinogenic pellet is deposited within a ventricle, an ependymoma or ependymoblastoma can be expected. A pellet situated in the mature cerebellar cortex . . . results in the development of a medulloblastoma and if implanted in the subcortex of the parietal lobe results in a malignant astrocytoma. Placement in frontal white matter results in a significant incidence of oligodendrogliomas . . . Though reproducible methods for the laboratory induction of brain tumors with carcinogenic chemicals are well established, the molecular mechanisms of induction and their relevance to human spontaneous tumors is only vaguely understood.

The types of tumors seen resemble those normally seen in spontaneous growth in rats (156).

Using the carcinogen methylnitrosourea (MNU), Swenberg et al. (157) found that in large part the route of administration determined the site of neoplastic development in rats—more central nervous system tumors developed following intravenous rather than oral administration.

In humans the greater frequency of brain tumors in males and the change in the sex ratio of incidence of these tumors at the age of puberty suggests that hormonal factors may influence the development of these tumors. Avtsyn and Yablonovskaya (158) tested this possibility in mice. Ependymoblastoma, oligodendroglioblastoma, and glioblastoma multiforme were induced in mice with 9-10-dimethyl-12-benzanthracene pellets introduced into the brain. These tumors were then transplanted to male mice, after which the testes of the animals were removed. Castration performed 19 days after transplantation prevented 59% of the tumors from developing and growing. In the few animals where the tumor had developed, there was regression. The only tumor type that failed to change with castration was the oligodendroglioblastoma. However, the protective effect of castration disappeared after administration of testosterone. This experimental evidence supports the hypothesis that hormonal factors may play a role in susceptibility to or induction of brain tumors.

Several experimental studies have been conducted to determine if transplacental carcinogenesis occurs in animals, a model which might have particular applicability to brain tumors in children. Intravenous injection of pregnant rats in the latter half of pregnancy with ethylnitrosourea (ENU) a derivative of dimethylnitrosamine, shows a dose-response effect of increasing incidence of nervous system tumors (gliomas and neurinomas) in offspring with increasing dose, reaching 100% incidence with doses over 20 mg ENU/kg body weight (159–162). These findings were also confirmed in hamsters in which oligodendrogliomas were the most frequently induced tumors, occurring most frequently in the hippocampus and adjoining periventricular tissues of the offspring. Further experiments indicated that the nervous system of fetal rats was about 50 times more sensitive to ENU than the nervous system of adult rats (163). In addition, following oral administration, ethylurea and nitrite formed sufficient quantities of ethylnitrosourea in the stomachs of gravid mothers to produce cancer in all descendents. Ethylnitrosourea also was absorbed through the skin of the pregnant rat in sufficient quantities to produce neurogenic tumors in the offspring. Because ENU converts to harmless endproducts with a half-life of about 90 minutes (164), pregnant rats given ENU and allowed to deliver and nurse their young, probably do not store and subsequently secrete ENU in the colostrum. This lends supportive evidence for the carcinogenic potential of transplacental exposure and tumor induction.

Transplacental carcinogenesis is dependent on the point in time of gestation at which the carcinogen is administered (165). Zulch and Mennel (166) found that no nervous system tumors could be induced with administration of the carcinogen prior to the twelfth day of gestation. Laqueur and Spatz (167) found that, in pregnant rats treated intraperitoneally or intravenously with the alkylating agent methylazomethanol (MAM), oligodendrogliomas were produced in 0.7% of the offspring only when administered on the twentieth or twenty-first day of gestation. Prior to that, MAM produced disorganization and destruction of the brain tissue (167,168).

The results of animal experiments investigating chemical carcinogenesis of brain tumors led Rice (164,165) to comment:

> Ependymomas, which in man have a peak incidence between two and five years of age, have been seen rather frequently in rats exposed transplacentally to ENU, but rarely are encountered in animals treated after birth. This fact, together with the greater apparent sensitivity to ENU of the fetal and neonatal nervous system in this species, has been cited as evidence supporting the hypothesis of perinatal chemical induction of brain tumors of childhood and infancy in man.

Viral Induction of Tumors

Brain tumors have been induced in a variety of species of animals by many types of oncogenic viruses. In addition, particles resembling viruses have been found in the brains of animals in whom tumors have been induced by chemical carcinogens (146,169).

One of the early studies demonstrated that 75% of mongrel dogs inoculated intracerebrally with Rous Sarcoma Virus (RSV) developed brain tumors—gliomas and sarcomas (170). Ogawa and co-workers (171) found that, following intracerebral inoculation of hamsters and mice with adenovirus type 12, 37% of hamsters and 30% of mice observed until death developed central nervous system tumors, primarily glioblastoma and medulloblastoma. Eight of 29 hamsters sacrificed at varying times after inoculation had tumors, although no tumors were found in mice sacrificed at varying times or in control animals. Mancini and colleagues (172) inoculated two litters of newborn hamsters intracerebrally with chicken-embryo-lethal-orphan virus (CELO) and found that 15 of 17 animals who survived the inoculation and developed neurologic symptoms had papillary ependymomas of the lateral ventricles similar to ependymomas induced by Simian virus 40 (SV40). SV40 has induced ependymomas upon intracerebral injection into hamsters (173), while intracerebral inoculation of JC papovavirus into hamsters has produced medulloblastomas, glioblastomas, ependymomas, and pineocytomas (174–177). In a study by Greenlee et al. (178), however, cell cultures from brain tumors of 80 human patients failed to show intranuclear tumor (T) antigen common to cells transformed by SV40, BK, or JC viruses.

Gliomas have been induced in rats using murine sarcoma virus (179), and intracranial astrocytomas have been induced in rats with avian sarcoma virus, with virus-like particles found in the tumor cells (180,181). C-type viruses morphologically resembling RNA-containing avian, feline, and murine leukemia and sarcoma viruses have been detected by electron microscopy in human brain tumors as well as in neurofibromas of patients with von Recklinghausen's disease (173).

The main routes of virus spread to the central nervous system are hematogenous, neural, and olfactory (182). The first is probably the most common. Blood-borne viruses probably cross the blood-brain barrier by passive transport through membranes and from the blood into the cerebrospinal fluid through the capillaries of the choroid plexus. From the cerebrospinal fluid the viruses may move across the meningeal and ependymal cells into the brain either by diffusion or active multiplication in the cells. Viruses also may be spread from the small blood vessels of the brain directly into the surrounding neurons and glial cells. This susceptibility of brain tissue to viral infection tends to decrease with age.

GENETIC FACTORS

Genetic factors have been implicated as predisposing factors in the occurrence of some types of tumors (53). According to Brain (19): "In a minority of cases congenital abnormality appears to play an important part in causation . . . It is uncertain whether the primitive character of the cells of which some gliomas are composed should be regarded as an indication that they are derived from embryonic cell rests, or should be considered as a cellular regression." The major areas of investigation into the association of childhood brain tumors with genetic factors include: (1) distribution of ABO blood groups in patients with brain tumors, (2) familial aggregation of brain tumors, and (3) the occurrence of brain tumors in persons with known genetic disorders.

Blood Groups

Studies of distributions of ABO blood types of patients with brain tumors have yielded conflicting results. In 1970, Choi and co–workers (94) reported blood types of 157 patients of all ages with histologically proved or clinically suspected central nervous system neoplasms seen in four hospitals in Minneapolis during an 18-month period from 1963 to 1964. Hospital controls were matched to cases for hospital, sex, age, race, and area of residence. No significant differences were found between cases and controls in frequencies of ABO or Rh blood groups. Garcia and his colleagues (183) also found no differences in blood group distribution in a comparison of 132 patients of all ages with intracranial astrocytoma, 279 patients with other brain tumors, 124 patients with brain trauma, and 95 patients with nonneoplastic neurosurgical lesions. Carter et al. (184) also found no significant differences in ABO blood group distributions between 160 patients admitted to Radcliffe Infirmary with histologically proven glioblastoma multiforme and a control group of blood donors.

Selverstone and Cooper (185), however, did observe differences in blood group distributions at the New England Medical Center when they studied 139 patients diagnosed between August 1949 and March 1960 with histologically verified astrocytomas and glioblastomas and 657 patients hospitalized for conditions other than brain tumors. Cases and controls did not differ by race, national origin, or religion. Significantly fewer cases than controls were blood group 0, and significantly more were blood group A. There was also a tendency for fewer cases to be blood group B and more to be group AB, although the numbers in these groups were small. The authors suggested that these observations might reflect an anti-A factor in the blood which might be associated with protection from astrocytomas.

In a study involving only children under age 15 years, Yates and Pearce (186) compared 473 patients with astrocytoma to 843 hospital patients with burns. The controls had blood group distributions corresponding to that of the adult population. Cases diagnosed before 1945 also had the expected blood group distribution. However, after 1945 a significant reduction in cases with blood group 0 were apparent. Selverstone and Cooper (185) also confirmed this observation in a study of patients of all ages who had astrocytomas. Strang et al. (187) examined this phenomenon further. The first 200 patients of all ages diagnosed with astrocytomas after 1940 and the first 700 such patients diagnosed after 1955 were compared to a control group consisting of blood donors, conscripts and paternity case subjects. No differences were found in ABO blood group distributions in cases and controls when all patients or females alone were considered. However, when male cases were analyzed separately, a significant excess of blood group A was found. There were no significant differences, however, in blood group distributions between patients diagnosed before and those diagnosed after 1945. In summary, the issue of the possible association of brain tumors with particular blood groups remains unsettled.

Familial Aggregation

The literature is replete with anecdotal reports of individual families in which two or more members have been afflicted with intracranial tumors, some of which have been presented in Table 6. In addition, in 1960 Kjellin et al. (207) reported seven families with a total of fifteen adults and children, including a

TABLE 6. Selected Case Reports of Familial CNS Tumors Since 1960

Findings	Date	Authors
Glioblastoma in two brothers; in another family astrocytoma in two first cousins	1972	Kaufman and Brisman (188)
Optic glioma in two sisters; in another family spinal ependymoma in a mother and astrocytoma of the vermis in her son	1971	Bromowicz et al. (189)
Meningioma and hemangioblastoma in sister and brother, respectively	1971	Chateau et al. (190)
Cerebellar medulloblastoma and small-cell parietal tumor in identical twins at 3 and 7 years, respectively	1971	Fairburn and Urich (191)
Meningioma in two brothers	1970	Grunert et al. (192)
Malignant astrocytoma in three siblings	1969	Armstrong and Hanson (193)
Cerebellar medulloblastoma in two of three newborn hydrocephalic sisters	1969	Belamaric and Chau (194)
Eight out of 17 family members having CNS neoplasms, including four children and five additional members with evidence of neurofibromatosis	1969	Lee and Abbott (195)
Cerebellar medulloblastoma in two brothers	1967	Bickerstaff et al. (196)

set of identical twins, afflicted with brain tumors. In six of the seven families, the same tumor types were found in the affected members. Lynch et al. (208) also reported 34 families in which two or more first and/or second degree relatives had histologically confirmed breast cancer. Eleven of these families had 21 of 275 first and second degree relatives who had developed soft tissue sarcomas, leukemia, or brain tumors, or combinations of these neoplasms. There were five individuals in five of these families with brain tumors, about 2.5 times the numbers expected from the frequency in the general population.

Anecdotal reports of familial aggregation, however, have serious limitations for drawing etiologic inferences. First, unusual instances of more than one member of a family having cancer tend to attract the attention of physicians and are thus more likely to be reported in the literature. More important, such anecdotal reports do not usually explore the possibility that such occurrences might well be expected on the basis of chance. Finally, even well-designed, controlled studies that report occurrence of familial aggregation of tumors do not necessarily implicate genetic factors, as family members share exposure to environmental factors, as well as genes.

Population-based studies of familial aggregation of relatively low incidence

TABLE 6. *(continued)*

Findings	Date	Authors
Meningioma in a mother and daughter	1965	Joynt and Perret (197)
Papilloma of choroid plexis in brother and sister	1965	Komminoth et al. (198)
Meningioma in two brothers and a female second cousin	1965	Sahar (199)
Frontal oligodendroglioma in two brothers	1962	Parkinson and Hall (200)
Glioblastoma and glioma in brother and sister, respectively	1960	Grosz and Plaschkes (201)
Glioblastoma multiforme in three sisters	1960	Koch and Middendorf (202)
Glioblastoma and oligodendroglioma in a brother and sister, respectively	1960	Symonds (203)
Cerebellar hemangioblastoma in a father, daughter, and three members of father's family; cerebellar hemangioblastoma in brother and sister whose two brothers and father died from brain tumors	1953	Adams (204)
Cerebellar hemangioblastoma in a brother and two sisters who all had Lindau's Syndrome	1952	Tonning et al. (205)
Cerebellar hemangioblastoma in a father, two sons and daughter	1944	Grossman and Kesert (206)

tumors are understandably scarce, though a few have been conducted. One of the first was by Harvald and Hauge (209). One hundred sixty-nine patients of all ages with histologically confirmed glioblastomas, seen at the Copenhagen University Clinic Neurosurgical Department from 1945 to 1953, were compared to control patients without cancer seen at the Univeristy Institute for Human Genetics and matched by sex and age. Parents, siblings, children, parents' siblings, and half siblings of probands were examined, and death certificates and hospital records were reviewed for intracranial tumors and cancer in the relatives. There were no significant differences in familial occurrence of intracranial tumors, cancer in general or of particular sites (except leukemia), epilepsy, or in age at onset of cancer. Similar results were found later by these investigators in a larger study of 5700 relatives over age 10 of 535 patients of all ages with histologically confirmed intracranial tumors and 2288 relatives of 250 controls "recruited from various social groups" (210).

However, two other retrospective studies did find a significant increase in frequency of central nervous system tumors, particularly gliomas, in families of patients of all ages who had brain tumors ($P < 0.01$ with 157 cases and $P < 0.03$ with 100 cases) compared to families of controls (94,211).

The major population-based studies of familial aggregation in children with brain tumors and other cancers were part of a larger investigation of the occurrence of cancer in siblings and twins of children with cancer (212–214). Miller (213) obtained the death certificates of all children under the age of 15 years who died of cancer in the United States between 1960 and 1964. He then identified siblings by matching the mother's maiden name and home address. The expected number of sibs with cancer was roughly estimated by assuming an average of two sibs per index case, each at risk of developing cancer for the 5-year interval. In the 21,659 death certificates, there were 26 sibships in which two siblings had died of cancer. Five of these sets were twins who had died of leukemia. Six pairs of siblings who were not twins died of brain tumors, compared to an expected number of 0.4—a highly significant difference. In 6 families, one child died of brain tumor and one child of another cancer, compared to two such deaths expected. In a later study, Miller (212) added death certificates of children under 20 years of age, who died of cancer from 1965 to 1975, and again identified sibships. In this additional group, one pair of female twins was found in which both had died at age 14—one of glioblastoma multiforme and the other of leukemia after removal of a limb for osteosarcoma. In the two studies, a total of eight pairs of siblings had died of brain tumors, compared to 0.9 expected pair.

In a longitudinal study, Norris and Jackson (214) followed twins and singletons born in California between 1940 and 1964 until they were 15 years old in order to determine their cancer death rates from 1940 to 1967. Based on cancer-specific mortality rates for single-born children who died during the same period, there were seven fewer cancer deaths than expected in twins for cancer other than leukemia. There were three twin pairs in which both twins died. In two of these one twin had died of a brain tumor and the other from some cause involving the central nervous system—probable epilepsy resulting in drowning and cerebral hemorrhage.

Association with Genetic Disorders

As with reports of familial aggregation, most of the literature about genetic disorders associated with brain tumors consists of case reports, several of which are shown in Table 7. However, there have also been a few controlled studies of genetic disorders associated with an increased incidence of brain tumors. The genetically determined disorders that have been reported most frequently to be associated with an increased incidence of brain tumors are von Recklinghausen's disease (neurofibromatosis), tuberous sclerosis, Down's Syndrome and immunodeficiency diseases (227,228).

Von Recklinghausen's disease is an autosomal dominant disorder that occurs about once in every 2000 to 3000 live births and has been associated with the development of intracranial or intraspinal tumors, including acoustic neuromas in adults, as well as meningiomas, astrocytomas, ependymomas and glioblastomas (220,223,226,229,230). Von Recklinghausen's disease is a slowly progressive disease characterized by cafe-au-lait spots and diffuse proliferation of the sheaths and enveloping membranes of the nervous system and supporting structures (221,226,231,232). The individual neurofibroma is composed primarily of hyperplasia of the Schwann sheath cells and fibroblastic proliferation of the supporting structures (231). Peripheral, spinal, or cranial nerves—particularly the optic, trigeminal and vagus nerves in children—may be involved. The association of neurofibromatosis with brain tumors appears to be documented largely by case reports, such as those in Table 7. However, in a small, hospital-based study, Pearce (233) reviewed the autopsy files of Massachusetts General Hospital for the period 1955–1965 and found 9 cases, all adults, of histologically confirmed neurofibromatosis. Six of these cases had intracranial tumors or malformations, including 3 astrocytomas, 1 hemorrhage, and 1 aneurysm. A comparison group without neurofibromatosis was not included. In a multicentered study of meningiomas in childhood and adolescence, Merten et al. (234) found that 23% of the 48 examined cases of meningioma had associated neurofibromatosis. However, it was not stated whether the observed frequency of neurofibromatosis differed from that of the general population.

Tuberous sclerosis is an autosomal dominant, progressive disease characterized by sebaceous adenomas of the skin, a "butterfly rash" on the face, muscle tumors, epileptic seizures, retinal tumors, malformations of the brain, and mental retardation (235,236). The brain may be studded with many nodules or tubers, usually composed of nests of glial fibers and abnormal ganglion cells. As with neurofibromatosis, the reported association of tuberous sclerosis with intracranial tumors is largely anecdotal, although one small hospital-based study has been conducted. Kapp et al. (219) reviewed 48 patients with tuberous sclerosis who were in hospitals in North Carolina. Of the 48, 7 had intracranial tumors of unspecified histology, 5 of whom were verified at autopsy. All of the patients with tumors were children, and all had tumors involving the ventricles of the brain.

Down's Syndrome, or trisomy 21, is a genetic disorder resulting primarily from nondisjunction in the maternal first meiotic division and occurs with an incidence of about 1.6/1000 live births (237). Clinically, the disorder is characterized by mental retardation, abnormal brain development, and characteristic facies. One of the first studies of the risk of malignancy in children with Down's Syndrome was conducted by Carter (238). Seven hundred twenty-five children admitted to an English hospital with Down's Syndrome between 1944 and 1955 were followed until 1955. One hundred thirty-six of the children died, including 3 from leukemia and 1 from a brain tumor, which was not in excess of what would have been expected. In a study of 2033 children with Down's Syndrome followed from 1 to 15 years in England, Holland and associates (239) found seven children who developed leukemia (18 times the expected number calculated from national vital statistics) and 2 who developed brain tumors, one a glioma and one an angioma. In a later study, Jackson et al., (240) followed 2100 individuals admitted with Down's Syndrome to 7 state hospitals in California from 1952 through 1962, for a total of 12,499 person-years. A total of 269 deaths occurred, 5 from leukemia a 12-fold excess over expected based on California mortality rates. There were no deaths from brain tumors.

In a more recent study, De Weerdt and Schut (241) determined the frequency of spina bifida and Down's Syndrome in 85 patients, most of whom were adults, with gliomas, medulloblastomas, or meningiomas. One child in the patient group with an astrocytoma also had spina bifida occulta, and two

TABLE 7. Selected Case Reports of Genetically Determined Disorders Associated With Brain Tumors in Children

Findings	Date	Authors
Tuberous sclerosis in an 8-year-old white female and 7-year-old white male with supratentorial giant-cell astrocytoma	1971	Cooper (215)
Tuberous sclerosis diagnosed at age 4 in a male who was then diagnosed with a third ventricle astrocytoma at age 14	1970	Huberland and Perou (216)
Familial neurofibromatosis in a 8–year-old male with cerebellar medulloblastoma, irradiated and found to have an enlarged thyroid gland, a spinal subarachnoid cyst, and numerous neurofibrosarcomas in the chest at age 17	1969	Corkill and Ross (217)
Multiple meningiomas in a 30-year-old female with neurofibromatosis and prior acoustic neurinoma	1968	Jamieson (218)
Tuberous sclerosis in seven children with astrocytomas of the third or lateral ventricles, near the foramen of Monro	1967	Kapp et al. (219)
Von Recklinghausen's disease in a 20-year-old white male with spinal and cranial meningiomas, and schwannoma of the eighth cranial nerve. Review of reports of tumors associated with von Recklinghausen's disease in patients 16 to 52 years old showed acoustic neurinomas, meningiomas, gliomas, and syringomyelia	1966	Rodriquez and Berthrong (220)

men in the patient group had brothers who had died in infancy from spina bifida. This was found not to be significantly different from the expected numbers of cases of spina bifida, based on population statistics. These authors also questioned relatives of 73 patients with spina bifida and found "many" cases of spina bifida in relatives but only one brain tumor in a sibling. When the relatives of a larger group of patients with brain tumors were studied, none were found to have Down's Syndrome and no more than the expected had spina bifida. In summary, it would seem that the association between Down's Syndrome or spina bifida and brain tumors, if it exists at all, is probably not a strong one.

Some authors have suggested a possible association between genetically determined immunodeficiency diseases and brain tumors. Gatti and Good (242) reviewed the literature on malignancies in patients with immunodeficiencies. They found astrocytomas associated with the Wiskott-Aldrich syndrome, an X-linked disorder characterized by low IgM levels, normal IgG levels, normal

TABLE 7. *(continued)*

Findings	Date	Authors
Neurofibromatosis in six cases, including three children, with intracranial lesions including a cervical plexiform neuroma, astrocytoma of the optic nerve and surrounding areas, and spongioblastoma polare of the optic nerve	1966	Davidson (221)
Ataxia telangiectasia in a brother and sister, with cerebellar medulloblastoma in the sister	1966	Shuster et al. (222)
Familial neurofibromatosis in monozygous male twins with brain stem gliomas which were diagnosed about 16 years apart and an optic glioma in one twin and neurofibromatosis and brain stem astrocytoma in their brother	1962	Brady (223)
Tuberous sclerosis in an 18-year-old white male with a grade II astrocytoma of the frontal lobe	1961	Rudnick et al. (224)
Two patients with intracranial hemangioma with pheochromocytoma, one of whom had a family history of neurofibromatosis	1959	Chapman et al. (225)
Familial neurofibromatosis in an 8-year-old white female with an optic glioma	1955	Marshall (226)

or high IgA and IgE levels, eczema, thrombocytopenic purpura, and increased susceptibility to infection (243). Medulloblastoma was also found to be associated with ataxia telangiectasia, an autosomal recessive disorder in which the thymus fails to grow and mature and IgA levels are low. Kersey et al. (244) collected reports from over 100 physicians and from the literature available on the development of cancer in patients with immunodeficiency. In 24 cases with Wiskott-Aldrich syndrome, one child had a cerebellar astrocytoma and two had malignant reticuloendotheliosis of the brain. In 52 cases of ataxia telangiectasia, one patient had a mixed glioma and one a medulloblastoma. In 41 cases of common variable immunodeficiency, one patient had a medulloblastoma. In seven cases of IgA deficiency, one patient had a pleiomorphic cerebral glioma. Overall, 4% of patients who had immunodeficiency diseases and a malignancy had malignancies in the nervous system.

In summary, the role of genetic factors in the etiology of brain tumors remains suggestive and provides an area for further active investigation using well-designed, well-controlled studies, which should ideally be population-based studies. The many case reports and the few inadequate studies thus far conducted tend to suggest that genetic factors play an etiologic role but the findings thus far cannot be considered by any means to be definitive.

Cytogenetics

The few reports in the literature, concerning the existence of any abnormal chromosome patterns in brain tumors, consist largely of studies of small numbers of patients. Bicknell (245) studied brain tumors from three patients, one of whom was a 16-year-old male with a fourth ventricle ependymoma. The cells in this tumor were found to have chromosome numbers ranging from 56 to 90, with extra chromosomes mainly in group C and to a lesser degree in groups D through G. Hansteen (246) studied ten glial tumors from ten adult patients and found mitoses to be scarce, but chromosomes from astrocytomas were in the diploid range in groups C, D, E, and G—particularly C and E. Lubs and Salmon (247) studied the karyotype of a medulloblastoma from a 8-year-old female. There were some double fragments of chromosomes, but no loss of chromosomes. The karyotype was largely normal, although there were some chromosome losses in various groups, which were also seen in blood and bone marrow specimens from the patient.

Congenital Brain Tumors

Congenital tumors, those which are present at birth or become symptomatic within three months of birth, have been reported in numerous case reports, several of which are summarized in Table 8. In some instances, these tumors occur in conjunction with a congenital malformation of some type, as shown in the table. In a review of case reports of congenital brain tumors in the literature, Solitare and Krigman (254) found reports of 26 "definitely congenital" (producing symptoms at birth), 3 "probably congenital" (producing symptoms in the first week of life), and 16 "possibly congenital" (producing symptoms in the first few months of life). Twenty percent of the congenital tumors were mesodermal, 30% were teratomas, and 30% were gliomas—a distribution of tumor types quite different from that usually seen in older children. In addition, unlike brain tumors in older children, the vast majority of congenital brain tumors were supratentorial. The risk of brain tumors developing is thus clearly present before birth; however, it is unclear whether congenital brain tumors are genetically or environmentally induced. Moreover, the differences in distributions of cell types and locations of congenital tumors and tumors occurring later in childhood suggest that different mechanisms of tumor induction may be operating in the two age groups.

QUALITY OF LIFE

Although some patients with brain tumors survive over 5 years following treatment, the majority of such patients have significant residual disability (6,22). Of 200 children with brain tumors treated from 1950 to 1967 in the Ra-

TABLE 8. Selected Case Reports of Congenital Brain Tumors

Findings	Year	Authors
Cerebellar medulloblastomas in 1-month-old Chinese female and her sister at birth	1969	Belamaric and Chau (194)
Fourth ventricle ependymoma in 6-week-old white male	1968	Abbott and Namiki (248)
Frontal fibrillar grade I astrocytoma in 4-week-old infant	1968	Barsky (249)
Cerebral astrocytoma in stillborn infant at 28 weeks gestation	1967	Cooperman et al. (250)
Oligodendroglioma of the pons in a full-term stillborn negro female. Mother's uterus at delivery found to have leiomyoma, and placenta had two cysts	1967	Fuste et al. (251)
Cerebellar medulloblastoma in newborn with multiple digestive and genitourinary system anomalies, who died 20 hours after delivery at 36 weeks gestation	1966	Duckett et al. (252)
Third ventricle astrocytoma in premature female; papilloma of choroid plexus in female with RH incompatibility: glioblastoma multiforme of choroid plexus in male with pregnancy complicated by severe fall in eighth month	1964	Raskind and Beigel (254)
Mixed hemangiopericytoma and fibroma of the meninges between the upper brain stem and right temporal lobe in a stillborn infant of 32-week gestation	1964	Solitare and Krigman (254)
Astrocytoma of the supratentorial basal ganglia in a full-term new-born who died 24 hours after delivery	1962	Sandbank (255)

diotherapy Department of the Christie Hospital in Manchester, England, 32% survived more than 5 years. In a sample of 30 of these long-term survivors, only 20% were found to have no residual problems, while 20% were "profoundly disabled." The remaining children had disabilities ranging from substantial emotional problems to impaired growth, vision, hearing, motor ability, and intelligence, and cranial nerve palsies. Gol and McKissock (66) reported similar frequencies of disability in children with cerebellar astrocytomas, as did Gold and Smith (22) for all types of brain tumors, consisting of a 5-year survival of only about 45%, accompanied by the prospect of impaired functioning even with survival, emphasizes the need for improved knowledge of the etiology of the tumors so that they can be prevented.

SUMMARY

While brain tumors have been induced experimentally in a variety of animals using numerous chemical and viral carcinogenic agents, relatively few population-based epidemiologic studies of brain tumors in humans have been conducted. The possibility that environmental factors are involved in the etiology of brain tumors is suggested by geographic variations in incidence and mortality, time and space clustering, urban-rural differences, and increased incidence of brain tumors following skull irradiation and certain infections. These observations are consistent in animals given intracerebral inoculations of chemical carcinogens and oncogenic viruses.

A role for genetic factors in the etiology of brain tumors has been suggested based on possible differences in the distribution of ABO blood groups between brain tumor patients and controls, anecdotal reports of familial aggregation of brain tumors, and the association of brain tumors with genetically determined disorders.

Factors that have been implicated in the etiology of brain tumors are summarized in Table 9. Among the possible etiologic factors for brain tumors which remain to be further studied in systematically well-designed epide-

TABLE 9. Summary of Characteristics of and Risk Factors for Patients with Brain Tumors

Characteristic	Adults	Children
Cell types and Sites		
Astrocytoma	Frequent	Frequent
Medulloblastoma	Rare	Frequent
Glioblastoma multiforme	Frequent	Rare
Infratentorial tumors	Rare	Frequent
Risk Factors		
Age peak in incidence	65–69 years	5–9 years
Male:female ratio	Over 1	Over 1
White race	Frequent	Frequent
International variation in mortality	Highest in Israel, lowest in Mexico	?
Domestic variation in mortality	Little variation	Highest in Pacific states
Association with religious affiliation	Highest in Jews	No association
Association with prior radiation exposure	High	High
Prior toxoplasma infection	Increased	?
Prior tuberculosis infection	Increased	?
Prenatal exposure to chickenpox	?	Increased
Blood group O	Decreased	Decreased
Blood group A	Increased	Increased in males
Familial aggregation	No	Yes
Neurofibromatosis	Yes	?
Tuberous sclerosis	?	Yes
Down's Syndrome	?	No

miologic investigations are socioeconomic differences, familial aggregation of brain tumors, trauma, hormonal factors, association with congenital or genetic disorders, prenatal exposures (e.g., infections, chemicals, or radiation), and exposure to animals, radiation, and environmental (e.g., occupational) chemicals. Thus, etiologic certainties regarding brain tumors are few, but the possibilities and opportunities for investigation remain vast and challenging.

REFERENCES

1. Cutler, S. J., Young, J. L. (1975) Third National Cancer Survey: Incidence Data, DHEW Publication No. (NIH) 75–787. Bethesda, Md.: National Cancer Institute, National Institutes of Health, Public Health Services, U.S. Department of Health, Education and Welfare.
2. Levin, D. L., Devesa, S. S., Godwin II, J. D., Silverman, D. T. (1974) Cancer Rates and Risks. 2d edition. DHEW Publication No. (NIH) Washington, D. C.: Superintendent of Documents, pp. 75–691.
3. Gold, E., Gordis, L. (1979) Determinants of survival in children with brain tumors. Ann. Neurol. 5, 569–574.
4. Gjerris, F. (1978) Clinical aspects and long-term prognosis in supratentorial tumors of infancy and childhood. Acta Neurol. Scand. 57, 445–470.
5. Axtell, L. M., Cutler, S. J., Myers, M. H. (1972) End Results in Cancer, Report No. 4 DHEW Publication No. (NIH) Bethesda, Maryland: National Cancer Institute, pp. 73–272.
6. Bamford, F. N., Jones, P. M.; Pearson, D., Ribeiro, G. G., Shalet, S. M., Beardwell, C. G. (1976) Residual disabilities in children treated for intracranial space occupying lesions. Cancer 37, 1149–1151.
7. Zulch, K. J. (1971) Atlas of the Histology of Brain Tumors. New York: Springer-Verlag, Inc.
8. Doll, R., Payne, P., Waterhouse, J. (1966) Cancer Incidence in Five Continents. New York: Springer-Verlag, Inc. (for the International Union Against Cancer).
9. Cushing, H. (1931) Experiences with the cerebellar astrocytomas, a critical review of seventy-six cases. Surg. Gynec. Obstet. 52, 129–191.
10. Green, J. R., Waggener, J. D., Kreigsfeld, B. A. (1976) Classification and incidence of neoplasms of the central nervous system. *In*: Advances in Neurology. Thompson, R. A., Green, J. R. (eds.). Neoplasia in the Central Nervous System. New York: Raven Press, pp. 51–55.
11. Bloom, H. J. G., Walsh, L. S. (1975) Tumours of the central nervous system. *In* Cancer in Children: Clinical Management. Bloom, H. J. G., Lemerle, J., Neidhardt, M. K., Voute, P. A. (eds.). New York: Springer-Verlag, Inc., pp. 93–119.
12. Shapiro, W. R. (1975) Chemotherapy of primary malignant brain tumors in children. Cancer 35, 965–972.
13. Committee on Professional Education, UICC International Union Against Cancer (1973) Clinical Oncology: A Manual for Students and Doctors. New York: Springer-Verlag, Inc., pp. 251–255.
14. Zimmerman, H. M. (1971) The ten most common types of brain tumor. Sem. Roentgenol. 6, 48–58.
15. Ford, F. R. (1960) Diseases of the Nervous System in Infancy, Childhood and Adolescence. 4th edition. Springfield, Illinois: Charles C. Thomas Publisher.
16. Ingraham, F. D., Matson, D. D. (1960) Tumors of the central nervous system. *In*: Cancer and Allied Diseases of Infancy and Childhood. Ariel, I. M., Pack, G. T. (eds.). Boston, Little, Brown and Co.
17. Schoenberg, B. S., Christine, B. W., Whisnat, J. P. (1976) The descriptive epidemi-

ology of primary intracranial neoplasms: the Connecticut experience. Am. J. Epidemiol. 104, 499–510.

18. Bailey, P. (1927) Further remarks concerning tumors of the glial group. Bull. Johns Hopkins Hosp. 40, 354–389.
19. Brain, W. R. (1962) Diseases of the Nervous System. London: Oxford University Press.
20. Bell, W. E., McCormick, W. F. (1972) Increased Intracranial Pressure in Children. Philadelphia: W. B. Saunders Co.
21. Arnold, A., Burrows, D. (1975) Scanning electron microscopy of cerebral tumors and glial cells. *In*: Gliomas: Current Concepts in Biology Diagnosis and Therapy, Recent Results in Cancer Research. Hekmatpanah, J. (ed.). New York: Springer-Verlag, Inc., vol. 15, pp. 52–62.
22. Gold, J. A. Smith, K. K. (1975) Childhood brain tumors: A 15-year survey of treatment in a university pediatric hospital. South Med. J. 68, 1337–1344.
23. Hendrick, E. G., Hoffman, Humphreys, R. P. (1975) Treatment of infratentorial gliomas in childhood. *In*: Gliomas: Current Concepts in Biology, Diagnosis and Therapy, Recent Results in Cancer Research. Hekmatpanah, J. (ed.). New York: Springer-Verlag, Inc., vol. 15, pp. 102–106.
24. Emery, E. W. (1972) Intracranial tumours. *In*: Tumours of Childhood: A Clinical Treatise. Williams, I. G. (ed.) New York: Appleton-Century-Crofts.
25. Bucy, P. C., Thieman, P. W. (1968) Astrocytomas of the cerebellum: a study of a series of patients operated upon over 28 years ago. Arch. Neurol. 18, 14–19.
26. Elvidge, A. R. (1968) Long-term survival in the astrocytoma series. J. Neurosurg. 28, 399–404.
27. Geissinger, J. D., Bucy, P. C. (1971) Astrocytomas of the cerebellum in children: long-term study. Arch. Neurol. 24, 125–135.
28. Takeuchi, K., Hoshina, K. (1977) Statistical analysis of factors affecting survival after glioblastoma multiforme. Acta. Neurochir. 37, 57–73.
29. Gerard-Marchant, R. (1975) Pathology. *In*: Cancer in Children: Clinical Management. Bloom, H. J. G., Lemerle, J., Neidhardt, M. K., Voute, P. A. (eds.). New York: Springer-Verlag, Inc., pp. 9–22.
30. Cushing, H. (1927) The intracranial tumors of preadolescence. Am. J. Dis. Child. 33, 551–584.
31. Schoenberg, B. S., Schoenberg, D. G., Christine, B. W., Gomez, M. R. (1975) The epidemiology of primary intracranial neoplasms of childhood: a population study. Neurology 25, 356.
32. Schaper, A. (1897) Die frühesten Differenzierungs vorgänge im Central-nervensystem. Arch. F. Entwklugsmechn. 5, 81.
33. Cruz, B. L. (1958) Medulloblastoma. Springfield, Illinois: Charles C. Thomas.
34. Bailey, P., Cushing, H. (1925) Medulloblastoma cerebelli: a common type of midcerebellar glioma of childhood. Arch. Neurol. Psychiatr. 14, 192–224.
35. Walker, M. D. (1976) Diagnosis and treatment of brain tumors. Ped. Clin. North Am. 23, 131–146.
36. Wilson, C. B. (1975) Diagnosis and surgical treatment of childhood brain tumors. Cancer 35, 950–956.
37. Waterhouse, J. A. H. (1974) Cancer Handbook of Epidemiology and Prognosis. Edinburgh: Churchill Livingstone.
38. McFarland, D. R., Horwitz, H., Saenger, E. L., Bahr, G. K. (1969) Medulloblastoma—a review of prognosis and survival. Br. J. Radiol. 42, 198–214.
39. Willis, R. A. (1962) The Pathology of the Tumours of Children. Springfield, Illinois: Charles C. Thomas.
40. Hooper, R. (1976) Intracranial tumours in childhood. Med. J. Aust. 1, 624–627.
41. Sheline, G. E. (1975) Radiation therapy of tumors of the nervous system in childhood. Cancer 35, 957–964.

42. Smith, C. E., Long, D. M., Jones, T. K., Levitt, S. H. (1973) Medulloblastoma: an analysis of time-dose relationships and recurrence patterns. Cancer 32, 722–728.
43. Hope-Stone, H. F. (1970) Results of treatment of medulloblastomas. J. Neurosurg. 32, 83–88.
44. Wilson, C. B. (1970) Medulloblastoma: current views regarding the tumor and its treatment. Oncology 24, 273–290.
45. Cuneo, H. M., Rand. C. W. (1952) Brain Tumors of Childhood. Springfield, Illinois: Charles C. Thomas.
46. Walker, M. D. (1973) Brain and peripheral nervous system tumors. *In*: Cancer Medicine. Holland, J. F., Frie III, E. (eds.). Philadelphia: Lea and Febiger, pp. 1385–1407.
47. Koos, W. T., Miller, M. W. (1971) Intracranial Tumors of Infants and Children. St. Louis: C. V. Mosby Co.
48. Leibowitz, U., Yablonski, M., Alter, M. (1971) Tumors of the nervous system: incidence and population selectivity. J. Chron. Dis. 23, 707–721.
49. Marsden, H. B., Steward, J. K. (1968) Tumors in children. *In*: Recent Results in Cancer Research. New York: Springer-Verlag, Inc. Vol. 13.
50. Aron, B. S. (1969) Twenty years' experience with radiation therapy of medulloblastoma. Am. J. Roentgenol. 105, 37–42.
51. Shuman, R. M., Alvord, E. C., Leech, R. W. (1975) The biology of childhood ependymonas. Arch. Neurol. 32, 732–739.
52. Bloom, H. J. G., Wallace, E. N. K., Henk, J. M. (1969) The treatment and prognosis of medulloblastoma in children. Am. J. Roentgenol. 105: 43–62.
53. Fishman, R. A. (1975) Intracranial tumors and states causing increased intracranial pressure. *In*: Textbook of Medicine, Beeson, P. B., McDermott, W. (eds.). 14th edition. Philadelphia: W. B. Saunders Co., pp. 734–747.
54. Gjerris, F. (1976) Clinical aspects and long-term prognosis of intracranial tumours in infancy and childhood. Develop. Med. Child Neurol. 18, 145–159.
55. Gjerris, F., Klee, J. G., Klinken, L. (1976) Malignancy grade and long-term survival in brain tumours of infancy and childhood. Acta Neurol. Scand. 53, 61–71.
56. Panitch, H. S., Berg. B. O. (1970) Brain stem tumors of childhood and adolescence. Am. J. Dis. Child. 119, 465–472.
57. Lassman, L. P., Arjona, V. E. (1967) Pontine gliomas of childhood. Lancet 1, 913–915.
58. Marsa, G. W., Probert, J. C., Rubinstein, L. J., Bagshaw, M. A. (1973) Radiation therapy in the treatment of childhood astrocytic gliomas. Cancer 32, 646–655.
59. Abramson, N., Raben, M., Cavanaugh, P. J. (1974) Brain tumors in children: analysis of 136 cases. Radiology 112, 669–672.
60. Starr, A. M. (1889) Tumors of the brain in childhood. Med. News, 54, 29–37.
61. Heiskanen, O. (1977) Intracranial tumors of children. Child's Brain 3, 69–78.
62. Stewart, A. M., Lennox, E. L., Sanders, B. M. (1973) Group Characteristics of children with cerebral and spinal cord tumours. Br. J. Cancer 28, 568–574.
63. Dastur, D. K., Lalitha, V. S. (1968) Pathological analysis of intracranial space-occupying lesions in 1000 cases including children. Part 2. Incidence, types, and unusual cases of glioma. J. Neurol. Sci. 8, 143–170, 1968.
64. MacKay, E. M., Seller, A. H. (1968) Malignant neoplasms of the central nervous system, Ontario Cancer Foundation Clinics, 1950–1964. Can. Med. Assoc. J. 99, 1245–1253.
65. Odom, G. L., Davis, C. H., Woodhall, B. (1956) Brain tumors in children: clinical analysis of 164 cases. Pediat. 18, 856–870.
66. Gol, A. McKissock, W. (1959) The cerebellar astrocytomas: a report on 98 verified cases. J. Neurosurg. 16, 287–296.
67. Hopewell, J. W., Edwards, D. N., Wiernik, G. (1976) Sex dependence of human intracranial gliomata. Br. J. Cancer 34, 666–670.

68. Silverberg, E., Holleb, A. I. (1975) Major trends in cancer: 25-year survey. Ca. Cancer. J. Clin. 25, 2–21.
69. Miller, R. W. (1969) Fifty-two forms of childhood cancer: United States mortality experience, 1960–1966. J. Pediat. 75, 685–689.
70. Mulcahy, G. M., Harlan, W. L. (1976) Occurrence of central nervous system tumors with special reference to relative genetic factors. *In*: Cancer Genetics. Lynch, H. T. (ed.). Springfield, Illinois: Charles C. Thomas, pp. 263–325.
71. Innis, M. D. (1970) Possible genetic basis of neoplasia. Med. J. Aust. 2, 1187–1189.
72. Handy, V. H., Goldberg, I. D. (1956) The occurrence of malignancies in children. N. Y. State J. Med. 56, 258–260.
73. Gold, E., Gordis, L. (1979) Patterns in the incidence of brain tumors in children. Ann. Neurol. 5, 565–568.
74. Munoz, N. (1976) Geographical distribution of pediatric tumors. Tumori 62, 145–156.
75. Lilienfeld, A. M., Levin, M. L., Kessler, I. I. (1972) Cancer in the United States. Cambridge, Mass.: Harvard University Press.
76. Gordon, I., Crittenden, M., Haenszel. W. (1961) Cancer mortality trends in the United States, 1930–1955. Part II. *In*: End Results and Mortality Trends in Cancer, No. 6. Washington, D. C.: J. Natl. Cancer. Inst.
77. Devesa, S. S., Silverman, D. T. (1978) Cancer incidence and mortality trends in the United States: 1935–1974, J. Natl. Cancer Inst. 60, 545–571.
78. Dorn, H. F., Cutler, S. J. (1959) Morbidity from Cancer in the United States. Washington, D. C.: U.S. Government Printing Office.
79. Schoenberg, B. S., Schoenberg, D. G., Christine, B. W., Gomez, M. R. (1976) The epidemiology of primary intracranial neoplasms of childhood: a population study. Mayo Clin. Proc. 51, 51–56.
80. Ederer, F., Miller, R. W., Scotto, J. (1965) U.S. childhood cancer mortality patterns, 1950–1959, JAMA 192, 97–100.
81. Quinn, R. J. M., Scragg, J. N., Rubidge, C. J. (1978) Primary intracranial tumours in black and Indian children, 1960–1975. So. Afr. Med. J. 53, 211–213.
82. Fan, K., Kovi, J., Earle, K. M. (1977) The ethnic distribution of primary central nervous system tumors: AFIP, 1958 to 1970. J. Neuropathol. Exp. Neurol. 36, 41–49.
83. Heshmat, M. Y., Kovi, J., Simpson, C., Kennedy, J., Fan, K. J. (1976) Neoplasms of the central nervous system: incidence and population selectivity in the Washington, D. C., metropolitan area. Cancer 38, 2135–2142.
84. Cohen, A., Modan, B. (1968) Some epidemiologic aspects of neoplastic diseases in Israeli immigrant population. III. Brain tumors. Cancer 22, 1323–1328.
85. Spiers, P. S. (1971) Sex ratio by age in childhood malignancies, J. Chron. Dis. 23, 907–911.
86. Leibowitz, U., Yablonski, M., Alter, M. (1971) Epidemiology of tumors of the nervous system in Israel. Israel J. Med. Sci. 7, 1491–1499.
87. Michael, P. (1964) Tumors of Infancy and Childhood. Philadelphia: J. B. Lippincott Co.
88. Choi, N. W., Schuman, L. M., Gullen, W. H. (1970) Epidemiology of primary central nervous system neoplasms. I. Mortality from primary central nervous system neoplasms in Minnesota. Am. J. Epidemiol. 91, 238–259.
89. Goldberg, I. D., Kurland, L. T. (1962) Mortality in 33 countries from diseases of the nervous system. World Neurol. 3, 444–465, 1962.
90. Kurland, L. T., Myrianthopoulos, N. C., Lessell, S. (1962) Epidemiologic and genetic considerations of intracranial neoplasms. *In*: The Biology and Treatment of Intracranial Tumors. Fields, W. S., Sharkey, P. C. (eds.). Springfield, Illinois: Charles C. Thomas, pp. 5–48.

91. Dohrmann, G. J., Farwell, J. R. (1976) Intracranial neoplasms in children: a comparison of North America, Europe, Africa and Asia. Dis. Nervous Sys. 37, 696–697.
92. Kurtzke, J. F. (1969) Geographic pathology of brain tumors, Acta Neurol. Scand. 45, 450–555.
93. MacMahon, B. (1957) Geographic variation in leukemia mortality in the United States. Public Health Rep. 72, 39–46.
94. Choi, N. W., Schuman, L. M., Gullen, W. H. (1970) Epidemiology of primary central nervous system neoplasms. II. Case-control study. Am. J. Epidemiol. 91, 467–485.
95. Brooks, W. H. (1972) Geographic clustering of brain tumors in Kentucky. Cancer 30, 923–926.
96. Kurtzke, J. F., Stazio, A. (1967) Geographic distribution of brain tumors. Trans. Am. Neurol. Assoc. 92, 253–254.
97. Maroun, F. B., Jacob, J. C. (1973) The frequency of intracranial neoplasms in Newfoundland. Can. J. Public Health 64, 53–57.
98. MacMahon, B. (1960) The ethnic distribution of cancer mortality in New York City, 1955. Acta Unio Internat. Contra Cancrum 16, 1716–1724.
99. Newill, V. A. (1961) Distribution of cancer mortality among ethnic subgroups of the white population of New York City, 1953–58. J. Natl. Cancer Inst. 26, 405–417.
100. Hirayama, T. (1973) Strategy for cancer epidemiology. *In*: Proceedings of the Third International Symposium of the Princess Takamatsu Cancer Research Fund. Analytic and Experimental Epidemiology of Cancer. Nakahar, W., Hirayama, T., Nishioka, K., Sugano, H. (eds.). Tokyo: University Park Press, pp. 393–420.
101. MacMahon, B., Newill, V. A. (1962) Birth characteristics of children dying from malignant neoplasms. J. Natl. Cancer Inst. 28, 231–244.
102. Gold, E., Gordis, L., Tonascia, J., Szklo, M. (1979) Risk factors for brain tumors in children. Am. J. Epidemiol. 109, 309–319.
103. Selvin, S., Garfinkel, J. (1972) The relationship between parental age and birth order with the percentage of low birth-weight infants. Hum. Biol. 44, 501–510.
104. Smith, D. W. (1977) Growth and Its Disorders: Basics and Standards, Approach and Classifications, Growth Deficiency Disorders, Growth Excess Disorders, Obesity. Philadelphia: W. B. Saunders Co.
105. Aronson, S. M., Aronson, B. D. (1965) Central nervous system in diabetes mellitis. Arch. Neurol. 12, 390–398.
106. Graham, S., Gibson, R., Lilienfeld, A., Schuman, L., Levin, M. (1970) Religion and ethnicity in leukemia. Amer. J. Public Health 60, 266–274.
107. Seidman, H. (1970) Cancer death rates by site and sex for religious and socioeconomic groups in New York City. Environ. Res. 3, 234–250.
108. Stewart, A., Kneale, G. W. (1968) Changes in the cancer risk associated with obstetric radiography. Lancet 1, 104–107.
109. Stewart, A., Webb, J., Hewitt, D. (1958) A survey of childhood malignancies. Br. Med. J. 2, 1495–1508.
110. MacMahon, B., Hutchison, G. B. (1964) Prenatal x-ray and childhood cancer: a review. Acta Unio. Intern. Contra Cancer 20, 1172–1174.
111. MacMahon, B. (1962) Prenatal x-ray exposure and childhood cancer. J. Natl. Cancer Inst. 28, 1173–1191.
112. Modan, B., Baidatz, D., Mart, H., Steinitz, R., Levin, S. G. (1974) Radiation-induced head and neck tumours. Lancet 1, 277–279.
113. Shore, R. E., Albert, R. E., Pasternack, B. S. (1976) Follow-up study of patients treated by x-ray epilation for tinea capitis. Arch. Environ. Health 31, 17–24.
114. Traynor, J. L., Casey, H. W. (1971) Five-year follow-up of primates exposed to 55 mev proton. Radn. Res. 47, 143–148.
115. Munk, J., Peyser, R., Gruszkiewicz, J. (1969) Radiation induced intracranial meningiomas. Clin. Radiol. 20, 90–94, 1969.

116. Haymaker, W., Rubinstein, L., Miguel, J. (1972) Brain tumors in irradiated monkeys. Acta Neuropathol. 20, 267–277.
117. Berry, C. L. (1976) Aetiological factors in childhood neoplasia. J. Clin. Patol. 29, 1032–1037.
118. Schuman, L. M., Choi, N. W., Gullen, W. H. (1967) Relationship of central nervous system neoplasms to toxoplasma Gondii infection. Am. J. Pub. Hlth. 57, 848–856.
119. Sigismund, P. (1960) Cancer in Childhood and Youth. Bristol: J. Wright and Sons, Ltd.
120. Ward, D. W., Mattison, M. L., Finn, R. (1973) Association between previous tuberculous infection and cerebral glioma. Br. Med. J. 1, 83–84.
121. Bithell, J. F., Draper, G. J., Gorbach, P. D. (1973) Association between malignant disease in children and maternal virus infections. Br. Med. J. 1, 706–708.
122. Fedrick, J., Alberman, E. D. (1972) Reported influenza in pregnancy and subsequent cancer in the child. Br. Med. J. 3, 485–488.
123. Adelstein, A. M., Donovan, J. W. (1972) Malignant disease in children whose mothers had chickenpox, mumps, or rubella in pregnancy. Br. Med. J. 4, 629–631.
124. Salonen, T. (1976) Prenatal and perinatal factors in childhood cancer. Ann. Clin. Res. 7, 27–42.
125. Salonen, T., Saxen, L. (1975) Risk indicators in childhood cancer. Int. J. Cancer 15, 941–946.
126. Clemmesen, J., Fuglsang-Frederiksen, V., Plum, C. M. (1974) Are anti-convulsants oncogenic? Lancet 1, 705–707.
127. Clemmesen, J., Hjalgrim-Jensen, S. (1977) On the absence of carcinogenicity to man of phenobarbitol. *In*: Statistical Studies in the Aetiology of Malignant Neoplasms. V. Trends and Risks, Denmark 1943–1972, Clemmesen, J. (ed.). Acta Pathol. Microbiol. Supplementium 261, Kobenhaven: Scand. Munksgaard, pp. 38–50.
128. Gold, E., Gordis, L., Tonascia, J., Szklo, M. (1978) Increased risk of brain tumors in children exposed to barbiturates. J. Natl. Cancer Inst. 61, 1031–1034.
129. Peraino, C., Fray, R. J., Staffeldt, E., Kisieleski, W. E. (1973) Effects of varying the exposure to phenobarbitol on its enhancement of 2-acetylaminofluorene-induced hepatic tumorigenesis in the rat. Cancer Res. 33, 2701–2705.
130. Takamiya, K., Chen, S. H., Kitagawa, H. (1973) Effect of phenobarbitol and DL-ethionine of 4-(dimethylamino) azobenzene-metabolizing enzymes and carcinogenesis. Gann. 64, 363–372.
131. International Agency for Research on Cancer (1977) Phenobarbital and phenobarbital sodium. IARC Monogr. Eval. Carcinog. Risk. Chem. Man. 13, 157–182.
132. Thorpe, E., Walker, A. I. (1973) The toxicology of dieldrin (HEOD). II. Comparative long-term oral toxicity studies in mice with dieldrin, DDT, phenobarbitone, β-BHC, and γ-BHC. Food Cosmet. Toxicol. 11, 433–442.
133. Ponomarkov, V., Tomatis, L., Turusov, V. (1976) The effect of long-term administration of phenobarbitone in CF-1 mice. Cancer Lett. 1, 165–172.
134. Nelson, M. M., Forfar, J. O. (1971) Associations between drugs administered during pregnancy and cogenital abnormalities of the fetus. Br. Med. J. 1, 523–527.
135. Meadow, S. R. (1968) Anticonvulsant drugs and congenital abnormalities. Lancet 2, 1296.
136. Speidel, B. D. Meadows, S. R. (1972) Maternal epilepsy and abnormalities of the fetus and newborn. Lancet 2, 839–843.
137. Napalkov, N. P. (1973) Some general considerations on the problems of transplacental carcinogenesis. IARC Sci. Publ. 4, 1–13.
138. Gunderson, C. H., Henry, J., Malamed, N. (1971) Plasma globulin determinations in patients with microglioma. J. Neurosurg. 35, 406–415.
139. Schneck, S. A., Penn, K. (1971) De novo brain tumours in renal-transplant recipients. Lancet 2, 983–986.

140. Brooks, W. H., Netsky, M. G., Normansell, D. E., Horwitz, D. A. (1972) Depressed cell-mediated immunity in patients with primary intracranial tumors. J. Exp. Med. 136, 1631–1647.

141. Lim, R., Kluskens, L. (1972) Immunological specificity of astrocytoma antigens. Cancer Res. 32, 1667–1670.

142. Levy, N. L., Mahaley, M. S., Day, E. D. (1972) In vitro demonstration of cell-mediated immunity to human brain tumors. Cancer Res. 32, 477–482.

143. Mitts, M. G., Walker, A. E. (1965) Autoimmune response to malignant glial tumors. Neurology 15, 474–476.

144. Scheinberg, L. C., Levy, A., Edelman, F. (1965) Is the brain an immunologically privileged site? Arch. Neurol. 13, 283–286.

145. Cowdry, E. V. (1968) Etiology and Prevention of Cancer in Man. New York: Appleton-Century-Crofts.

146. Rubin, R., Ames, R. P., Sutton, C. H., Zimmerman, H. M. (1969) Virus-like particles in murine ependymoblastoma. J. Neuropathol. Exp. Neurol. 28, 371–387.

147. Zimmerman, H. M. (1962) Experimental brain tumors. *In*: The Biology and Treatment of Intracranial Tumors. Fields, W. S., Sharkey, P. C. (eds.) Springfield, Illinois: Charles C. Thomas, pp. 49–74.

148. Zimmerman, H. M., Arnold, H. (1941) Experimental brain tumors. I. Tumors produced with methylcholanthrene. Cancer Res. 1, 919–938.

149. Peers, J. H. (1939) The response of the central nervous system to the application of the carcinogenic hydrocarbons. II. Methylcholanthrene. Am. J. Pathol. 16, 799–816.

150. Seligman, A. M., Shear, M. J. (1939) Studies in carcinogenesis. VIII. Experimental production of brain tumors in mice with methylcholanthrene. Am. J. Cancer 37, 364–395.

151. Gershbein, L. L., Benuck, I. (1975) Cortical implantation of hydrocarbons in rats and mice. Oncology 31, 76–82.

152. Augenlicht, L. H., Biessmann, H., Rajewsky, M. F. (1975) Chromosomal proteins of rat brain: increased synthesis and affinity for DNA following a pulse of the carcinogen ethylnitrosoureau in vivo. J. Cell Physiol. 86, 431–438.

153. Ishida, Y., Tamura, M., Kanda, H., Okamoto, K. (1975) Histopathological studies of the nervous system tumors in rats induced by N-nitroso-methyl-urea. Acta Pathol. Jap. 25, 385–401

154. Weiss, J. F., Cravioto, H., Ransohoff, J. (1975) Desmosterol in rat central and peripheral nervous systems during normal and neoplastic growth, J. Natl. Cancer Inst. 54, 781–783.

155. Kirsch, W. M., Schultz, D. (1972) The chemical induction of brain tumors with carcinogenic hydrocarbons and miscellaneous agents. *In*: The Experimental Biology of Brain Tumors. Kirsch, W. M., Grossi-Paoletti, E., Paoletti, P. (eds.). Springfield, Illinois: Charles C. Thomas, pp. 181–193.

156. Fitzgerald, J. E., Schardein, J. L., Kurtz, S. M. (1974) Spontaneous tumors of the nervous system in albino rats. J. Natl. Cancer Inst. 52, 265–273.

157. Swenberg, J. A., Koestner, A., Wechsler, W., Brunden, M. N., Abe, H. (1975) Differential oncogenic effects of methylnitrosourea. J. Natl. Cancer Inst. 54, 89–96.

158. Avtsyn, A. P., Yablonovskaya, L. Y. (1964) Effects of disturbances in the hormonal status on experimental brain tumors. Acta Union Intern. Contra Cancer 20, 1519–1522.

159. Druckrey, H., Ivankovic, S., Preussmann, R., Zulch, K. J., Mennel, H. D. (1972) Selective induction of malignant tumors of the nervous system by resorptive carcinogens. *In*: The Experimental Biology of Brain Tumors. Kirsch, W. M., Grossi-Paoletti, E., Paoletti, P. (eds.). Springfield, Illinois: Charles C. Thomas, pp. 85–147.

160. Swenberg, J. A., Koestner, A., Wechsler, W., Denlinger, R. H. (1972) Quantitative

aspects of transplacental tumor induction with ethylnitrosourea in rats. Cancer Res. 32, 2656–2660.
161. Koestner, A., Swenberg, J. A., Wechsler, W. (1971) Transplacental production with ethylnitrosourea of neoplasms of the nervous system in Sprague-Dawley rats, Am. J. Pathol. 63, 37–59.
162. Druckrey, H. (1973) Chemical structure and action in transplacental carcinogenesis and teratogenesis. *In*: Transplacental Carcinogenesis. Tomatis, L., Mohr, U. (eds.). Lyon: International Agency for Research in Cancer, IARC Scientific Publication No. 4, pp. 45–55.
163. Zeller, W. J. (1975) Problems in transplacental carcinogenesis, Indian J. Cancer 12, 12–29.
164. Rice, J. M. (1973) An overview of transplacental chemical carcinogenesis. Teratology 8, 113–126.
165. Druckrey, J., Ivankovic, S., Preussman, R. (1966) Teratogenic and carcinogenic effects in the offspring after single injection of ethylnitrosourea to pregnant rats. Nature 210, 1378–1379.
166. Zulch, K. G., Mennel, H. D. (1973) Recent results in new models of transplacental carcinogenesis in rats. *In*: Transplacental Carcinogenesis. Tomatis, L., Mohr, U. (eds.). Lyon: International Agency for Research on Cancer, IARC Scientific Publication No. 4, pp. 29–44.
167. Laquer, G. L., Spatz, M. (1973) Transplacental induction of tumors and malformations in rats with cycasin and methylazomethanol. *In*: Transplacental Carcinogenesis. Tomatis, L., Mohr, U. (eds.). Lyon: International Agency for Research on Cancer, IARC Scientific Publication No. 4, pp. 59–64.
168. Napalkov, N. P. (1973) Some general considerations on the problem of transplacental carcinogenesis. *In*: Transplacental Carcinogenesis. Tomatis, L., Mohr, U. (eds.). Lyon: International Agency for Research on Cancer, IARC Scientific Publication No. 4, pp. 1–13.
169. Ikuta, F., Zimmerman, H. M. (1965) Virus particles in reactive cells induced by intracerebral implantation of dibenzanthracene. J. Neuropathol. Exp. Neurol. 24, 225–243.
170. Grove, A. S., CiChiro, G., Rabotti, G. F. (1967) Experimental brain tumors, with a report of those induced in dogs by Rous sarcoma virus. J. Neurosurg. 26, 465–477.
171. Ogawa, K., Hamaya, K., Fujii, Y., Matsuura, K., Endo, T. (1969) Tumor induction adenovirus type 12 and its target cells in the central nervous system. Gann. 60, 383–392.
172. Mancini, L. O., Yates, V. J., Jasty, V., Anderson, J. (1969) Ependymomas induced in hamsters inoculated with an avian adenovirus (CELO). Nature 222, 190–191.
173. Yohn, D. S. (1972) Oncogenic viruses: expectations and applications in neuropathology. Prog. Exp. Tumor Res. 17, 74–92.
174. Corallini, A., Barbanti-Brodano, G., Bortoloni, W., et al. (1977) High incidence of ependymomas induced by BK virus, a human papovavirus. J. Natl. Cancer Inst. 59, 1561–1564.
175. Padgett, B. L., Walker, D. L., Zurhein, G. M., et al. (1977) JC papovavirus neurooncogenicity of strains of JC virus on human polyoma virus in newborn syrian hamsters. Cancer Res. 37, 718–720.
176. Padgett, B. L., Walker, D. L. (1976) New human papovaviruses. Prog. Med. Virol. 22, 1–35.
177. Walker, D. L., Padgett, B. L., Zurhein, G. M., et al. (1973) Human papovavirus (JC): induction of brain tumors in hamsters. Science 181, 674–676.
178. Greenlee, J. E., Becker, L. E., Narayan, D., Johnson, R. T. (1978) Failure to demonstrate papovavirus tumor antigen in human cerebral neoplasms. Ann. Neurol. 3, 479–481.
179. Ida, N., Ikawa, Y., Ogawa, K., Takada, M., Sugano, H. (1974) Cell culture from a rat

brain tumor induced by intracerebral inoculation with murine sarcoma virus, J. Natl. Cancer Inst. 53, 431–447.

180. Cloyd, M. W., Burger, P. C., Bigner, D. D. (1975) R-type virus-like particles in avian sarcoma virus-induced rat central nervous system tumors. J. Natl. Cancer Inst. 54, 1479–1482.

181. Vick, N. A., Bigner, D. D. (1975) Gliomas induced by avian sarcoma virus (ASV): early and sequential structural events of the neoplastic transformation in vivo. J. Neuropathol. Exp. Neurol. 34, 99–100.

182. Thormar, H., Lin, F. H., Karl, S. C. (1973) Effects of viral infections on the brain. *In*: Biology of Brain Dysfunction. Gaull, G. E. (eds.). New York: Plenum Press, vol. 1, pp. 191–228.

183. Garcia, J. H., Okazaki, H., Aronson, S. M. (1963) Blood-group frequencies and astrocytomata. J. Neurosurg. 20, 397–399.

184. Carter, R. L., Hitchcock, E. R., Sato, F. (1964) Malignant glioma and ABO blood group. Br. Med. J. 1, 122.

185. Selverstone, B., Cooper, D. R. (1961) Astrocytomas and ABO blood groups. J. Neurosurg. 18, 602–604.

186. Yates, P. O., Pearce, K. M. (1960) Recent change in blood-group distribution of astrocytomas. Lancet 1, 194–195.

187. Strang, R. R., Rovi, D., Lopez, J. (1966) Astrocytomas and the ABO blood groups. J. Med. Genet. 3, 274–275.

188. Kaufman, H. H., Brisman, R. (1972) Familial gliomas: report of four cases. J. Neurosurg. 37, 110–112.

189. Bromowicz, J., Araszkiewiza, H., Kinderman, B. (1971) Familial occurrence of neoplasms of the central nervous system. Neurol. Neurochir. Pol. 5, 721–725, 1971. *Cited in*: Cancer Genetics (1976) Lynch H. T. (ed). Springfield, Illinois: Charles C. Thomas, pp. 263–325.

190. Chateau, R., deRougemont, J., Groslamberg, R., Barge, M., Pasqlier, B., Faure, H. (1971) A propos des trimeurs cerebrales familiales (mengiome fibroblastique et hemangioblastome solitaire de cerbelet). J. Med. Lyon 52, 675–678. *Cited in*: Cancer Genetics (1976) (Lynch, H. T. (ed.). Springfield, Illinois: Charles C. Thomas Publisher, pp. 263–325.

191. Fairburn, B., Urich, H. (1971) Malignant gliomas occurring in identical twincs. J. Neurol. Neurosusurg. Psychiat. 34, 718–722.

192. Grunert, B., Horcajada, J., Sunder-Plassman, M. (1970) Familiares Auftreten intrakranieller meningeome. Wien Med. Wochenschr 120, 807–808. *Cited in*: Cancer Genetics (1976) Lynch, H. T. (ed.). Springfield, Illinois: Charles C. Thomas Publisher, pp. 263–325.

193. Armstrong, R. M., Hanson, C. W. (1969) Familial Gliomas. Neurology 19, 1061–1063.

194. Belamaric, J., Chau, A. S. (1969) Medulloblastoma in newborn sisters: report of two cases. J. Neurosurg. 30, 76–79.

195. Lee, D. K., Abbott, M. L. (1969) Familial gliomas. Arch. Neurol. 20, 154–160.

196. Bickerstaff, E. R., Connolly, R. C., Woolf, A. L. (1967) Cerebellar medulloblastoma occurring in brothers. Acta Neuropathol. 8, 104–107.

197. Joynt, R. J., Perret, G. E. (1965) Familial meningiomas. J. Neurosurg. Psychiat. 28, 163–164.

198. Komminoth, R., Woringer, E., Baumgartner, J., Braun, J. P., LeMaistre, D. (1965) Papillome intraventriculaire familial: caracteristique angiographiques. Neurochir. 11, 267–272. *Cited in*: Cancer Genetics (1976) Lynch, H. T. (ed.) Springfield, Illinois: Charles C. Thomas Publisher, pp. 263–325.

199. Sahar, A. (1965) Familial occurrence of meningiomas. J. Neurosurg. 23: 444–445.

200. Parkinson, D., Hall, C. W. (1962) Oligodendrogliomas: simultaneous appearance in frontal lobes of siblings. J. Neurosurg. 19, 424–426.

201. Grosz, K., Plaschkes, S. J. (1960) The occurrence of cerebral tumors in a brother and sister. Isr. Med. J. 19, 302–305.
202. Koch, G., Middendorf, E. (1960) Vorkommen von Glioblastoma Multiforme bei 3 Schwestern in Alter von 50 Bis 54 Jahren (Neuere Betrachtungen zur Ätiologie dysontogenetischer Geschwulste). Med. Welt 2, 2541–2544. *Cited in*: Cancer Genetics (1976) Lynch, H. T. (ed.). Springfield, Illinois: Charles C. Thomas Publisher, pp. 263–325.
203. Symonds, C. (1960) Disease of mind and disorder of brain. Br. Med. J. 2, 1–5.
204. Adams, J. E. (1953) Familial hemangioblastoma of the cerebellum: pedigree of two families. J. Neurosurg. 10, 421–423.
205. Tonning, H. O., Warren, R. F., Barrie, H. J. (1952) Familial hemangiomata of the cerebellum. J. Neurosurg. 9, 124–132.
206. Grossman, M. O., Kesert, B. H. (1944) Familial incidence of tumors of the brain: cerebellar hemangioblastoma. Arch. Neurol. Psychiatr. 52, 327–328.
207. Kjellin, K., Muller, R., Astrom, K. E. (1960) The occurrence of brain tumors in several members of a family. J. Neuropathol. Exp. Neurol. 10, 528–537.
208. Lynch, H. T., Krush, A. J., Harlan, W. L., Sharp, E. A. (1973) Association of soft tissue sarcoma, leukemia, and brain tumors in families affected with breast cancer. Am. Surg. 39, 199–206.
209. Harvald, B. Hauge, M. (1956) On the heredity of glioblastoma. J. Natl. Cancer Inst. 17, 289–296.
210. Hauge, M., Harvald, B. (1957) Genetics in intracranial tumors, Acta Genet. 7, 573–591.
211. Van de Wiel, H. J. (1960) Inheritance of Glioma. Amsterdam: Elsevier Publishing Co.
212. Miller, R. W. (1971) Deaths from childhood leukemia and solid tumors among twins and other sibs in the United States, 1960–67. J. Natl. Cancer Inst. 46, 203–209.
213. Miller, R. W. (1968) Deaths from childhood cancers in sibs. N. Engl. J. Med. 279, 122–126.
214. Norris, F. D. and Jackson, E. W. (1970) Childhood cancer deaths in California-born twins: a further report on types of cancer found. Cancer 25, 212–218.
215. Cooper, J. R. (1971) Brain tumors in hereditary multiple system hamartomatosis (tuberous sclerosis). J. Neurosurg. 34, 194–202.
216. Huberland, C., Perou, M. (1970) Glioma with nuclear inclusions in tuberous sclerosis. Acta Neuropathol. 16, 73–76.
217. Corkill, A. G. L., Ross, C. G. (1969) A Case of neurofibromatosis complicated by medulloblastoma. neurogenic sarcoma, and radiation-induced carcinoma of the thyroid. J. Neurol. Neurosurg. Psychiat. 32, 43–47.
218. Jamieson, K. G. (1968) Multiple intracranial tumors in neurofibromatosis: report of a case. Aust. N. Z. J. Surg. 38, 51–54.
219. Kapp, J. P., Paulson, G. W., Odom, G. L. (1967) Brain tumors with tuberous sclerosis. J. Neurosurg. 26, 191–202.
220. Rodriguez, H. A., Berthrong, M. (1966) Multiple primary intracranial tumors in von Recklinghausen's neurofibromatosis. Arch. Neurol. 14, 467–475.
221. Davidson, K. (1966) Cranial and intracranial lesions in neurofibromatosis. Am. J. Roentgenol. Radium Ther. Nucl. Med. 98, 550–556.
222. Shuster, J., Hart, Z., Stimson, C. W., Brough, A. J., Poulek, M. D. (1966) Ataxis telangiectasia with cerebellar tumor. Pediatrics 37, 776–786.
223. Brady, W. J., (1962) Brain stem gliomas causing hydrocephalus in twins with von Recklinghausen's disease, J. Neuropathol. Exp. Neurol. 21, 555–565.
224. Rudnick, P. A., Hoshino, N., Kitaoka, T., Miura, M. (1961) Tuberous sclerosis complex and astrocytoma: report of a case with successful removal of the neoplams. J.A.M.A. 178, 73–75.

225. Chapman, R. L., Kemp, V. E., Taljaferro, I. (1959) Pheochromocytoma associated with multiple neurofibromatosis and intracranial hemangioma. Am. J. Med. 26, 883–890.

226. Marshall, D. (1955) Glioma of the optic nerve: as a manifestation of von Recklinghausen's disease. Am. J. Ophthal. 37, 15–36.

227. Miller, R. W. (1968) Relation between cancer and congenital defects: an epidemiologic evaluation. J. Natl. Cancer Inst. 40, 1079–1085.

228. Miller, R. W. (1966) Relation between cancer and congenital defects in man. N. Engl. J. Med. 275, 87–93.

229. Holt, J. F. (1978) Neurofibromatosis in children, Am. J. Roentgenol. 130, 615–639.

230. Aita, J. A. (1967) Genetic aspects of tumors of the nervous system. *In* Recent Results in Cancer Research. Lynch, H. T. (ed.). New York: Springer-Verlag, Inc., vol. 12, pp. 86–110.

231. Chao, D. H. (1959) Congenital neurocutaneous syndromes in childhood. J. Pediat. 55, 189–199.

232. Lichtenstein, B. W. (1949) Neurofibromatosis (von Recklinghausen's disease of the nervous system). Arch. Neurol. Psychiat. 62, 822–839.

233. Pearce, J. (1967) The central nervous system pathology in multiple neurofibromatosis. Neurology 17, 691–697.

234. Merten, D. F., Gooding, C. A., Newton, T. H., Malamud, N. (1974) Meningiomas of childhood and adolescence. J. Pediat. 84, 696–700.

235. Reis, D. J. (1975) Degenerative and heredofamilial diseases of the central nervous system. *In*: Textbook of Medicine. Beeson, P. B., McDermott, W. (eds.). 14th edition. Philadelphia: W. B. Saunders Co., pp. 759–769.

236. Thompson, J. S., Thompson, M. W. (1973) Genetics in medicine. 2nd edition. Philadelphia: W. B. Saunders Co.

237. Gerald, P. (1975) Chromosomes and their disorders. *In*: Textbook of Medicine. Beeson, P. B., McDermott, W. (eds.). 14th edition. Philadelphia: W. B. Saunders Co., pp. 31–36.

238. Carter, C. O. (1958) A Life-table for Mongols with the Causes of Deaths, J. Ment. Def. Res. 2, 64–74.

239. Holland, W. W., Doll, R., Carter, C. O. (1962) The Mortality from Leukemia and Other Cancers Among Patients with Down's Syndrome (Mongols) and Among Their Parents, Br. J. Cancer 16, 177–186.

240. Jackson, E. W., Turner, J., Howard, K., Melville, R., Norris, F. D. (1968) Down's Syndrome: Variation of Leukemia Occurrence in Institutionalized Populations, J. Chron. Dis. 21, 247–253.

241. DeWeerdt, C. J., Schut, T. (1972) Some Aspects of Heredity of Brain Tumors, Psychiat. Neurol. Neurochir. 75, 293–298.

242. Gatti, R. A., Good, R. A. (1971) Occurrence of malignancy in immunodeficiency diseases. Cancer 28, 89–98.

243. Good, R. A. (1975) The primary immunodeficiency diseases. *In*: Textbook of Medicine. Beeson, P. B., McDermott, W. (eds.). 14th edition. Philadelphia: W. B. Saunders Co., pp. 106–109.

244. Kersey, J. H., Spector, B. D., Good, R. A. (1973) Primary immunodeficiency diseases and cancer: the immodeficiency cancer registry, Int. J. Cancer 3, 333–347.

245. Bicknell, J. M. (1967) Chromosome studies of human brain tumors. Neurology 17, 485–490.

246. Hansteen, I. L. (1967) Chromosome studies in glial tumours, Eur. J. Cancer 3, 183–191.

247. Lubs, H. A., Salmon, J. A. (1965) The chromosomal complement of human solid tumors. J. Neurosurg. 22, 160–168.

248. Abbott, M., Namiki, H. (1968) Congenital ependymoma. J. Neurosurg. 28, 162–165.

249. Barsky, P. (1968) Congenital astrocytoma: definitive diagnosis at 30 days of age, with survival. Can. Med. Assoc. J. 98, 216–217.

250. Cooperman, E., Marshall, K. G., Haust, M. D. (1967) Congenital astrocytoma. Can. Med. Assoc. J. 97, 1405–1407.

251. Fuste, F. G., Snyder, D. E., Price, A. (1967) Congenital spongioblastoma of the pons. Am. J. Clin. Pathol. 47, 790–796.

252. Duckett, S., Claireaux, A. E., Pearse, A. G. E. (1966) Histoenzymatic study of fetal medulloblastoma with associated congenital malformations. Neurology 16, 283–287.

253. Raskind, R., Beigel. F. (1964) Brain tumors in early infancy—probably congenital in origin, J. Pediat. 65, 727–732.

254. Solitaire, G. G., Krigman, M. R. (1964) Congenital intracranial neoplasm, J. Neuropathol. Exp. Neurol. 23, 280–292.

255. Sanbank, U. (1962) Congenital astrocytoma. J. Pathol. Bact. 84, 226–228.

CANCER AND OCCUPATIONAL EXPOSURE TO CHROMIUM CHEMICALS

RICHARD B. HAYES, PH.D.

CONTENTS

INTRODUCTION

Unlike many metals, chromium was unknown in antiquity. The first known chromium-containing mineral was crocoite, a brilliant, orange-red mineral; it was discovered in a Siberian gold mine about 1790. In 1797 Nicolas-Louis Vauquelin, a French chemist, described a new element found in crocoite. He emphasized that whatever reagents he used to extract the new element, the resulting filtrates were brilliantly colored: yellow, red, and green. From its colorful compounds, he named the new metallic element "chrome" from the Greek word *chroma* meaning color.

In 1798 another mineral containing chromium was found in the Ural mountains. Called chromite, this mineral appears dull and black and contains chromic and iron oxides, together with some magnesium and aluminium oxides. Chromite ore soon became and remains the source of all commercially used chromium.

Chromite was first used to make chemicals about 1800 to 1816 and was first employed as a refractory in blast furnaces in France about 1879. Intensified use of chromium as an alloy component in steel started about 1908 to 1912. These metallurgic, refractory, and chemical applications constitute the main uses of chromium ore today (1). The major chrome bearing products and their uses are shown in Figure 1.

Although other adverse health effects have been reported, this review will be primarily concerned with epidemiologic studies of cancer in humans exposed to chromium in the industrial setting. The studies will be presented according to the type of industry: metallurgic, refractory, or chemical industry. The chemical industry, which has been most extensively studied with regard to occupational carcinogenesis, will be further subdivided into the primary chromium chemical production industry, often referred to as the chromate industry, and into the secondary "user" industries including the chromate pigment production, leather tanning and chrome plating industries. As a necessary background, the chemistry and biology of chromium, the industrial methods of production, and the health effects of exposure to chromium are briefly reviewed.

Chemistry of Chromium and Its Compounds

Chromium, symbol Cr, is a transition metal having the atomic number 24 and an atomic weight of 52.0. It can occur in every one of the valence states from −2 to +6 although only 0, +2, +3, and +6 are common. Chromium in the zero valence state has been suggested (6) as possibly being bound to ribonucleic acids in the form of "sandwich complexes." There is, however, no evidence for such a role. Divalent chromic compounds have such strong reducing power that they will oxidize unless protected from air. Only the tri-

From the Municipal Health Department, and The Study Center of Social Oncology, Rotterdam, Netherlands.

This research was supported in part by grant No. 5P01 CA11489 from the National Cancer Institute, Washington, D.C. The author was the recipient of a Cancer Epidemiology Research Fellowship (5T32CA09002-03) from the National Cancer Institute.

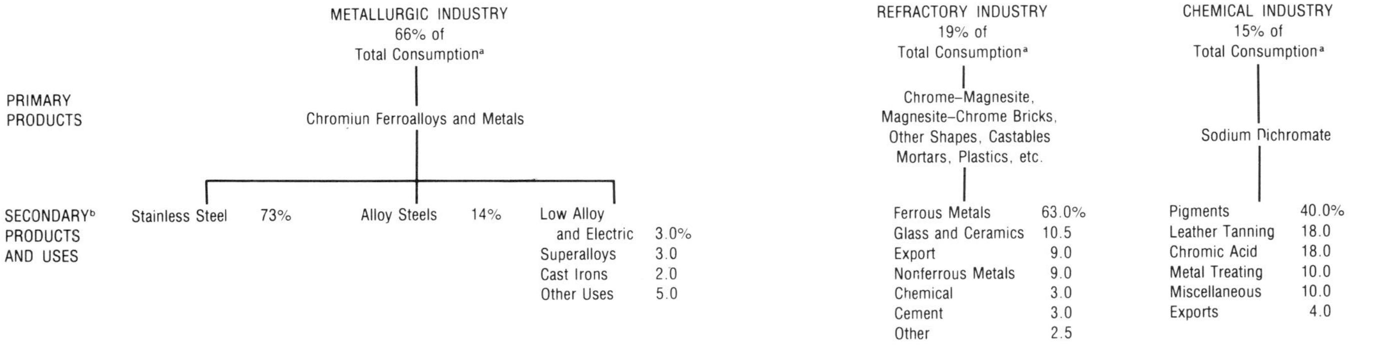

FIGURE 1. Major chrome-bearing products and their uses.

Source: Adapted in part from Charles River Associates, Inc., Economic Analysis of the Chromium Industry. Cambridge, Mass., 1970.

[a] Figures are percentages of gross weight consumption in 1973 from Minerals Yearbook, U.S. Bureau of Mines, United States Department of the Interior, Washington, D.C., 1975.

[b] Figures for secondary products and uses of ferroalloys are percentages of U.S. consumption, by end uses and consumer stocks, of chromium ferroalloys and metal in 1973, from reference 3. Figures for secondary products and uses of refractories are estimates for 1966 from Brick and Clay Record, January, 1968. Figures for secondary products and uses for the chemical industry are estimates from Chem. & Eng. News, December 3, 1962.

valent and hexavalent compounds are understood to play a role in biologic systems. The chemical and physical properties of selected trivalent and hexavalent chromium compounds are presented in Tables 1 and 2, respectively.

Trivalent Chromium. The trivalent form is the most stable oxidation state. The trivalent ion does not exist in aqueous solution due to the strong tendency of the element in this valence state to form coordination compounds, complexes and chelates. In aqueous solution, water serves as the ligand, or substrate, which combines with the trivalent chromium (10), forming octahedral complexes.

Other ligands include ammonia, urea, ethylendiamine, anions like halides and sulfate, as well as the anions of many organic acids. Many of these ligands tend to slowly replace the water from chromium. With time, the simple water-bound compounds form mixed complexes and chelates. In acidic solutions of $pH<4$, these complexes are quite stable.

Under alkaline pH conditions, OH^- will slowly replace water in the coordinated compound. Poly-nucleate complexing of chromium, formed by the bridging of hydroxo (ol) groups, is a process called olation. Because of the strong tendency of trivalent chromium for olation and consequent precipitation, Cr^{+3} can only be kept in solution when in an alkaline milieu by complex and chelate formation with ligands capable of competing with OH^- (10).

Hexavalent Chromium. The hexavalent form of chromium, almost always linked to oxygen, is a strong oxidizing agent. The important anions of hexavalent chromium are the chromates, CrO_4^{-2}, and the dichromates, $Cr_2O_7^{-2}$. The dichromates can be readily converted into monochromates in mildly alkaline solutions (11), such as blood or lymph at physiologic pH. Interconversion of these two forms reportedly (12) can also occur in the industrial environment.

The chromates appear to be relatively stable in pure water, probably due to the absence of reducing material (10). The chromates and dichromates are readily reduced to the trivalent form in acidic solution. Similarly, hexavalent forms are readily reduced after exposure to traces of organic matter. The kinetics of the oxidation potential of trivalent chromium compounds, such as chromite ore and metallic chromium dust, indicate that oxidation of these substances to the hexavalent state is unlikely.

Biologic Interactions of Chromium and Its Compounds

The biologic interactions of the chromium compounds can largely be understood in relation to their chemical properties. As typified by the process of leather tanning, hexavalent chromium when reduced to the trivalent form has the ability to extensively cross-link with proteins. The reaction of hexavalent chromium with skin also involves reduction to the trivalent form. This process of initial reduction of the hexavalent to the trivalent form and later complex formation is also thought to be the mechanism by which hexavalent chromium reacts with nucleic acids (13).

Chromium is found, in vivo, in high concentrations in nucleic acids. Although its function in nucleic acids is unknown, chromium has been shown,

TABLE 1. Chemical and Physical Properties and the Uses of Selected Trivalent Chromium Compounds

Chemical name	Synonyms	Molecular formula	Solubility		Physical properties	Uses
			Cold water	Other		
Chromium acetate	Chromic acetate	$Cr(C_2H_3O_2)_3 \cdot H_2O$	Soluble	Insoluble in alcohol	Grayish-green powder or bluish green pasty mass	Textile mordant; tanning
Chromium carbonate	Chromous carbonate	$Cr_2O_3 \cdot xCO_2 \cdot 4H_2O$	Slight	Soluble in mineral acids, insoluble in alcohol	Grayish-green amorphous mass	
Chromium oxide	Chromic oxide Chromia Chromium sequioxide Green cinnabar Chromium (III) oxide	Cr_2O_3	Insoluble	Insoluble in acids, and alkalies	Bright green crystalline powder	Metallurgy; green paint pigment; ceramics; catalyst in organic synthesis; green granules in asphalt roofing; component of refractory brick
Chromium phosphate	Chromic phosphate	a) $CrPO_4 \cdot 6H_2O$ b) $CrPO_4 \cdot 4H_2O$	Insoluble	Soluble in acids	(a) Violet crystals (b) Green crystals	Paint pigment
Chromium sulfate	Chromic sulfate Koreon	a) $Cr_2(SO_4)_3$ b) $Cr_2(SO_4)_3 \cdot 15H_2O$ c) $Cr_2(SO_4)_3 \cdot 18H_2O$	(a) Insoluble (b) Soluble (c) Soluble	Insoluble in acids Insoluble in alcohol Soluble in alcohol	(a) Violet or red powder (b) Dark green scales (c) Violet cubs	Textile industry; green paints and varnishes; green ink; ceramics; tanning

Source: Adapted from data in References 7–9.

TABLE 2. Chemical and Physical Properties and the Uses of Selected Hexavalent Chromium Compounds

Chemical name	Synonyms	Molecular formula	Solubility		Physical properties	Uses
			Cold Water	Other		
Ammonium chromate		$(NH_4)_4CrO_4$	Soluble decomposes	Insoluble in alcohol	Yellow crystals	Mordant in dyeing; photography; catalyst; corrosion inhibitor
Barium chromate	Lemon yellow Steinbuhl yellow	$BaCrO_4$	Very slight	Soluble in acids	Heavy yellow crystalline powder	Safety matches; paint pigments; ceramics; fuses; pyrotechnics; metal printers; ignition control devices
Calcium chromate		$Ca\ CrO_4{\cdot}2H_2O$ or $Ca\ CrO_4$	Moderate	Soluble in dilute acids	Bright yellow powder	Pigment; corrosion inhibitor; depolorizer for batteries; coating for light metal alloys
Chromium trioxide	Chromium (VI) oxide Chromic anhydride "Chromic acid"	CrO_3	Soluble	Soluble in acid	Dark-purplish red crystals	Chemicals (chromates, catalysts); chromium plating; medicine (caustic); process engraving; anodizing; ceramic glazes; colored glass; inks; tanning; paints; textile mordant
Lead chromate	Natural crocoite Chrome yellow	$Pb\ CrO_4$	Very slight	Soluble in strong acids	Yellow crystals	Paint pigment
Molybdenum orange	Molybdate orange	$Pb\ CrO_4$			Fine dark orange or light red powder	Pigment in printing inks, paints, plastics

Molybdenum orange (*cont.*)	Pb MoO_4 Pb SO_4			A solid solution of lead chromate, lead molybdate, and lead sulfate	
Chromium carbonyl	Cr $(CO)_6$	Insoluble		Colorless crystals, sublimes at room temperature	
Sodium chromate	$Na_2CrO_4 \cdot 10H_2O$	Soluble	Soluble in acid	Yellow, translucent, efflorescent crystals	Inks; dying; paint pigment; leather tanning; other chromates; anti-corrosive; wood preservative
Sodium chromate, tetrahydrate	$Na_2CrO_4 \cdot 4H_2O$	Soluble	Soluble in acid	Yellow crystals	Pigment manufacture; corrosion inhibitor; leather tanning; other chromium compounds
Sodium dichromate	$Na_2Cr_2O_7 \cdot 2H_2O$	Soluble	Soluble in acid	Red or red-orange deliquescent crystals	Chromic acid; corrosion inhibitor, tanning; electroplating; mordanting
Strontium chromate	$SrCrO_4$	Slight	Soluble in acid	Light yellow pigment	Metal protective coatings; polyvinyl chloride resins to produce pastel primrose yellows; pyrotechnics

(continued)

TABLE 2. Chemical and Physical Properties and the Used of Selected Trivalent Chromium Compounds (*continued*)

Chemical name	Synonyms	Molecular formula	Solubility		Physical properties	Uses
			Cold water	Other		
Potassium chromate	Yellow potassium chromate; Neutral potassium chromate	K_2CrO_4	Soluble	Soluble in acid	Yellow crystals	Reagents; aniline black; textile mordant; enamels; chromate pigments; inks; medicine; fungicide; leather finishing; chromium compounds
Potassium dichromate	Red potassium chromate; Potassium bichromate	$K_2Cr_2O_7$	Soluble	Soluble in acid	Yellowish red transparent crystals	Oxidizing agent; analytic reagent; brass pickling; electroplating; pyrotechnics; explosives; safety matches; textiles; dying and printing; tanning; poison fly paper; photography; synthetic perfumes; chrome alum; ceramics; alloys
Zinc chromate		$ZnCrO_4$	Insoluble	Soluble in acid	Yellow powder	Artists' color; varnishes; linoleum; pigment in rust-resistant primer and automative paints
Zinc potassium chromate	Zinc yellow; Zinc chrome; Citron yellow; Buttercup yellow	$4ZnO{\cdot}K_2O{\cdot}4Cr_2O_3{\cdot}3H_2O$ (approx.)	Partial	Soluble in acid	Greenish yellow pigment	Artists' color; rust-inhibiting paints

Source: Adapted from data in References 7–9.

among other transition elements, to stabilize, in vitro, the ordered structure of RNA (14).

Hexavalent chromium compounds have the ability to pass readily through biologic membranes, making the chromates useful compounds for the labeling of erythrocytes. After entering the cells, the chromate is reduced and bound to hemoglobin, forming a stable marker. Similarly, hexavalent compounds are readily absorbed from the lung, whereas trivalent compounds dissipate slowly from this site. The rate of dissipation is related to the solubility of the compounds.

Chromium compounds are stored in various organs. Chromium concentrations in the lungs are among the highest in the body and they do not decrease with age, as has been reported for other organs (13). Particularly high concentrations of chromium have been described in the lungs of men who had been employed in old chromium chemical manufacturing plants (15). It has been suggested (11) that such depots, of presumably trivalent chromium, may serve as a source of hexavalent chromium, although the kinetics of the necessary oxidation reaction, as mentioned above, would seem to make this unlikely.

Several authors (10,16) have suggested that chromium, in the trivalent form, may be a necessary substance utilized in the regulation of glucose metabolism. A relationship between chromium ingestion and lipid metabolism has also been suggested (17,18).

Industrial Methods of Production

Chromite ore is the only commercial source of chromium for the industrial production of chromium bearing products. The production of metallurgic products accounts for over 60% of the chromite ore consumed. Virtually all the chromium used in metallurgic applications is added in the smelting process to steel to form chromium ferroalloys. The chromium used in the metallurgic industry is mainly trivalent, or in the zero valence state.

The second major consumer of chromite ore is the refractory brick industry. The iron and steel industry are, in turn, the major consumers of refractory brick. Chromite is used in the production of bricks for the blast furnaces because of its high melting point (3600°F), stability at high temperatures and chemical neutrality. Because of the change from the open-hearth to the basic oxygen converter process in the steel industry, it is expected that there will be less demand for chrome refractory brick in the future (2).

The manufacture of refractory bricks consists of crushing and drying refractory grade chromite ore, milling and grinding the ore, mixing and mulling the finely divided ore with sulfuric acid, and then molding the mixture into bricks. The chromium used in the refractory industry is trivalent, in the form of chromite ore.

The third major use of chromite ore is in the primary production of chromium chemicals (see Figure 1). The products of the chromium chemical industry are derived from the treatment of chromite ore to produce hexavalent chromates and dichromates. Briefly, the industrial process consists of roasting a finely milled mixture of chromite ore, soda ash, and a variable proportion of lime to produce water soluble sodium chromate and a complex mixture of chromium-containing compounds as well as compounds of aluminum, iron, silicate, magnesium, and other trace compounds. Sodium chromate is separated from the residue materials by a water leaching process. The leachate is then converted by acidification and crystallization into crystalline sodium dichromate. Other chromium bearing products and by-products are produced by treatment and recovery from the primary process. The useful end-products include sodium chromate, sodium dichromate, potassium dichromate, chromium sulfate, chromic acid, and various other minor products.

The proportion of primary U.S. chromium chemical production which went to various secondary uses in 1962 is shown in Figure 1. Pigment production accounted for about 40% of the consumption of chromium chemicals. The chromate pigment industry uses hexavalent sodium dichromate as the primary chromium bearing raw material. Lead chromate and zinc chromate pigments are the major end-products, which are used mainly for exterior and interior paints.

Chemicals for the tanning of leather and the preparation of chromic acid, which is mainly used for electroplating, each accounted for an additional 18% of chromium chemical consumption in the United States in 1962 (see Figure 1). The tanning process starts with a solution of hexavalent chromium to which a reducing agent is added. Through a complex chemical reaction, the hide or skin is converted into leather. Electroplating is the process of electrodeposition of a metallic ion onto a metal. In chrome plating, a solution of hexavalent chromic acid with a trace of sulphuric acid as catalyst is used. The process was established on a commercial basis in 1935. Since then the industry has expanded considerably. Metal treating, for the prevention of corrosion, and other miscellaneous uses accounted for the remaining consumption of chromium chemicals (see Figure 1). Most of these chemicals are also of the hexavalent form.

Health Effects of Exposure to Chromium

Since the earliest period of its use, it has been recognized that workers exposed to chromium in the industrial setting have suffered adverse health effects. Of the three industries using chromium (the metallurgic, refractory, and chemical industries), the chromium chemical industry has been most strongly associated with health hazards. There are several conditions which occur frequently in workers who produce and handle chromium chemicals, including ulcerations of the skin and nose and perforation of the nasal septum. These effects have been attributed to the oxidative effects of hexavalent chromium compounds, particularly the chromates. Asthmatic reactions, contact dermatitis, and other conditions have also been reported (13,19).

Beginning with two cases of lung cancer diagnosed in 1911 and 1912, a series of cases of cancer of the respiratory system have been reported among chromium chemical production workers. Several later epidemiologic studies consistently demonstrated that workers in the production and handling of chromium chemicals do experience an increased risk of developing respiratory cancer. Although the exact identity of the compound or compounds responsible is still unknown, the evidence indicates that the carcinogenic compounds are all hexavalent compounds. Whether all or only a subclass of the hexavalent chromium compounds have carcinogenic properties is an unsettled point of considerable practical interest.

Hueper (20) in 1966 reviewed the evidence related to chromium exposure and cancers of the respiratory system. He listed in detail the population groups with occupational and environmental exposure to chromium. In 1974 an extensive review of the medical and biological effects of chromium was published (13). Reviews of the effects of occupational exposure to hexavalent chromium (21) and to chromic acid (22) were also published at about this time.

Recent studies in the chromium chemical production industry and in other industries where chromium is used, as well as recent experimental data, make a review of occupational exposure to chromium and carcinogenesis at this time pertinent. In this review, the emphasis will be on the epidemiologic evidence for the carcinogenicity of chromium and its various compounds. Experimental data as they relate to the interpretation of the epidemiologic studies will be discussed.

EPIDEMIOLOGIC STUDIES

The epidemiologic studies of occupational exposure to chromium and the risk of developing cancer are here reviewed by types of industry. In the interest of brevity, the major aspects of these studies are presented in tabular form. The study population, method of follow-up, comparison population and the results with regard to respiratory cancer and other cancers are described (see Tables 1–5).

Metallurgic Industry

Although more than half of the chromite ore used in industrial production is consumed by the metallurgic industry, until recently there have been no studies of the risk of cancer among workers employed in this industry. Interest in this had perhaps been lacking because the major exposure is to chromium in the trivalent, or in the zero valence state.

Pokrovskaya and Shabynina (23) in 1973 reviewed the causes of death among workers employed in a chromium ferroalloy plant of a Russian city. According to the city death rates for comparison, there was reported to be an excess of deaths due to malignancies of the lung and of all sites combined, for both men and women employees (see Table 3). Although these workers were mainly exposed to trivalent chromium compounds, there was also exposure to hexavalent chromium in concentrations exceeding the permissible quantity and to 3,4-benzpyrene, as contaminants in the industrial process.

Axelsson and Rylander (personal communication) in a preliminary report have described the mortality among employees of a Swedish ferrochromium industry (see Table 3). They found no increase in observed tumors in relation to the expected number for all workers. There was also no significant gradient in cancer risk with respect to place of work or calendar time of employ-

TABLE 3. Summary of Industry-Based Epidemiologic Studies of Cancer in Workers Employed in the Chromium Ferroalloy and Refractory Brick Industries

Author (reference)	Study population	Follow-up	Respiratory cancer: Number of cases	Respiratory cancer: Estimate of relative risk	Other cancers: Site	Other cancers: Number of cases	Other cancers: Estimate of relative risk	Comparison population
			CHROMIUM FERROALLOY INDUSTRY					
Pokrovskaya and Shabynina (23), 1973	Workers employed in a Russian chromium ferroalloy iron smelting plant between 1955 and 1969	Death certification from city archives	[a]	3.2	Stomach	[a]	6.6[b]	Cancer mortality rates for the city in which the plant was located
					Esophagus	[a]	2.0[b]	
					All sites	[a]	3.3[b]	
Axelsson and Rylander (personal communication)	Males employed for at least one year during 1930 to 1975 in a Swedish ferroalloy industry	Deaths reported since 1951 to the National Bureau of Statistics	5	0.7	All other sites	65	0.9	Cancer mortality rates for the county in which the plant was located
			CHROMIUM REFRACTORY BRICK INDUSTRY					
USPHS (24), 1952	Workers employed, between 1937 and 1950, in one plant which produced chromite refractory brick	Death certificates available from the plant. No further tracing	1	0.1	Stomach	1	n.r.[c]	Cancer mortality rates for U.S. males
					Testes	1	n.r.	

[a]Number of cases not reported. The results presented here are for males age 50–59.

[b]$P < 0.05$, calculated using an assumption that the observed number of deaths is distributed as a Poisson random variable.

[c]n.r. = not reported.

ment. These investigators also report that there was exposure to hexavalent chromium at this worksite, although the major exposure was to chromium of trivalent and zero valence.[1]

Refractory Brick Industry

The one available report of the health of workers in the refractory brick industry (24) is part of a larger study of workers in the chromium chemical producing industry. Actually, this mortality study of refractory brick workers was undertaken to serve as a control for the analysis of mortality among the chromium chemical workers. The death certificates of all employees of the plant were analysed. Forty-three deaths were recorded from 1937 to 1950. Three cases of cancer were identified: a cancer of the testes, a stomach cancer and a lung cancer. The authors state that 9 lung cancers would have been expected if the death rate for United States males had applied.

Little information was presented about the completeness of ascertainment of the worker population or of their mortal outcome. As only five deaths were found to have been due to diseases of the heart, whereas 27 would have been expected, the thoroughness of the follow-up or the means of data analysis may be open to question (see Table 3).

Chromium Chemical Industry

Early Reports of Cancer. The first two cases of lung cancer among workers exposed to chromium were observed in 1911 and 1912. These workers were employed at Ludwigshafen, Germany, where dichromates were produced to be used for oxidizing anthracene and its derivatives into compounds with a quinone structure, in the manufacture of alizarin dyes. These cases, however, were not reported until 1932 when Lehmann (25) concluded that the cases were too few to be significant, that isolated cases occurred in all classes of workers, and that the increase of cancers of all kinds was partly due to better diagnostic methods, to the increased proportion of the elderly in the population and to the successful lowering of other causes of death, especially tuberculosis. Several other cases, however, were reported in the German literature during subsequent years.

Baetjer (26), in reviewing the literature as of 1948, stated that "at least 52 cases of cancer of the respiratory tract have been reported among the workers in the chromate producing plants of Germany." The recorded evidence on the occurrence of these respiratory occupational cancer hazards in Germany up to 1952 was reviewed by Spannagel (27), who reported a total of 86 lung cancer cases and four nasal sinus cancers among German chromium chemical and chromate pigment workers.

The suggestion that some occupational factor, to which chromium chemical workers were exposed, was responsible for the development of bronchiogenic carcinoma first appeared in the German literature, but there was insufficient

[1] Langard et al. [Brit. J. Ind. Med. (in press)] have reported an excess of lung cancer among Norwegian ferrochromium workers.

information to compute incidence or mortality rates. The diagnosis of many cases was also incomplete, and a number of cases were exposed to other substances, some of which may have been carcinogenic, such as anthracene and its derivatives. The cases were reported sporadically, and there was no analysis of the prevalence of cancer in the industry as compared with other industrial workers of the same age and sex.

Epidemiologic Studies. The first case of lung cancer in a chromium chemical producer in the United States was recognized in 1946 as the result of litigation (20). In response, the chromium chemical production industry in the United States employed Willard Machle (28) to assess the problem in their plants. The study results indicated that chromium chemical production employees were at an excess risk of developing respiratory cancer (see Table 4).

One plant handling only dichromates, chromic acid, and a tanning compound, had an experience of 1,853 male-years of exposure with 33 deaths, none of which was due to cancer of the respiratory system. This experience suggested to the authors that the monochromates may be the compounds responsible for lung cancer.

Although the data used by Machle and Gregorius were the best available, they had certain inherent limitations: (1) the conclusions as to the cause of death for the study group were based in some cases on clinical findings only; (2) the control groups were not comparable in a number of respects to the study groups; (3) reliance on proportional mortality and crude death rates can be misleading; and (4) workers who left the chromate industry were not included.

Baetjer (29) compared the proportion of individuals having a recorded history of occupational exposure to chromates among histopathologically confirmed cases of lung cancer and several control series in two Baltimore hospitals. Eleven of the 290 lung cancer patients had had an occupational exposure to chromium compounds, whereas none of the 902 control series patients had had such an exposure reported. Ten of the 11 lung cancer cases with a history of exposure had been employed in the Baltimore chromium chemical production plant. When individuals who lived outside of Baltimore or who did not have an occupation specified in the medical record were excluded, seven of 75 cases and none of 88 controls had a history of chromate exposure. Possible differences between the case and control series with regard to race, differential rate of admission to the hospitals, and differential reporting of occupational history were considered and thought not to influence the conclusions. Other factors, such as smoking history and socioeconomic status, were not included in the analysis.

Mancusco (30) and Mancusco and Hueper (31) reported the results of a follow-up study of all employees who had worked for 1 year or more at a chromium chemical production facility in Ohio (see Table 4). The findings were based upon a proportionate mortality analysis. Apparently, differences in age distribution between the study population and the controls were not considered. From detailed job histories, they assigned a weighted average exposure to soluble and insoluble chromium compounds for the study group. As only a small proportion of all workers were predominantly exposed to soluble chromium and none of the lung cancer deaths had been predominantly

TABLE 4. Summary of Industry-Based Epidemiologic Studies of Cancer in Workers Employed in the Chromium Chemical Producing Industry

Author (reference)	Study population	Follow-up	Respiratory cancer: Number of cases	Respiratory cancer: Estimate of relative risk	Other cancers: Site	Other cancers: Number of cases	Other cancers: Estimate of relative risk	Comparison population
Machle and Gregorius (28), 1948	Employment records available for 4 to 17 years prior to 1948, for 6 of the 7 U.S. chromate plants	Mortality based upon life insurance claims of active workers. Those who left the industry were excluded	32	29[a]	Digestive tract	13	2[a]	Cancer mortality rates of male employees of an oil refining company, 1933–1938
					Oral region	3	5.4[a]	
Mancusco and Hueper (31), 1951	Workers employed 1 year or more, between 1931 and 1949, in an Ohio chromate plant	Mortality based upon death certificates for workers, including those who left the industry	6	15[a]	Not reported			Proportionate mortality, 1937–1947 among males 15 years of age and over, for county in which the plant was located
USPHS (24), 1952	Members of sick-benefit plans for 2 to 8 years prior to 1948, for 6 of the 7 U.S. chromate plants	Mortality based upon death certification for death benefits. Disabled workers remained eligible for only 1 year. No further follow-up of workers who left the industry	26	29[a]	All other sites	6	1.0	Average cancer mortality rates for U.S. males, 1940–1948

TABLE 4. Summary of Industry-Based Epidemiologic Studies of Cancer in Workers Employed in the Chromium Chemical Producing Industry (*continued*)

Author (reference)	Study population	Follow-up	Respiratory cancer: Number of cases	Respiratory cancer: Estimate of relative risk	Other cancers: Site	Other cancers: Number of cases	Other cancers: Estimate of relative risk	Comparison population
Bidstrup and Case (34) 1956	Workers employed, in November 1949, in 3 chromate plants in Great Britain	Mortality, based upon death certification, until September 1955. Workers who left the industry (30%) were not followed	12	3.6[a]	All other sites	9	1.1	Cancer mortality rates for males in England and Wales, 1951–1959
Taylor (35), 1966	Workers employed, between 1937 and 1940, in 3 U.S. chromate plants and having earnings reported to OASDI	Mortality, based upon death certification, until December, 1960, of deceased who had death-benefit claims filed with OASDI	71	8.6[a]	All other sites	32	1.3	Cancer mortality rates for U.S. males, 1950 1953, 1958
Watanabe and Fukuchi (37), 1975	Workers employed more than 9 years in the Japanese chromate industry	Mortality, based upon death certification and hospital records. Follow-up from 1960–1973	5	15.1[a]	Not reported			Cancer mortality rates for Japan 1960–1971

Hayes et al. (40), 1979	Workers initially employed between 1945 and 1974 in a U.S. chromate plant, and employed 90 days or more	Mortality, based upon death certification, until July 1977, including those who left the industry	59	2.0[a]	All other sites	27	0.5	Cancer mortality rates for Baltimore, Maryland, the city in which the plant was located
	Employed 3 years or more in a new plant with improved hygiene standards		3	4.0[a]	Not reported			

[a] $P < 0.05$, calculated on the assumption that the observed number of deaths is distributed as a Poisson random variable.

exposed to soluble chromium, they concluded that the data "suggest that the inhalation of dust of chromite ore [i.e., insoluble chromium] might not be without importance in the causation of lung cancer (31)". This inference rests upon the observed predominance of exposure to insoluble chromium for both diseased and non-diseased study members rather than upon considerations of relative risk.

The U.S. Public Health Service (USPHS) reported upon the clinical and environmental findings of an investigation of the six U.S. plants producing chromates and dichromates in 1950 (24,32). Part of this study dealt with an analysis of the prior cancer morbidity and mortality of workers in these plants. Disability and death from cancer were based on assessment of the experience of members of sick and death benefit plans (see Table 4). Studying the same industry for part of the same time period and with a similar design, the conclusions with regard to mortality were similar to those of Machle and Gregorius (28).

The complete report of the USPHS (24) presented weighted average exposures by job classification to various suspected products in the chromate producing process. This information was only used in discussing the exposure experience of the ten lung cancer cases with known exposure. Several suggestions were made in that discussion. In contrast to the results reported by Mancusco and Hueper (31), the workers exposed to chromite ore were at low risk; exposure to the water soluble hexavalent compounds implied a low risk because of their rapid dissipation; exposure to the largely insoluble trivalent products implied low risk; but the acid-soluble, water-insoluble byproducts found in the roast and in the residue were largely responsible for the increased risk of lung cancer. As the distribution of job histories among noncases was not considered in the analysis of this study it is difficult to determine whether an excess risk was really associated with certain jobs. In any event, the suggestion that the excess risk was associated with acid-soluble, water-insoluble compounds was based upon theoretical considerations of chemical activity.

Bidstrup (33) interviewed and took chest x-rays of more than 90% of the 786 chromium chemical production workers in Great Britain, in 1949. Bidstrup and Case (34), in 1956, reported the results of a follow-up of the workers surveyed by Bidstrup (33). An attempt was made to follow the remaining 723 persons from the time of the original survey for a period of 5 years and 10 months. They concluded that workers in the chromium chemical production industry were at excess risk of carcinoma of the lung (see Table 4). They stated that the risk estimate should not be considered final, as the workers had only been followed for a short period of time. They also discussed the difficulty of explaining the increased risk by place of residence, social class and smoking habits, although no direct measurement of these variables was analysed.

Taylor (35) identified all males born after 1890 who had worked in one of three U.S. chromate plants between January 1, 1937, and December 1, 1940, and who had earnings reported to the Old-Age and Survivors Disability Insurance (OASDI) of the Social Security Administration. As the chromium chemical production plants were among the industries "covered" under the Social

Security Act of 1936, all workers who had been employed one or more calendar quarters were presumed to have been included (see Table 4).

Taylor attempted to relate survivorship to level of exposure, as approximated by the length of time worked. OASDI provided information on the length of employment of the employees from January 1, 1937, onward. Because no information was available concerning duration of work before 1937, he assumed that the unknown portion of employment in the chromate industry for older workers prior to January 1, 1937, could be estimated from the observed age at initial employment of the younger workers. Using this assumption, Taylor showed that age-specific survivorship decreased with increasing duration of work. The excess mortality was observed for "all causes" including, specifically, cardiovascular disease, respiratory disease, and cancer. Age-specific mortality from respiratory cancer contributed substantially to the increase in mortality with increase in duration of employment. However, the possibility that a bias had been introduced by the analytic procedures used is not adequately resolved in the report. The mortality of study members was based solely upon OASDI claims, whereas the comparison rates were based upon U.S. mortality experience. Discrepancies in the completeness of reporting may have biased the estimates of the excess mortality risk.

Enterline (36) in 1974 reported a reanalysis of the Taylor (35) study. He found that of 246 deaths, 99 were due to cancer, 69 of which were of the respiratory system. Two of these neoplasms were of the maxillary sinuses, a number greatly in excess of that expected based on the experience of the United States male population. Digestive cancers were reported to be slightly higher; 16 observed deaths where 10.4 were expected. Enterline pointed out that the data, "when examined by follow-up period, shows a great improvement in mortality as time since the cohort was first identified increased." This improvement in Standardized Mortality Ratios (SMR) may, in part, be artifactual as it was found for all causes of death, for respiratory cancer and "curiously this decline also shows up for some other causes. Mortality for heart disease, for example, declined from an SMR of 148.5 to 67.9." It should also be noted that this reported decrease in relative mortality can not directly be associated with changes in industrial hygiene conditions, as the members of the cohort may or may not have continued to work in the chromium chemical industry after 1940.

Watanabe and Fukuchi (37) briefly described a study of 136 workers employed in the Japanese chromate producing industry for more than 9 years. The period of observation was 1960 to 1973. The dates and confirmed causes of death were ascertained from death certificates and hospital records (see Table 4).

Maltoni (38) has reported that of 69 Italian chromate and dichromate production workers, 91% had signs of squamous metaplasia upon examination by sputum cytology. Twenty-two percent showed signs of squamous dysplasia. Little information was given in this brief report to corroborate these findings.

Bigaliev et al. (39) reported finding a significant increase of chromosome aberrations, as assayed in peripheral blood lymphocytes, among Russian workers engaged in chromium chemical production.

Hayes et al. (40) reported a study of workers newly employed between 1945 and 1974 in a U.S. chromium chemical production plant. An attempt was made to trace all males employed for 90 days of more. The vital status ascertainment was about 88 percent. The major purpose of the study was to determine whether workers exclusively employed in a newly constructed facility, designed to reduce exposure to hazardous chemicals, were at a reduced risk of respiratory cancer as compared to workers employed at about the same period of time in an old production facility. As compared to previous studies in the U.S. chromium chemical industry, which had included this study plant (24,28,29,35), the risk for respiratory cancer among the entire study sample was considerably lower, although the observed rate was still significantly higher than that expected based upon comparison population mortality rates. With regard to employment in the new production facility, the results indicate that the occupational environment in the study plant was not sufficiently changed by the improved hygiene measures to eliminate the excess risk of lung cancer. This particular result is based upon small numbers (see Table 4).

Comparisons were made of the association between cancer of the lung and a history of ever having worked in specific job positions, for cases and matched controls. It was reported that workers who had ever been employed in the Soda-Bichromate and Special Products areas of the plant, where mainly water soluble hexavalent materials were handled, were at excess risk for lung cancer. However, many of these workers had not been employed exclusively in these areas.

Secondary User Industries of Chromium Chemicals

Although the carcinogenic effect of chromium compounds in the chromium chemical producing industry has been reported over the last several decades, there had been until recently a dearth of information about the situation in the user's side of the chromium chemical industry. Reports of epidemiologic studies of workers in the chromate pigment and in the chrome plating industry have recently become available.

Chromate Pigment Industry. Newman (41) in 1890 described an adenocarcinoma of the inferior turbinate of the nose in a worker producing chromate pigment. Baetjer (26) in 1950, in reviewing the literature, reported 11 cases of pulmonary carcinoma in the German chromate pigment industry.

Langard and Norseth (42) in 1975 published the first epidemiologic study of the carcinogenic effects of workers' exposure to chromate pigments. The company studied was established in Norway in 1948. From 1948 to 1951 production consisted of only lead chromate pigment. From 1951 to 1956 both lead chromate and zinc chromate were produced; since 1956 the only product has been zinc chromate pigment. Although the study sample was small, an excess of respiratory cancer was observed (see Table 5).

An epidemiologic study of workers in U.S. chromate pigment plants was conducted in 1976 by Equitable Environmental Health, Inc. (43), for the Dry Colors Manufacturing Association. A population of 577 male workers who had been exposed to the relatively insoluble lead chromate for at least 6 months at some time before 1974 was identified. These men had worked in three lead chromate production facilities, one of which also produced zinc chromate, an insoluble hexavalent compound. Mortality follow-up was ascertained only from death benefit claims to the Social Security Administration (see Table 5).

Maltoni (38,44) has reported the frequency of individuals with cellular atypias, among workers exposed to chromium pigment compounds in one Northern Italian factory. By cytological examination of the sputum, 89% of 47 examined workers were reported to have squamous metaplasia and 10% to have squamous dysplasia (38). Little information was given in these brief reports to corroborate the findings.

Davies (45) has recently reported the results of a mortality study in three English factories manufacturing chromate pigments. In two factories both lead and zinc chromate pigments were produced, whereas in the third factory only lead chromate pigments were manufactured (see Table 5). Exposure for as little as 1 year was found to be associated with increased mortality. The author stated that the absence of excess lung cancer at the factory where only lead chromate pigments were manufactured suggested that zinc chromate pigments may be the responsible carcinogens.

Chrome Plating Industry. Since this industry was established on a commercial scale it has grown considerably, yet the possible carcinogenic effect of repeated inhalation of the highly soluble hexavalent chromic acid has only recently been explored in epidemiologic studies.

Royle (46) in 1975 reported on a study of past and current workers in 54 British chromium plating plants. The workers to be followed were individually matched to non-exposed workers by sex, and age when last known to be alive, as evidenced, in the case of past workers, by the date of leaving their place of work. In addition, the results of the initial two years of a prospective study of identified workers was reported (see Table 6). The method of matching and the analytic technique used make the results difficult to interpret with regard to the extent of exposure and subsequent risk of cancer. The prospective study is being continued (personal communication).

Waterhouse (47) in a brief note in 1975 described interim results from an ongoing study of some 5,000 workers who had been employed by a single large British chromium plating factor since 1946. With about 80 percent of the workers traced, respiratory cancer appeared to be significantly in excess in male workers only, although the relative risk was only 1.4 (see Table 6). Unfortunately, the study had to be discontinued (personal communication).

Okubo and Tsuchiya (48) recently reported the results of a study of workers in 589 Tokyo chromium plating firms. Given incomplete reporting from the management of the firms and a short period of follow-up, it is difficult to draw conclusions from this study (see Table 6).

Chromium Exposure in Other Industrial Settings

Tsuchiya (49) reported on lung cancer mortality among workers in a large sample of Japanese industries; two hundred enterprises, with more than 1,000 employees each, were sampled. The total number of workers studied was about 400,000 each year, for the 3 year period 1957 to 1959. Health supervi-

TABLE 5. Summary of Industry-Based Epidemiologic Studies of Cancer in Workers Employed in the Chromate Pigment Industry

Author (reference)	Study population	Follow-up	Respiratory cancer: Number of cases	Respiratory cancer: Estimate of relative risk	Other cancers: Site	Other cancers: Number of cases	Other cancers: Estimate of relative risk	Comparison population
Langard and Norseth (42), 1975	24 workers with more than 3 years employment in a Norwegian chromate pigment plant which produced lead and zinc chromate	Norwegian cancer registry, 1951–1972	3	38.0[a]	Gastro-intestinal system	1	n.r.[b]	Cancer incidence rates for Norwegian males, 1955–1971
					Nasal	1	n.r.	
Equitable Environmental Health, Inc. (43), 1976	Workers hired before 1960, employed 10 years or more, and exposed to lead chromate only	Mortality, based upon death certification, as reported to OASDI	2	2	Digestive system	0	n.r.	Cancer mortality rates for U.S. males and for counties where plants were located
	Workers hired before 1960, employed 10 years or more, and exposed to lead and zinc chromate		6	2.5[a]	Digestive system	6	2.1	

Davies (45), 1978	Males initially employed at 3 chromate pigment plants at or after the time of beginning follow-up	Deaths reported to the N.H.S. Cancer registry, to mid-1977			Not reported	Cancer mortality rates for England and Wales, adjusted for area and social class
	Zinc and lead chromate					
	High and medium exposure		25	2.6[a]		
	Low exposure		2	1.0		
	Lead chromate exposure		2	0.7		

[a]$P < 0.05$, calculated using an assumption that the observed number of deaths is distributed as a Poisson random variable.

[b]n.r. = not reported.

TABLE 6. Summary of Industry-Based Epidemiologic Studies of Cancer in Workers Employed in the Chromium Plating Industry

			Respiratory cancer		Other cancers			
Author (reference)	Study population	Follow-up	Number of cases	Estimate of relative risk	Site	Number of cases	Estimate of relative risk	Comparison population
Royle (46), 1975	Current and former workers, employed greater than 3 months, in 54 British chromium plating plants	"Retrospective" tracing of deaths of current and former workers	17	1.7[a,b]	Gastro-intestinal	9	2.4[a,b]	Non-exposed workers individually matched on age sex, and when last known to be alive
					Other sites	13	1.9[a,b]	
		"Prospective" analysis for 2 years of identified population	7	2.3[a,b]	Gastro-intestinal	2	[c]	
					Other sites	3	[c]	

Waterhouse (47), 1975	About 5000 male and female workers employed since 1946 in a British chromium plating factory	Incomplete, about 80% traced	49[d]	1.4[b]	Not reported			Mortality analysis, method not specified
Okubo and Tsuchiya (48), 1977	Workers with 6 or more months of employment in the Tokyo chromium plating industry and registered with a health insurance society between 1970 and 1976	Reports from management of the plating firms (70% response) and follow-up of retirees	0	[e]	Other sites	5	0.5	Tokyo mortality rates. Also compared experience of "non exposed" clerical and unskilled workers

[a]Relative risk based upon the ratio of deaths observed in the exposed and non-exposed groups.

[b]$P < 0.05$, calculated using an assumption that the observed number of deaths is distributed as a Poisson random variable.

[c]No cases observed in the non-exposed group.

[d]Male employees only.

[e]Expected 1.2 cases.

sors at the individual plants were asked to report all deaths from cancer and to specify the major products of the company and other chemical substances used by the company, with special reference to carcinogens used in appreciable amounts. During the studied time period, 22 cancer deaths were reported for persons in industries using chromium and nickel. There was no way of ascertaining whether the individual lung cancer deaths were actually exposed to these compounds, only whether the compounds were reported to be used in the companies where they were employed (see Table 7).

Korallus et al. (50) studied the causes of death of men working in German plants involved in the production of trivalent chromium compounds. Because of the limited methods of case ascertainment and analysis, the findings are difficult to assess (see Table 7).

Summary

All of the studies summarized in the tables are basically similar in design. Workers employed in specific plants have been identified, their health outcomes have been determined, and these outcomes have been compared to an "expected" outcome. In evaluating the conclusions of the individual studies these aspects of study design and execution should be considered.

With regard to the identification of the study group, workers have generally been identified from plant records, although lists of membership in sick benefit plans (24,48) and records of reported earnings to the OASDI of the Social Security Administration (35) have also been used. Most of the studies have included both employees active as of a certain date and subsequent new employees as eligible members of the study group. In the study by Hayes et al. (40), and apparently in the one by Davies (45), only workers newly employed after a certain date were included in the study group. Several of the studies only included workers who had been employed for at least a specified period of time, ranging in the various studies from 90 days to 10 years. The definition of the study groups is important in regard to the generalizations which can be drawn from their findings.

The method of follow-up and case ascertainment has varied considerably among the studies reviewed. Some studies have only followed workers during their period of employment or for limited periods of time thereafter (24,28,34,49,50). In other studies, a single limited source of information has been used (35,43). In some of these studies (40,47), follow-up was incomplete. Often the percent follow-up is not specified, or it is assumed to be complete, such as when national registry systems were used for case finding. This latter assumption relies upon the completeness of the respective registries. Disease outcome has been ascertained by identification of incident disease cases and/or by identification of deaths. Various forms of verification of ascertained cases have been used. The length of time for follow-up, considering disease latency, and the thoroughness of case ascertainment have a direct bearing on the estimates of the risk of developing disease.

The health experience of workers has been compared to that of individuals in special health surveys (28) and to that of other industrial workers (28,46). The suitability and stability of the comparison rates should be considered. Local and national morbidity and mortality data have generally been used for

TABLE 7. Summary of Industry-Based Epidemiologic Studies of Cancer in Workers Employed in "Other" Industries

Author (reference)	Study population	Follow-up	Respiratory cancer: Number of cases	Respiratory cancer: Estimate of relative risk	Other cancers: Site	Other cancers: Number of cases	Other cancers: Estimate of relative risk	Comparison population
Tsuchiya (49), 1965	Workers employed between 1957 and 1959 in 200 large Japanese industries. Chemical use determined by questionnaire to factory "health supervisors"	Report of cancer deaths by plant "health supervisors"	22[a]	2.0[b]				Cancer mortality rates, Japan 1958. Crude rates for age 20–59
Korallus et al. (50), 1974	Workers employed in German factories where only trivalent chromium is handled	Factory records of illness. No further follow-up of workers who left the industry	3	—	Stomach	4	—	None

[a]Deaths reported among workers employed in industries where chromium and nickel was reported to be handled.

[b]$P < 0.05$, calculated using an assumption that the observed number of deaths is distributed as a Poisson random variable.

analytic purposes which again raises issues of comparability. Statistical analyses were generally performed using proportionate mortality or standardized mortality analyses. While both of these methods have their limitations, the latter is generally to be preferred to the former.

Two additional variables that may have affected the risk of lung cancer in the study populations are the smoking habits of the workers and the history of other cancer related occupational exposures. Some consideration has been given to the influence of smoking habits upon the development of lung cancer among chromium chemical production workers. As recently as the 1960s, Oettel [cited in (20)] alleged that cancers of the lung occur only in chromium chemical workers who smoke. The fact that smoking habits do not account for the high lung cancer rate in these workers has been adequately demonstrated (24,51,34), although the interrelationship between smoking and chromium chemical exposure has not been well examined. The possible exposure of workers to carcinogens at other places of employment has not been accounted for in the reported studies.

SELECTED ASPECTS OF THE RELATIONSHIP OF CHROMIUM EXPOSURE AND CANCER

In the previous section, the epidemiologic studies of occupational exposure to chromium were reviewed, with particular emphasis given to the methods of study. In this section, several aspects of the relationship between occupational exposure to chromium and cancer will be considered. The nature of the etiologic relation will be discussed in terms of strength and consistency, latency period, and dose-response effect. The experimental evidence will be briefly reviewed as it relates to the carcinogenicity of specific chromium compounds and intermediate production products. Finally, the evidence concerning specific etiologic agents and the biologic plausibility of chromium carcinogenesis will be considered.

Strength and Consistency

The strength of the association between a factor and a disease indicates how important this factor is in the production of the disease. The consistent finding of an association between a factor and a disease in several populations, under different circumstances of study, increases the plausibility that the observed association is causal in nature.

The two studies (23; Axelsson and Rylander, personal communication) in the chromium ferroalloy industry had different results. The one study (24) of the chromium refractory brick industry was not well executed (see Table 3). Based upon the available studies, there is a lack of a strong and consistent relationship between exposure to chromium in these industries and the development of cancer.

The risk of lung cancer has been shown consistently to be high for chromium chemical production workers, although the strength of the relationship in the reported studies has varied (see Table 4). This variation may in part be due to differences in worker exposure related to method of production and in part to differences in methods of study, including criteria for study eligibility and thoroughness of the follow-up effort.

The health of workers in the chromate pigment industry has been reported upon in 3 studies. In one study (42), based upon 3 cases, a relative risk of 38 was reported for those employed 3 years or more. In two larger studies (43,45) about a 2–fold elevation in risk was reported. Employees in this industry appear to be at an excess risk for lung cancer, although the risk may be lower than that experienced by chemical production workers (see Table 5).

The possibility that there may be an increased risk for lung cancer among chromium platers has been suggested in two studies (46,47), although the reported risks were considerably lower than those generally shown for chromium chemical production workers. The results for chromium platers should however be considered tentative due to the methodological problems of the reviewed studies (see Table 6).

The strength and consistency of the association of risk of cancer and occupational exposure in "other" industries, where chromium chemicals are handled, has not been well studied (see Table 7).

An excess of cancers at sites other than the respiratory system has been reported in the ferrochromium alloy industry (23), the chromium chemical production industry (28), the chromate pigment industry (43) and in the chromium plating industry (46). Such findings have not been consistently found in all studies (24,34,40,48).

Latency Period

An important consideration in studies of occupational cancer is the latency period between exposure to the carcinogenic stimulus and appearance of the clinically diagnosable cancer. This period is a summation of the time periods required for the initiation of a malignant change and for the growth of a malignancy to a size that permits recognition and diagnosis. In occupational mortality studies, this period is approximated by the length of time between first exposure and the date of death. In considering latency periods it is important to recognize that the observed mean latency period will be effected by the criteria used for defining a case, the duration of the follow-up and by any possible bias in the method of ascertainment of cases.

For the studies reviewed, the mean latency period for lung cancer ranged between 15 and 27 years. Given the differences in methods of study, it would appear that the mean latency period may be somewhat shorter in the chromate pigment industry than it is in the chromium chemical production industry (see Table 8).

Dose-Response Relationship

Exposure to a substance may be defined both in terms of the quantity and the duration of that exposure. An hypothesis of disease causality is strengthened by the demonstration of a relationship between an increasing degree of exposure to the possible causative agent and an increasing risk of disease.

Several studies have reported air concentrations of chromium in the work-

TABLE 8. Latency Period: Mean and Standard Deviation in Years of the Interval from Initial Exposure to the Date of Cancer Diagnosis for Workers in Chromium Producing and Using Industries

Author (reference)	Country	Type of production	Number of cases	Latency in years Mean	SD	Case definition
Baetjer (26), 1950	Germany	Chromates	39	27	10	Diagnosis of lung cancer
	United States	Chromates	49	17	9	Diagnosis of lung cancer
Bidstrup and Case (34), 1956	Great Britain	Chromates	12	21	10	Death due to lung cancer
Watanabe and Fukuchi (37), 1975	Japan	Chromates	7	24	9	Diagnosis of lung cancer
Hayes et al. (40), 1979	United States	Chromates	59	20	6	Death due to lung cancer
Baetjer (26), 1950	Germany	Pigments	7	15	4	Diagnosis of lung cancer
Langard and Norseth (42), 1975	Norway	Pigments	3	15	5	Diagnosis of lung cancer

place. The studies reporting air concentrations of chromium in chemical production facilities are summarized in Table 9 and those reporting air concentrations of chromium in other workplaces are summarized in Table 10.

The reported results are of only limited usefulness with regard to discerning possible associations between the level of exposure and risk. Aside from the difficulties in comparing the air concentration values between locations due to variations in methods of sampling and analysis, the published data are generally of a cross-sectional nature and therefore do not provide information about average exposures or changes in exposure over time. Consequently, the information is not sufficient for attempting to relate an increasing gradient in concentration to an increasing gradient in risk, or for attempting to determine maximum allowable exposures in the work setting.

Another approach to assessing risk is to consider the duration of employment as a proxy measure of the degree of exposure. Several studies have reported on the duration of years worked for those who developed lung cancer. When compared to the length of exposure of other employees, these results show that cases have been exposed longer (24), although the results may be biased if the follow-up procedure did not include those who left the industry.

In a few studies it was possible to calculate the duration of employment as related to the risk of developing cancer. Axelsson and Rylander (personal

TABLE 9. Concentration in the Air of Chromium (as Total Cr, Cr^{+3}, Cr^{+6}) at Specific Sites in Chromium Chemical Production Facilities

Country (year)	Author (reference)	Operations	Cr^{+3} (mg/m^3)	Cr^{+6} (mg/m^3)	Cr total (mg/m^3)
United States (1948)	Machle and Gregorius (28)	Chromate production			
		Kiln and mills			0.01–2.8
		Packing			0.20–21.0
		General area			0.03–1.0
France (1951)	Spannagel (27)	Chromate production			
		Ore crushing			8.0
		Sodium chromate barreling			0.16
Great Britain (1951)	Buckell and Harvey (12)	Chromate production			
		Chromite and lime mixing	2.14	0.005	2.145
		Roast	0.17	0.029	0.199
		Filtering	0.037	0.52	0.557
		Shipping	0.0053	0.88	0.8853
United States (1950)	Bourne and Yee (52)	Chromate production			
		Chromite and lime mixing	1.52	0.03	1.53
		Roast	0.26	0.39	0.65
		Filtering	0.08	0.12	0.2
		Shipping	0.3	0.2	0.5
United States (1947)	Allied Chemical (53)	Chromate production			
		Dry process—dust		0.34[a]	
		Wet process—mist		0.36[a]	
		Product—dust		1.37[a]	
United States (1973/1975)	Allied Chemical (53)	Chromate production			
		Dry process—dust		0.01[a]	
		Wet process—mist		0.008[a]	
		Product—dust		0.005[a]	

[a]Reported as "the mean average."

communication) found a consistent absence of excess risk in ferrochromium workers, when the results were analysed with respect to the length of employment. For the chromium chemical production industry, Taylor (35), using estimates of work experience, reported that the greatest relative increase in mortality occurs for persons having between 9 and 14 years of cumulative work experience. Further, Hayes et al. (4) reported an SMR of 1.6, with respect to lung cancer, for workers employed 90 days to 2 years, and an SMR of about 3.2 for those employed 3 years or more.

Davies (45) reported an absence of excess risk of lung cancer for those employed less than 1 year, and an excess risk for those employed more than 1 year, in the chromate pigment industry. Two other reports (42,43) indicate that the excess risk in chromate pigment workers is concentrated in the longer

TABLE 10. Concentration in the Air of Chromium (as Total Cr) in Facilities Other Than Chromium Chemical Production Facilities

Country (year)	Author (reference)	Operations	Cr Total (mg/m^3)
		CHROMIC ACID USING	
United States (1928)	Bloomfield and Blum (54)	Chromium plating	
		Plant A	2.1
		Plant B	0.7
		Plant C	0.4
		Plant D	1.3
		Plant E	0.06
		Plant F	0.9
United States (1944)	Gresh (55)	Anodizing	
		Original exhaust	0.3
		Revised exhaust	neg.
United States (1965)	Kleinfeld and Rosso (56)	Chromium plating	
		Original exhaust	0.09–0.72
		Revised exhaust	< 0.006
Brazil (1972)	Gomes (57)	Electroplating	
		Hard chrome	0.08[a]
		Brilliant chrome	< 0.05[a]
		CHROMATE PIGMENT PRODUCTION	
Norway (1974)	Langard and Norseth (42)	Chrome pigment production	
		Mixing raw materials	0.01–0.35
		Sack filling	0.08–0.43
		Foreman	0.04–0.19
United States (1976)	Equitable Environmental Health, Inc. (43)	Chrome Pigment Production	
		Lead chromate	
		Plant A	0.05
		Plant B	0.06
		Lead and zinc chromate	
		Plant C	0.19
		TRIVALENT CHROMIUM COMPOUNDS	
Germany (1974)	Korallus et al. (50)	Chromium oxide and Chromium (III) sulphate producton (trivalent compounds)	
		Filter	0.92
		Revolving filter	0
		Dryer	0.53
		Packing	2.36
		Packing	0.62
		Spraying apparatus	0.11

[a]Median of reported values.

term workers. From the descriptive evidence of case histories and the analytic evidence, it would appear that longer employment in the hazardous industries is associated with a higher risk of respiratory cancer.

Experimental Support

There is extensive experimental support for the epidemiologic association between exposure to chromium compounds and the development of cancer. In the experimental situation it is possible to select specific chemicals for study using specified test systems. Consequently, much effort has been expended in attempting to determine experimentally which chromium compounds and classes of compounds are associated with an elevated cancer risk.

Attention has been focused on several of the intermediate products of the chromium chemical production process and upon specific chromium compounds. The valence state and the solubility properties of the various substances have been considered as being related to their carcinogenicity. This work has already been reviewed (9,13,21,22). In this section, only selected reports including recent findings will be considered.

The carcinogenicity of various intermediate products of the chromium chemical production process, particularly of the residue of the roast process, has been demonstrated. The carcinogenicity of these products for bronchial tissues has recently been shown by tracheal pellet implantation (58,59) and by dust inhalation (60). This finding is of considerable importance for industrial hygiene. However, from this evidence it is not possible to determine which chemicals of the complex intermediate products are the responsible carcinogens.

With respect to valence state, there is little experimental support that exposure to trivalent chromium causes cancer. It has, however, been demonstrated (61) that exposure to divalent chromous chloride, presumably a trivalent chromium compound under the conditions of study, was associated with misincorporation of nucleotides in nucleic acid synthesized in vitro.

Within the group of hexavalent chromium compounds, solubility of the respective compounds has been considered to be related to the carcinogenic effect. Moderately soluble compounds, such as calcium chromate, have most consistently been shown to cause cancer including squamous cell carcinoma of the respiratory tract, in experimental studies (59,60,62,63).

Compounds of low solubility, such as lead, barium, and zinc chromate, have not been shown to be carcinogenic as consistently. Negative studies (64,65) and studies showing a low incidence among exposed test animals (66), compared to the effects of the moderately soluble compounds, have been reported. Other studies have shown the development of sarcomas in rats after exposure to lead chromate (38,67) and to molybdenum orange (38), a mixture of lead chromate, lead molybdenate, and lead sulfate. Recently, Lane and Mass (68), using a syngeneic transplant technique, have produced squamous cell carcinomas of the trachea, in the presence of the insoluble hexavalent compound, chromium carbonyl. This compound may, however, be moderately unstable.

The highly soluble compounds have not been shown to be carcinogenic in the mammalian animal model. Given the problems of their rapid dissipation due to their high solubility and their high toxicity, the question may be raised whether doses of sufficient quantity and duration, which would be analogous to the level and duration of exposure among workers, have been employed.

Recent in vitro studies of the effects of highly soluble hexavalent chromium compounds on chromosome structure have been reported. Tsuda and Kato (69) have reported increased chromatid breaks and chromatid exchanges in embryonic hamster cells exposed, in vitro, to potassium dichromate. Interestingly, at concentrations higher than 1 ug/ml, no metaphase cells were detected due to the cytotoxicity of the chemical; and, conversely, the ability to induce chromosomal aberrations was lost when the hexavalent salt was reduced to the trivalent form. Bigaliev et al. (70) showed chromosome aberrations in the bone marrow of rats, after exposure to potassium dichromate. Chromosome aberrations in cultured human leukocytes exposed to chromium trioxide have also been reported (71). The author also reports chromosome aberrations in cells exposed to trivalent chromium chloride, but at concentrations of chromium of about 100 times those required for such effects with the hexavalent chromium trioxide.

Using recently developed mutation assay systems, several authors (72–74) have shown hexavalent chromium compounds of moderate and of high solubility to be mutagenic. Trivalent compounds (73,74) and a reduced dichromate (72) showed no such effect, supporting the noncarcinogenicity of forms other than the hexavalent. In one study (75), trivalent chromium compounds were reported to be mutagenic at concentrations 10^3 times those used for hexavalent compounds.

The results of the experimental studies may be summarized as follows: (1) intermediate products of the chromium chemical production process, particularly the roast residue, have been shown to be carcinogenic in the animal model; (2) trivalent compounds appear not to be carcinogenic although their effects upon in vitro DNA synthesis and upon chromosome structure and their mutagenicity at high concentrations need further investigation; (3) medium solubility hexavalent chromates have been consistently shown to be carcinogenic; (4) the evidence for the carcinogenicity of the low solubility hexavalent products is not strong or consistent, although recent evidence indicates a carcinogenic role and (5) the highly soluble hexavalent compounds have not been shown to be carcinogenic, perhaps due to technical difficulties, although they have recently been shown to cause chromosomal aberrations and mutations in experimental test systems.

Etiologic Agents in the Industrial Setting

The evidence reviewed shows that there is an association between exposure to chromium compounds and an excess risk of developing lung cancer. This, however, does not indicate that the specific substance(s) which cause cancer in the industrial setting, have been identified. Several investigators have proposed hypotheses to explain the association with lung cancer.

Mancusco and Hueper (31) proposed that exposure to the trivalent forms, such as chromite ore, may be associated with the excess risk for lung cancer among workers in the chromium chemical production industry. Grogan (11) pointed out that body stores of trivalent chromium may operate as a depot chromium which is gradually transformed into the hexavalent form through the oxidative action of biologic processes. Definitive epidemiologic studies of workers exposed exclusively to trivalent compounds have not been conducted. The experimental studies give little support to the hypothesis.

Machle and Gregorius (28) have suggested that the hexavalent monochromates, such as sodium chromate, may be the carcinogenic agents in the chromium chemical production industry. They based this conclusion on the fact that one of the plants studied, which dealt with production from the sodium dichromate stage onward, had no reported deaths from respiratory cancer. This hypothesis has not again been suggested and it is difficult to support, given the likelihood of conversion of monochromates to dichromates in the atmosphere under industrial conditions (12).

Within the group of hexavalent chromium compounds there is diversity with regard to solubility in water and other substances. This factor has been posited as influencing their carcinogenicity. The authors of the U.S. Public Health Service report (24) argued that in the chromium chemical production industry the acid soluble water-insoluble compounds may be the causative agents of pulmonary carcinoma. These compounds are produced in the roast and remain in the residue which is recirculated in the roasting process. As small amounts remain in the leach liquor and are to be found as airborne dust, they could be spread widely throughout a chromate plant but would not likely be found in appreciable amounts in plants which produced end-products from sodium dichromate. Studies do suggest an elevated risk of cancer among workers who are concerned with the production of agents from the dichromate stage onward (42–47).

Recent evidence from the chromate pigment industry (42–45) indicates that workers involved in the production of these compounds of low solubility, are at excess risk for respiratory cancer, and possibly other forms of cancer. The evidence (see Table 3) is not sufficient to determine whether an excess risk of cancer can be attributed to the production of any one type of chromate pigment. Additionally, the primary raw materials for chromate pigment production are the highly soluble hexavalent chromates.

Highly soluble hexavalent chromium compounds have generally not been considered to be carcinogenic. In a literature review designed to establish a recommended standard for occupational exposure to hexavalent chromium, highly soluble chromium compounds, including the monochromates and dichromates of hydrogen, lithium, sodium, potassium, rubidium, cesium and ammonium and chromium (VI) oxide, were designated as "noncarcinogenic chromium" (21). The recent experimental evidence reviewed earlier concerning chromosomal aberrations and mutations as well as the suggestive epidemiologic evidence (40,46,47) with regard to carcinogenesis indicate that this conclusion should be modified until further research has been conducted.

It has not been possible to specify a particular chromium compound as being the carcinogenic agent in the chromium chemical production industry or in the other industries where chromium is handled. In the light of the present evidence it would seem prudent to assume that the hexavalent chromium compounds, as a class, have the potential for carcinogenic activity. That some compounds may be more carcinogenic than others may well be a result of the chemical activity and rate of dissipation of the specific compounds.

Mechanism of Carcinogenesis

The mechanism of chromium carcinogenesis is not known. Several hypotheses have been suggested. Schoental (76) suggested that the carcinogenicity of the chromates may be related to their ability to tan leather. He proposed that tanning depends on the formation of glycidal, an epoxyaldelyde derived from neutral fats by hydrolysis and subsequent oxidation of glycerol. Glycidal, in turn, is reported to be carcinogenic for rats and mice (77). This suggestion has not been further developed.

Mutagenicity testing is considered to have predictive value for carcinogenicity. Nucleic acid base-pair substitutions and frame shift errors have been reported to be the mutagenic mechanisms in the studies reviewed, perhaps indicating a direct effect upon the genome as the carcinogenic mechanism. These errors have occurred predominantly upon exposure to hexavalent chromium compounds.

Gruber and Jennette (78) have suggested a role for the trivalent chromium compounds in carcinogenesis, citing the study of Sirover and Loeb (61) as indicating that a trivalent chromium compound was more efficient than hexavalent compounds in causing nucleic acid coding errors during in vitro DNA synthesis. They present evidence that the intracellular reduction of hexavalent chromium to trivalent chromium may, in part, be under the control of microsomal enzymes such as the mixed function oxidases. They also hypothesize that the reduced form, being a good electrophile, may be carcinogenic by binding with proteins and nucleic acids. The possibility that the trivalent forms may be the ultimate intracellular carcinogens does not negate the evidence that it is exposure to the hexavalent forms which is predominantly associated with carcinogenesis. However, it does illustrate that the mechanism of carcinogenesis is complex and presently not well understood.

The recent in vitro studies have provided interesting hypotheses concerning the molecular mechanism of carcinogenesis. The analogies between in vitro DNA synthesis and eukaryotic mutagenesis, on the one hand, and human carcinogenesis, on the other hand, may, of course, not be entirely appropriate. Additionally, caution should be exercised in attributing quantitative differences in biologic effects of the various chromium chemicals, based upon these essentially qualitative assay systems.

SUMMARY AND CONCLUSIONS

In this study, the chemistry and biologic activity of the trivalent and hexavalent chromium compounds were first reviewed. Trivalent chromium compounds are of stable valence state and have a strong tendency to form coordination compounds, complexes, and chelates. They are deposited in the body, apparently in a very stable form. The hexavalent compounds are highly oxidative, pass through biologic membranes and are easily reduced to the trivalent form allowing them to bind with a variety of cellular constituents, including the information macromolecules. The chemical and biological activity of the two valence forms lends theoretical consistency to the epidemiologic and experimental evidence for the carcinogenicity of chromium compounds.

Next, the methods of production in the chromium industry were described for the metallurgic, refractory, and chemical industries. The secondary "user" industries of chromium chemicals were also briefly considered. The epidemiologic studies of occupational exposure to chromium were emphasized and it was pointed out that the conclusions which could be drawn from the respective studies are dependent upon the methods of study.

Studies of workers in the ferroalloy industry have been inconsistent and those of refractory brick workers incomplete. Given the variety in the methods of study, a strong and consistent relationship has been shown between employment in the chromium chemical production industry and the development of lung cancer. An elevated risk of lung cancer was also consistently reported for workers in the chromate pigment industry, although the risks may not be as high as that shown for the chromium chemical production industry. A moderate excess of cancer may also exist for workers in the chrome plating industry. The risk associated with occupational exposure to chromium, and its compounds in other industries has not been adequately studied.

With regard to ascertaining specific chemical compounds as etiologic agents, the results of the epidemiologic studies have not been completely satisfactory. Ferroalloy workers are exposed mainly to trivalent compounds, yet hexavalent chromium exposure also occurs. Chromium chemical production workers are exposed to a complex variety of chromium compounds. Chromate pigment workers produce relatively insoluble hexavalent compounds, yet the raw material is a highly soluble compound. Chromium platers are exposed to only a highly soluble compound, but the studies available on this industry are not sufficient to draw firm conclusions.

The experimental evidence generally supports the conclusion that exposure to the trivalent chromium compounds does not cause cancer. Concerning the hexavalent compounds, the medium solubility compounds have been shown conclusively to be carcinogenic. The evidence for carcinogenicity of the low solubility compounds is not as strong, yet it is highly suggestive. Although the high solubility compounds have not been shown to be carcinogenic, they appear to have strong mutagenic properties in experimental test systems. The combined epidemiologic and experimental evidence indicates a definite carcinogenic role for the hexavalent chromium compounds, with perhaps a variation in carcinogenic potential based upon the solubility of the individual compounds. This evidence should be considered in the development of standards for occupational and environmental exposure.

Several areas remain which will require further research. It has not been demonstrated that improved industrial hygiene conditions in newer production facilities removes the excess risk of lung cancer for chromium chemical production workers; and continued follow-up of workers employed in these facilities is indicated. Further information is also needed concerning the risk of cancer in the chromium chemical "user" industries, particularly the chromium plating industry. More definitive results for this industry would have implications for workers in several other industries, where the highly soluble compounds are used. The exposure to chromium compounds in other occupational settings also needs to be documented and the risk of disease evaluated. For example, there is very little known about the carcinogenic hazards in the organic chemical industry where such products as chromium carbonyl are produced.

Although it is generally agreed that exposure to the trivalent form does not cause cancer, it has been suggested that small amounts from deposits in the body may be oxidized to the hexavalent state to cause cancer at a later time. This hypothesis has not been widely accepted, yet it deserves further consideration and clarification because of its potential etiologic importance.

The identification of the specific chromium compounds that are carcinogens and the understanding of the mechanism by which they act may help to provide a better understanding of the carcinogenic process and a safer working environment.

REFERENCES

1. Udy, M. S. (ed). (1956) Chemistry of Chromium and its Compounds. Am. Chem. Soc. Monogr. 132, Rheinghold, New York.
2. Economic Analysis of the Chromium Industry (1970). Cambridge, Mass.: Charles River Associates.
3. U.S. Department of the Interior (1975) Bureau of Mines Minerals. Yearbook 1973, Vol. 1. Metals, Minerals and Fuels. Washington, D.C.: U.S. Government Printing Office.
4. Brick and Clay Record. January 1968.
5. Chrome chemicals' 1962 jump won't repeat. (1962) Chem. & Eng. News, December 3, pp. 30–31.
6. Wacker, W. E. C., Vallee, B. L. (1959) Nucleic acids and metals. I. Chromium, manganese, nickel, iron and other metals in ribonucleic acids from diverse biological sources. J. Biol. Chem. 234, 3257–3262.
7. Weast, R. C. (ed). (1971) Physical constants of inorganic compounds. *In*: Handbook of Chemistry and Physics—A Ready Reference Book of Chemical and Physical Data. 52nd ed. Cleveland, Ohio: Chemical Rubber Co.
8. Hawley, G. G. (ed) (1971) The Condensed Chemical Dictionary. 9th ed. New York: Van Nostrand Reinhold Co.
9. International Agency for Research on Cancer (1972) Monographs on the Evaluation of Carcinogenic Risk of Chemicals to Man. Lyon, France: Monograph No. 2.
10. Mertz, W. (1969) Chromium occurrence and function in biological systems. Physiol. Rev. 49, 163–239.
11. Grogan, C. H. (1957) Experimental studies in metal cancerigenesis. VIII. On the etiological factor in chromate cancer. Cancer 10, 625–638.
12. Buckell, M., Harvey, D. G. (1951) An environmental study of the chromate industry. Br. J. Ind. Med. 8, 298–301.
13. Committee on Biologic Effects of Atomospheric Pollutants. (1974) Chromium Medical and Biological Effects of Environmental Pollutants. Washington, D. C.: National Academy of Sciences.
14. Fuwa, K., Wacker, W. E. C., Druyan, R., et al. (1960) Nucleic acids and metals. II. Transition metals as determinants of the conformation of ribonucleic acids. Proc. Nat. Acad. Sci., U.S.A. 46, 1298–1307.

15. Baetjer, A. M., Damron, C., Budacz, V. (1959) The distribution and retention of chromium in men and animals. Arch. Industr. Hlth. 20, 136–150.

16. Doisy, R. J., Streeten, D. H. P., Freiberg, J. M., Schneider, A. J. (1976) Chromium metabolism in man and biochemical effects. *In*: Trace Elements in Human Health and Disease. Vol. II, Essential and Toxic Elements. Prasad, A. S. (ed). New York: Academic Press.

17. Punsar, S., Wolf, W., Mertz, W., Karvonen, M. J. (1977) Urinary chromium excretion and atherosclerotic manifestations in two Finnish male populations. Ann. Clin. Res. 9, 79–83.

18. Boyle, E., Mondschein, B., Dash, H. H. (1977) Chromium depletion in the pathogenesis of diabetes and atherosclerosis. South. Med. J. 70, 1449–1453.

19. Barborik, M. (1970) The problem of harmful exposures to chromium compounds. Industr. Med. 39, 221–224.

20. Hueper, W. C. (1966) Occupational and Environmental Cancers of the Respiratory System. New York: Springer-Verlag.

21. National Institute for Occupational Safety and Health (1975) Criteria for a Recommended Standard: Occupational Exposure to Chromium (VI). Washington, D.C.: U.S. Department of Health, Education and Welfare.

22. National Institute for Occupational Safety and Health (1973) Criteria for a Recommended Standard: Occupational Exposure to Chromic Acid. Washington, D.C.: U.S. Department of Health, Education and Welfare.

23. Pokryovskaya, L. V., Shabynina, N. K. (1973) Carcinogeneous hazards in the production of chromium ferroalloys. Gig. Trud. Prof. Zabol 10, 23–26 (Russian, Engl. abstr.).

24. Public Health Service. (1953) Health of Workers in Chromate Producing Industry. Gafafer, W. M. (ed). U.S.P.H.S. Public 192. Washington, D.C.: U.S. Department of Health, Education and Welfare.

25. Lehmann, K. B. (1932) Ist Grund zu einer besonderen Beunruhigung wegen des Auftretens von Lungenkrebs bei Chromatarbeitern Vorhanden? Zentralbl. Gewerbehyg. 9, 168–170.

26. Baetjer, A. M. (1950) Pulmonary carcinoma in chromate workers. I. A review of the literature and report of cases. Arch. Ind. Hyg. Occup. Med. 2, 487–504.

27. Spannagel, H. (1953) Lungenkrebs und andere Organschaden durch Chromverbindungen. Arbeitsmedizin, Heft 28. Leipzig: Johann Ambrosius Bart.

28. Machle, W., Gregorius, F. (1948) Cancer of the respiratory system in the United States chromate-producing industry. Publ. Hlth. Rep. 63, 1114–1127.

29. Baetjer, A. M. (1950) Pulmonary carcinoma in chromate workers. II. Incidence on basis of hospital records. Arch. Ind. Hyg. Occup. Med. 2, 505–516.

30. Mancusco, T. F. (1949) Occupational cancer survey in Ohio. Proc. Publ. Hlth. Cancer Assoc. Am., pp. 57–70.

31. Mancusco, T. F., Hueper, W. C. (1951) Occupational cancer and other health hazards in a chromate plant: A medical appraisal. I. Lung cancer in chromate workers. Ind. Med. Surg. 20, 358–363.

32. Brinton, H. P., Frasier, E. S., Koven, A. L. (1952) Morbidity and mortality experience among chromate workers. Publ. Hlth. Rep. 67, 835–847.

33. Bidstrup, P. L. (1951) Carcinoma of the lung in chromate workers. Br. J. Ind. Med. 8, 302–305.

34. Bidstrup, P. L., Case, R. A. M. (1956) Carcinoma of the lung in workermen in dichromates-producing-industry in Great Britain. Br. J. Ind. Med. 13, 260–264.

35. Taylor, F. H. (1966) The relationship of mortality and duration of employment as reflected by a cohort of chromate workers. Am. J. Publ. Hlth. 56, 218–229.

36. Enterline, P. E. (1974) Respiratory cancer among chromate workers. J. Occup. Med. 16, 523–526.

37. Watanabe, S., Fukuchi, Y. (1975) An epidemiologic survey on lung cancer in workers of a chromate producing industry in Hokkaido, Japan. Brighton, England: XVII International Congress on Occupational Health, pp. 149–150.

38. Maltoni, C. (1974) Occupational carcinogenesis. *In*: Proceedings, Second International Symposium on Cancer Detection and Prevention, Bologna, 1973. Amsterdam: Excerpta Medica, pp. 19–26.

39. Bigaliev, A. B., Turabaev, M. N., Bigalieva, R. K., Elemesova, M. Sh. (1977) Tsitogeneticheskoe obsledovanie lits, zaniatykb v sfere krhomovogo proizvadstva. Genetika 13, 545–547.

40. Hayes, R. B., Lilienfeld, A. M., Snell, L. M. (1979) Mortality in chromium chemical production workers: a prospective study. Int. J. Epidemiol 8, 365–374.

41. Newman, D. (1890) A case of adenocarcinoma of the left inferior turbinated body and perforation of the nasal septum in the person of a worker in chrome pigments. Glasgow Med. J. 33, 469–470.

42. Langard, S., Norseth, T. (1975) A cohort study of bronchial carcinomas in workers producing chromate pigments. Br. J. Ind. Med. 32, 62–65.

43. The Dry Color Manufacturers Association (1976) An Epidemiologic Study of Lead Chromate Plants: Final Report. Berkeley, California: Equitable Environmental Health.

44. Maltoni, C. (1976) Precursor lesions in exposed populations as indicators of occupational cancer risk. Ann. N.Y. Acad. Sci. 271, 444–447.

45. Davies, J. M. (1978) Lung cancer mortality of workers making chrome pigments (Letter) Lancet 1, 384.

46. Royle, H. (1975) Toxicity of chromic acid in the chromium plating industry. Environ. Res. 10, 39–53.

47. Waterhouse, J. A. H. (1975) Cancer among chromium platers. Br. J. Cancer 32, 262.

48. Okubo, T., Tuscuhiya, K. (1977) An epidemiological study in lung cancer among chromium plating workers. Keio J. Med. 26, 171–177.

49. Tsuchiya, K. (1965) The relation of occupation to cancer, especially cancer of the lung. Cancer 18, 136–144.

50. Korallus, U., Ehrlicher, H., Wüstefeld, E. (1974) Dreiwertige Chromverbindungen. Ergebnisse einer arbeitsmedizinischen Untersuchung. Arbeitsmed. Sozialmed. Präventivmed. 9, 51–54.

51. Fisher, R. S., Rieckert, P. W. (1959) Lung cancer in chromate workers. Am. J. Pathol. 35, 699.

52. Bourne, H. G., Jr., Yee, H. T. (1950) Occupational cancer in a chromate plant—an occupational appraisal. Ind. Med. Surg. 19, 563–567.

53. Allied Chemical Corporation (1976) Response to OSHA FR Notice (29 CFR Part 1910) (Docket H-054), June 14.

54. Bloomfield, J. J., Blum, W. (1928) Health hazards in chromium plating. Publ. Hlth. Rep. 43, 2330–2347.

55. Gresh, J. T. (1944) Chromic acid poisoning from inhalation of mist developed from five percent chromic acid solution. II. Engineering aspects of chromic acid poisoning from anodizing operations. J. Ind. Hyg. Toxicol. 26, 127–130.

56. Kleinfeld, M., Rosso, A. (1965) Ulcerations of the nasal septum due to inhalation of chromic acid mist. Ind. Med. Surg. 34, 242–243.

57. Gomes, E. R. (1972) Incidence of chromium induced lesions among electroplating workers in Brazil. Ind. Med. 41, 21–25.

58. Kuschner, M., Laskin, S. (1971) Experimental models in environmental carcinogenesis. Am. J. Pathol. 64, 183–199.

59. Laskin, S., Kuschner, M. Drew, R. T. (1970) Studies in pulmonary carcinogenesis. *In*: Inhalation Carcinogenesis. Hanna, M. G., Jr., Nettesheim, P., Gilbert, J. R. (eds.) Proceedings of an Oak Ridge National Laboratory, Biology Division, Conference. Washington, D.C.: U.S. Atomic Energy Commission, pp. 321–351.

60. Kuschner, M., Laskin, S. (1976) Studies in Pulmonary Carcinogenesis. Summary Progress Report: Inhalation Studies with Industrial Chrome Compounds. Washington, D.C.: Department of Health, Education and Welfare, National Cancer Institute.
61. Sirover, M. A., Loeb, L. A. (1976) Infidelity of DNA synthesis in vitro: Screening for potential metal mutagens or carcinogens. Science 194, 1434–1436.
62. Levy, L. S., Venitt, S. (1975) Carcinogenic and mutagenic activity of chromium containing materials. Br. J. Cancer 32, 254–255.
63. Laskin, S., Capiello, V. P., Isola, D., et al. (1973) Chronic inhalation exposures with calcium chromate aerosols. *In*: A.I.H.A. Industrial Health Conference. Boston, Mass.: Abstract 164, pp. 175.
64. Hueper, W. C., Payne, W. W. (1962) Experimental studies in metal carcinogenesis. Arch. Environ. Hlth. 5, 445–462.
65. Stefee, C. H. and Baetjer, A. M. (1965) Histopathologic effects of chromate chemicals. Report on studies in rabbits, guinea pigs, rats and mice. Arch. Environ. Hlth. 11, 66–75.
66. Hueper, W. C. (1961) Environmental carcinogenesis and cancers. Cancer Res. 21, 842–857.
67. Furst, A., Schlauder, M., Sasmore, D. P. (1976) Tumorigenic activity of lead chromate. Cancer Res. 36, 1779–1783.
68. Lane, B. P. and Mass, M. J. (1977) Carcinogenicity and cocarcinogenicity of chromium carbonyl in heterotopic tracheal grafts. Cancer Res. 37, 1476–1479.
69. Tsuda, H., Kato, K. (1977) Chromosomal aberrations and morphological transformation in hamster embryonic cells treated with potassium dichromate in vitro. Mut. Res. 46, 87–94.
70. Bigaliev, A. B., Elemesova, M. Sh., Bigalieva, R. K. (1976) Khromosomnye aberratsii v somaticheskikh kletok mickopilaiushchikh, vyzvannye soedineniiami khroma. Tsitol. Genet. 10, 222–224.
71. Kaneko, T. (1976) Chromosome damage in cultured human leukocytes induced by chromium chloride and chromium trioxide. Jap. J. Ind. Hlth. 18, 136–137.
72. Nishioka, H. (1975) Mutagenic activities of metal compounds in bacteria. Mut. Res. 31, 185–189.
73. Petrelli, F. L., de Flora, S. (1977) Toxicity and mutagenicity of hexavalent chromium on Salmonella typhimurium. Appl. Environ. Microbiol. 33, 805–809.
74. Venitt, S., Levy, L. S. (1974) Mutagenicity of chromates in bacteria and its relevance to chromate carcinogenesis. Nature 250, 493–494.
75. Lofroth, G., Ames, B. (1977) Abstracts Environmental Mutagen Society. Colorado Springs, Colorado (cited in ref. 78), p. 30.
76. Schoental, R. (1975) Chromium carcinogenesis, Formation of Epoxyaldehydes and tanning. Br. J. Cancer 32, 403–404.
77. Van Duuren, B. L. (1969) Carcinogenic epoxides, lactones, and halo-ethers and their mode of action. Ann. N.Y. Acad. Sci. 163, 633.
78. Gruber, J. E., Jennette, K. W. (1978) Metabolism of the carcinogen chromate by rat liver microsomes. Biochem. Biophys. Res. Comm. 82, 700–706.

INDEX

F

G

H

I

L

M

N

O

P

R

S

T

V